The Long-Term Impact of Medical Complications in Pregnancy

SERIES IN MATERNAL-FETAL MEDICINE

Published in association with the
Journal of Maternal-Fetal & Neonatal Medicine

Edited by
Gian Carlo Di Renzo and Dev Maulik

Howard Carp, *Recurrent Pregnancy Loss*, ISBN 9780415421300

Vincenzo Berghella, *Obstetric Evidence Based Guidelines*,
ISBN 9780415701884

Vincenzo Berghella, *Maternal-Fetal Evidence Based Guidelines*,
ISBN 9780415432818

Moshe Hod, Lois Jovanovic, Gian Carlo Di Renzo, Alberto de Leiva,
Oded Langer, *Textbook of Diabetes and Pregnancy, Second Edition*,
ISBN 9780415426206

Simcha Yagel, Norman H. Silverman, Ulrich Gembruch,
Fetal Cardiology, Second Edition, ISBN 9780415432658

Fabio Facchinetti, Gustaaf A. Dekker, Dante Baronciani,
George Saade, Stillbirth: *Understanding and Management*,
ISBN 9780415473903

Vincenzo Berghella, *Maternal–Fetal Evidence Based Guidelines,
Second Edition*, ISBN 9781841848228

Vincenzo Berghella, *Obstetric Evidence Based Guidelines, Second Edition*,
ISBN 9781841848242

Howard Carp, *Recurrent Pregnancy Loss: Causes, Controversies, and
Treatment, Second Edition*, ISBN 9781482216141

Moshe Hod, Lois G. Jovanovic, Gian Carlo Di Renzo, Alberto De Leiva,
Oded Langer, *Textbook of Diabetes and Pregnancy, Third Edition*,
ISBN 9781482213607

Vincenzo Berghella, *Maternal–Fetal Evidence Based Guidelines,
Third Edition*, ISBN 9781841848228

Vincenzo Berghella, *Obstetric Evidence Based Guidelines, Third Edition*,
ISBN 9781841848242

Eyal Sheiner, *The Long-Term Impact of Medical Complications in Pregnancy:
A Window into Maternal and Fetal Future Health*, ISBN 9781498764674

The Long-Term Impact of Medical Complications in Pregnancy

A Window into Maternal and Fetal Future Health

Edited by

Eyal Sheiner, MD, PhD

Professor and Chairman, Department of Obstetrics and Gynecology B, Soroka University Medical Center, and Vice Dean, Student Affairs, Faculty of Health Sciences, Ben-Gurion University of the Negev, Be'er Sheva, Israel

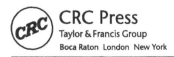

CRC Press
Taylor & Francis Group
Boca Raton London New York

CRC Press is an imprint of the
Taylor & Francis Group, an **Informa** business

CRC Press
Taylor & Francis Group
6000 Broken Sound Parkway NW, Suite 300
Boca Raton, FL 33487-2742

© 2017 by Taylor & Francis Group, LLC
CRC Press is an imprint of Taylor & Francis Group, an Informa business

No claim to original U.S. Government works

Printed on acid-free paper
Version Date: 20161111

International Standard Book Number-13: 978-1-4987-6467-4 (Paperback)

Visit the Taylor & Francis Web site at
http://www.taylorandfrancis.com

and the CRC Press Web site at
http://www.crcpress.com

Printed and bound in the United States of America by
Edwards Brothers Malloy on sustainably sourced paper

The book is dedicated with love to my wife, Einat, who has stood beside me and given me strength all these years, and our four children, the joy of my life: Ofir, Yonathan, Lior, and Yuval.

Contents

Preface

In general, most women are medically screened (or even just examined) on three occasions throughout their lives: as infants soon after birth, during pregnancy, and then usually only years later when diagnosed with an illness. As risk assessment for atherosclerotic disease is suboptimal, especially in women, pregnancy should be viewed by physicians not only as a stress test that provides a unique glimpse into the future, but also as an opportunity to counsel women and influence their destiny. Accordingly, I was pleased to have the opportunity to participate in the creation of this book. I thank all the authors for their excellent chapters and hope that this work does justice to their contributions.

Eyal Sheiner
Ben-Gurion University of the Negev
Be'er Sheva, Israel

Contributors

Oren Barak
Department of Obstetrics and Gynecology
Kaplan Medical Center
Rehovot, Israel

Jennifer M. Beale
King Edward Memorial Hospital
Subiaco, Western Australia

Ruthy Beer-Weisel
Soroka University Medical Center
School of Medicine
Ben-Gurion University of the Negev
Be'er Sheva, Israel

Howard Berger
Department of Obstetrics and Gynecology
Saint Michael's Hospital
Institute for Health Policy, Management and
    Evaluation
University of Toronto
Toronto, Canada

Tal Biron-Shental
Meir Medical Center
Tel Aviv University
Tel Aviv, Israel

Ron Charach
Department of Obstetrics and Gynecology
Soroka University Medical Center
School of Medicine
Ben-Gurion University of the Negev
Be'er Sheva, Israel

Sharon Davidesko
Department of Obstetrics and Gynecology
Soroka University Medical Center
School of Medicine
Ben-Gurion University of the Negev
Be'er Sheva, Israel

Offer Erez
Maternity Department D and Obstetrical Day
    Care Unit
Division of Obstetrics and Gynecology
Soroka University Medical Center
School of Medicine
Faculty of Health Sciences
Ben-Gurion University of the Negev
Be'er Sheva, Israel

Idit Erez-Weiss
Department of Family Medicine
School of Medicine
Ben-Gurion University of the Negev
Be'er Sheva, Israel

Salvatore Gentile
Department of Mental Health
ASL Salerno
Mental Health Centre n. 63
Cava de' Tirreni, Italy
and
Medical School "Federico II"
Department of Neurosciences
Division of Psychiatry–Perinatal Psychiatry
University of Naples
Naples, Italy

Hannah Glinter
Medical School for International Health
Ben-Gurion University of the Negev
Be'er Sheva, Israel

Walter H. Gotlieb
Division of Gynecologic Oncology
Segal Cancer Center
Jewish General Hospital
McGill University
Montreal, Canada

Shirley Greenbaum
Soroka University Medical Center
School of Medicine
Ben-Gurion University of the Negev
Be'er Sheva, Israel

Avi Harlev
Department of Obstetrics and Gynecology
Soroka University Medical Center
School of Medicine
Ben-Gurion University of the Negev
Be'er Sheva, Israel

Roger Hart
School of Women's and Infant's Health
and Fertility Specialists of Western Australia,
    Bethesda Hospital
Claremont, Western Australia
and
King Edward Memorial Hospital
University of Western Australia
Subiaco, Western Australia

Aaron Herzog
Medical School for International Health
Ben-Gurion University of the Negev
Be'er Sheva, Israel

Zeva Daniela Herzog
Medical School for International Health
Ben-Gurion University of the Negev
Be'er Sheva, Israel

Roy Kessous
Division of Gynecologic Oncology
Segal Cancer Center
Jewish General Hospital
McGill University
Montreal, Canada

Vered Klaitman
Soroka University Medical Center
School of Medicine
Ben-Gurion University of the Negev
Be'er Sheva, Israel

Jonah Susser Kreniske
Department of Obstetrics and Gynecology
Soroka University Medical Center
Ben-Gurion University of the Negev
Be'er Sheva, Israel

Grace Eunjin Lee
The Medical School for International Health
Ben-Gurion University of the Negev
Be'er Sheva, Israel

Tom Leibson
Department of Clinical Pharmacology and
    Toxicology
The Hospital for Sick Children
University of Toronto
Toronto, Canada

Hanns-Ulrich Marschall
Department of Molecular and Clinical Medicine
Sahlgrenska Academy, Institute of Medicine
University of Gothenburg
Gothenburg, Sweden

Salvatore Andrea Mastrolia
Department of Obstetrics and Gynecology
University of Bari "Aldo Moro"
Bari, Italy
and
Soroka University Medical Center
School of Medicine
Ben-Gurion University of the Negev
Be'er Sheva, Israel

Samantha Meltzer-Brody
Department of Psychiatry
University of North Carolina
Chapel Hill, North Carolina

Shelly Meshel
Leah Shalev Internal Medicine Department
Soroka University Medical Center
School of Medicine
Ben-Gurion University of the Negev
Be'er Sheva, Israel

Gali Pariente
Department of Clinical Pharmacology and
    Toxicology
The Hospital for Sick Children
University of Toronto
Toronto, Canada

Jennifer C. Pontré
King Edward Memorial Hospital
Subiaco, Western Australia

Gal Rodavsky
Soroka University Medical Center
School of Medicine
Ben-Gurion University of the Negev
Be'er Sheva, Israel

Kira Nahum Sacks
Department of Public Health
Ben-Gurion University of the Negev
Be'er Sheva, Israel

Leah Shalev
Internal Medicine F
Soroka University Medical Center
Ben-Gurion University of the Negev
Be'er Sheva, Israel

Eyal Sheiner
Department of Obstetrics and Gynecology
Soroka University Medical Center
School of Medicine
Ben-Gurion University of the Negev
Be'er Sheva, Israel

Edi Vaisbuch
Department of Obstetrics and Gynecology
Kaplan Medical Center
Rehovot, Israel

Asnat Walfisch
Department of Obstetrics and Gynecology
Soroka University Medical Center
School of Medicine
Ben-Gurion University of the Negev
Be'er Sheva, Israel

Judah Weiss
Department of Obstetrics and Gynecology
Soroka University Medical Center
School of Medicine
Ben-Gurion University of the Negev
Be'er Sheva, Israel

Kent Willis
Department of Neonatal–Perinatal
    Medicine
University of Tennessee Health Science
    Center
Memphis, Tennessee

Talya Wolak
Internal Medicine D and Hypertension Unit
Soroka University Medical Center
School of Medicine
Ben-Gurion University of the Negev
Be'er Sheva, Israel

Yoav Yinon
Department of Obstetrics and Gynecology
Sheba Medical Center
Tel Aviv University
Tel Aviv, Israel

Yariv Yogev
Department of Obstetrics, Gynecology and
    Fertility
Tel Aviv Sourasky Medical Center
Sackler Faculty of Medicine
Tel Aviv University
Tel Aviv, Israel

Shiran Zer
Soroka University Medical Center
School of Medicine
Ben-Gurion University of the Negev
Be'er Sheva, Israel

1

Preeclampsia and Long-Term Maternal Atherosclerotic and Cardiovascular Disease

Yoav Yinon

Introduction

Preeclampsia is a multisystem disorder of pregnancy characterized by the new onset of hypertension, usually in the third trimester, and is sometimes associated with proteinuria. It is a major cause of both maternal and neonatal morbidity and mortality [1–3].

Despite the morbidity and mortality associated with preeclampsia, the underlying pathophysiology is not completely understood. It is currently believed that the initiating event is reduced placental perfusion due to shallow cytotrophoblast migration toward the uterine spiral arterioles, leading to inappropriate vascular remodeling and a hypoperfused placenta [4]. The placental ischemia results in the release of factors that cause maternal vascular endothelial dysfunction, which leads to many of the manifestations of preeclampsia including hypertension and proteinuria. Recently, the circulating antiangiogenic factors soluble fms-like tyrosine kinase (sFlt-1) and soluble endoglin (sEng) have been implicated in the pathogenesis of preeclampsia. The administration of adenovirus-expressing sFlt-1 to pregnant rats causes preeclampsia-like syndrome, exacerbated by the coadministration of sEng [5,6]. Moreover, a rise in sFlt-1 and sEng and a reduction in placental growth factor (PLGF) have been demonstrated in maternal serum 5–10 weeks before the onset of preeclampsia and are thought to contribute to maternal endothelial dysfunction [7,8]. Although many of the clinical and physiological manifestations associated with preeclampsia resolve soon after delivery, its impact persists years after pregnancy. Epidemiological studies provide evidence that women with a history of preeclampsia are more likely to develop cardiovascular disease later in life. The strength of these data has led to the American Heart Association (AHA) recommendation that a history of preeclampsia should be considered a major risk factor for cardiovascular disease and cerebrovascular disease [9]. The mechanism linking preeclampsia with future cardiovascular disease are unknown but may include preexisting risk factors common to both preeclampsia and cardiovascular disease such as insulin resistance, obesity, chronic hypertension, renal disease, and diabetes [10–12]. Endothelial dysfunction is an important indicator for subsequent cardiovascular disease and is a regular feature in preeclamptic pregnancies. Several studies have shown reduced maternal endothelial function months to years after a preeclamptic pregnancy [13–15].

In this chapter we will review the epidemiologic data on the increased risk of cardiovascular disease after preeclampsia and highlight the pathophysiologic mechanisms mediating the link between preeclampsia and future cardiovascular disease. Recommendations to optimize the clinical management of women with a history of preeclampsia will be discussed.

Preeclampsia and Long-Term Vascular Complications

Preeclampsia and Future Cardiovascular Disease

In recent years, a growing body of literature has clearly shown a link between preeclampsia and future vascular disease. An increased future risk of hypertension, cardiovascular disease, stroke, and end-stage renal disease has been noted in women with a history of preeclampsia [16–23]. In order to determine the association between preeclampsia and future cardiovascular disease, a systematic review and meta-analysis including 25 studies was carried out [16]. Overall, this meta-analysis included 3,488,160 women, of whom 198,252 had preeclampsia and over three million did not. The relative risk of later development of hypertension in women after preeclampsia was 3.7 (95% confidence interval [CI] 2.7–5.05) compared with women who did not have preeclampsia (Table 1.1). Analysis according to parity indicated a higher risk of hypertension after preeclampsia in any pregnancy compared with preeclampsia in the first pregnancy only [16]. Similarly, women with previous preeclampsia were at increased risk of developing ischemic heart disease (relative risk of 2.16, 1.86–2.52) as well as future fatal ischemic heart disease events (relative risk of 2.6, 1.94–3.49) compared with women with no history of preeclampsia. Moreover, the overall risk of stroke as well as venous thromboembolism in later life also increased among women with a history of preeclampsia, with a relative risk of 1.81 (1.45–2.27) and 1.79 (1.37–2.33), respectively (Table 1.1). However, no increased risk of any cancer, including breast cancer, was found 17 years after preeclampsia. Overall mortality after preeclampsia also increased after 14.5 years, with a relative risk of 1.49 (95% CI 1.05–2.14) [16]. In accordance with these findings, Shalom et al. have recently reported on a significantly higher rate of chronic hypertension in 2072 patients with previous preeclampsia compared with 20,742 patients without a history of preeclampsia (12.5% vs. 0.9%; odds ratio of 15.8, 95% CI 12.9–19.3) [24].

The risk of future vascular disease after preeclampsia seems to be related to the gestational age at delivery and to the severity of preeclampsia (Table 1.2). A Norwegian population-based cohort study has looked at the mortality from cardiovascular causes, cancer, and stroke of 626,272 mothers whose first delivery was registered between 1967 and 1992, with a median follow-up of 13 years [18]. They found that women who had preeclampsia had a 1.2-fold higher long-term risk of death (95% CI 1.02–1.37) than women who did not have preeclampsia, but this risk increased to 2.71 (1.99–3.68) in women with preeclampsia and preterm delivery at less than 37 weeks of gestation compared with women who did not have preeclampsia and whose pregnancies went to term. Furthermore, the risk of death from cardiovascular causes among

TABLE 1.1

Preeclampsia and Risk of Future Vascular Disease

Disease	Mean Follow-Up (Years)	Relative Risk	95% CI
Hypertension [14]	14.1	3.7	2.7–5.05
Ischemic heart disease [14]	11.7	2.16	1.86–2.52
Stroke [14]	10.4	1.81	1.45–2.27
Thromboembolism [14]	4.7	1.79	1.37–2.33
End-stage renal disease [19]	26.5	4.7	3.6–6.1

TABLE 1.2

Preeclampsia and Risk of Cardiovascular Mortality According to Gestational Age at Onset or Delivery

Reference	Definition of Early Preeclampsia	Early Preeclampsia: Hazard Ratio (95% CI) for Cardiovascular Death	Late Preeclampsia Hazard Ratio (95% CI) for Cardiovascular Death
Irgens et al. [18]	Delivery <37 weeks	8.12 (4.3–15.3)	1.65 (1.0–2.7)
Mongraw-Chattin et al. [25]	Onset <34 weeks	9.54 (4.5–20.2)	2.08 (1.2–3.4)
Cirillo and Cohn [26]	Onset <34 weeks	6.7 (2.7–16.2)	2.5 (1.3–3.8)
Skjaerven et al. [27]	Delivery <37 weeks	3.7 (2.7–4.8)	1.6 (1.4–2.0)

women with preeclampsia and preterm delivery was 8.12-fold higher (4.31–15.33) than women without preeclampsia who delivered at term, whereas women with preeclampsia who delivered at term had only a 1.65-fold (1.01–2.7) higher risk of cardiovascular death (Table 1.2) [18]. Therefore, women with a history of early-onset preeclampsia appear to be at a much higher risk of future cardiovascular disease compared with women who developed late-onset preeclampsia during their pregnancy. Likewise, in the California Health and Development Study, women with prior preterm preeclampsia (onset of preeclampsia <34 weeks) had a 9.5-fold increased risk of cardiovascular death compared with women with normotensive pregnancies, in contrast to a 2.1-fold risk among women with previous late-onset preeclampsia [25]. A recent study using the same cohort has shown that early-onset preeclampsia (<34 weeks) was not only a strong predictor of cardiovascular death, but also showed evidence of age dependence, as early-onset preeclampsia was associated with very high cardiovascular mortality by age 60 [26]. In a Norwegian study, the hazard ratio for cardiovascular death associated with preterm preeclampsia (delivery <37 weeks) compared with normotensive pregnancy was 3.7 compared with a 1.6-times higher risk among women with prior preeclampsia at term [27]. Moreover, among women with only one lifetime pregnancy, the increased risk of cardiovascular death was higher than for those with two or more children (hazard ratio of 9.44 after preterm preeclampsia and 3.4 after term preeclampsia compared with normotensive pregnancies) [27]. There is also evidence for an association between the severity of preeclampsia and the future risk of cardiovascular disease. Compared with women who had a normotensive pregnancy, women who had mild preeclampsia had a relative risk of future cardiovascular disease of 2 (95% CI 1.83–2.19), women who had moderate preeclampsia had a relative risk of 2.99 (2.51–3.58), and those who had severe preeclampsia had a relative risk of 5.36 (3.96–7.27) [28]. Similarly, Kessous et al. have recently shown a significant association between preeclampsia and cardiovascular morbidity (Figure 1.1). Moreover, they have shown a linear association between the severity of preeclampsia (no preeclampsia, mild preeclampsia, severe preeclampsia, and eclampsia) and the risk of future cardiovascular morbidity (2.75 vs. 4.5% vs. 5.2% vs. 5.7%, respectively; $p = .001$) [29].

Another question is the extent to which recurrent preeclampsia is associated with cardiovascular risk. Preeclampsia usually occurs only in first pregnancies and recurs in only 15% of second pregnancies following a first pregnancy complicated by preeclampsia. Less than 1% of parous women experience preeclampsia twice. However, those who do appear to be at especially high risk of cardiovascular disease. In a registry-based cohort study from Denmark, multiparous women had a 1.3-fold (95% CI 1.1–1.5) increased risk of future cardiovascular disease if their first pregnancy was preeclamptic, and a 2.8-fold (95% CI 2.3–3.4) increased risk after two pregnancies complicated by preeclampsia compared with multiparous women without hypertensive disease. The corresponding relative risks for stroke were 1.2 and 1.5 [30]. Likewise, Kessous et al. have recently demonstrated a significant linear association between the number of previous pregnancies with preeclampsia and the risk of future cardiovascular disease [29]. In a Norwegian study, the differences in

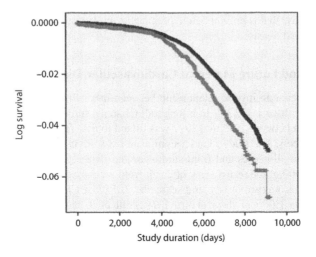

FIGURE 1.1 Cardiovascular disease following preeclampsia (survival curve). Dark gray line—controls and light gray line—preeclampsia.

cardiovascular risk were more subtle among women with nonrecurrent and recurrent preeclampsia: women with preeclampsia only in their first pregnancy had a relative risk of cardiovascular death of 1.5 (1.2–1.9), whereas women with two preeclamptic pregnancies had a relative risk of cardiovascular death of 2 (1.2–3.3) compared with multiparous women with normotensive pregnancies [27].

As opposed to preeclamptic mothers, the future cardiovascular risk of fathers of preeclamptic pregnancies did not increase. The aforementioned Norwegian population cohort study also looked at the mortality of fathers of preeclamptic pregnancies and found that the risk of death from cardiovascular disease was not higher than that of fathers of pregnancies in which preeclampsia did not occur [18].

Preeclampsia and End-Stage Renal Disease

Preeclampsia is more common in women with underlying renal disease, especially when associated with chronic hypertension [31]. In a study that was done more than 30 years ago, when hypertensive pregnant women often underwent postpartum renal biopsy, glomerular endotheliosis, the classic renal histology of preeclampsia, was associated with other renal diseases in 24% of primigravid preeclampsia and 76% of multiparous preeclampsia [32]. Microalbuminuria, which might indicate an underlying renal disease but also acts as a marker for cardiovascular disease, is more common after preeclampsia [33,34]. Bar et al. found that 58% of women with previous preeclampsia had microalbuminuria 2–4 months after delivery, and 42% of them had evidence of microalbuminuria 3–5 years after delivery. There was no difference in renal function between previous preeclamptic women and women with previous normal pregnancy, and within the study group the rate of microalbuminuria was similar among nulliparous and multiparous women [33]. In order to determine the association between preeclampsia and the subsequent development of end-stage renal disease, Viske et al. have linked the data from the Medical Birth Registry of Norway for women who had their first singleton birth between 1967 and 1991 with data from the Norwegian Renal Registry. Among women who had been pregnant one or more times, preeclampsia during the first pregnancy was associated with a relative risk of end-stage renal disease of 4.7 (95% CI 3.6–6.1) (Table 1.1) [21]. Among women who had been pregnant two or more times, preeclampsia during the first pregnancy was associated with a relative risk of end-stage renal disease of 3.2 (95% CI 2.2–4.9), and preeclampsia during the second pregnancy was associated with a relative risk of end-stage renal disease of 6.7 (95% CI 4.3–10.6). Moreover, preeclampsia during two or three pregnancies was associated with a relative risk of 15.5 (95% CI 7.8–30.8). Further analysis showed that having a low–birth weight infant or preterm infant increased the relative risk of end-stage renal disease [21]. Several mechanisms might explain the association between preeclampsia and subsequent renal disease. One hypothesis is that kidney disease and preeclampsia are caused by the same underlying factors, including hypertension, obesity, and insulin resistance [35,36]. A second possibility is that preeclampsia may exacerbate subclinical kidney disease that is present before pregnancy, or alternatively, preeclampsia may cause the later development of renal disease.

Low Birth Weight and Future Maternal Cardiovascular Disease

Several studies have shown an inverse relationship between infants' birth weight and mothers' mortality from cardiovascular disease [37,38]. In a longitudinal study, information from the birth registry in England of infants born between 1976 and 1997 was linked to data from the census and death registration for the study members. The study found a significant association between infants' birth weight and mothers' mortality from all causes and from cardiovascular disease. For mothers whose infants' birth weight was less than 2500 g, the relative risk of death from all causes was 3.06 (95% CI 2.15–4.35) and the relative risk of death from cardiovascular disease was 7.05 (95% CI 2.64–18.77) compared with mothers of offspring weighing 3500 g or above at birth [37]. Smith et al. have evaluated whether complications of pregnancy linked with low birth weight are associated with the mother's subsequent risk of ischemic heart disease by using discharge data on all singleton first births in Scotland between 1981 and 1985 and linking it to the mothers' subsequent admissions and deaths. They found that delivering a baby in the lowest birth weight quintile for gestational age, delivering preterm, and having preeclampsia were all associated with an increased risk of admission to hospital for ischemic heart disease or death from

TABLE 1.3

Pregnancy Complication and Risk of Death Due to Ischemic Heart Disease

Pregnancy Complication	Relative Risk	95% CI
Lowest birth weight quintile	2.4	1.3–4.4
Lowest birth weight quintile and preeclampsia	3.9	1.3–11.6
Lowest birth weight quintile and preterm labor	6.8	2.0–22.9
Lowest birth weight quintile, preeclampsia, and preterm labor	16.1	3.6–72.6

Source: Smith GC, Pell JP, and Walsh D. *Lancet.* 2001;357:2002–6.

ischemic heart disease during the subsequent 19 years [39]. Delivering a baby less than 2500 g resulted in a relative risk of death of 11.3 (95% CI 3.5–36.1) due to ischemic heart disease compared with women whose offspring's birth weight was 3500 g or above. Women who had pregnancies complicated by low birth weight and preeclampsia had a greater risk of future cardiovascular disease compared with women who had only preeclampsia. Moreover, women who had all three pregnancy complications—a low–birth weight infant, preeclampsia, and preterm labor—had the highest risk of cardiovascular disease in later life with a relative risk of 16.1 (95% CI 3.6–72.6) (Table 1.3) [39]. Likewise, Cirillo and Cohn have recently investigated the combination of pregnancy complications and the risk of cardiovascular death in women from the California Child Health and Development Study cohort. They found that the combination of small for gestational age (SGA) and preexisting hypertension, gestational hypertension and preterm delivery, preeclampsia and preexisting hypertension, and preterm delivery and preexisting hypertension conferred a 4- to 7-fold risk of cardiovascular death [26]. A recent study explored the mortality risk among women with placental abruption. Over two million women with a first singleton birth between 1967 and 2002 in Norway and 1973 and 2003 in Sweden were included. Women with placental abruption in their first pregnancy had an increased risk of cardiovascular death with a hazard ratio of 1.8 (95% CI 1.3–2.4). Results did not change even after the exclusion of women with pregestational hypertension or preeclampsia. Women with placental abruption in any pregnancy also had a 1.8-fold (1.5–2.2) increased risk of cardiovascular mortality compared with women who had never experienced this condition [40].

Endothelial Dysfunction: The Link between Preeclampsia and Future Cardiovascular Disease

The mechanisms that account for an increased risk of cardiovascular disease in women with a history of preeclampsia are not yet well understood. However, it appears that endothelial dysfunction might be the mechanism linking preeclampsia with future cardiovascular disease.

Several studies have shown that endothelial dysfunction is more common in women with a history of preeclampsia many years after the affected pregnancy compared with women with previous normal pregnancy [13,41–43]. Chambers et al. studied 113 women with previous preeclampsia, 35 of them with recurrent episodes and 78 with a single episode, and 48 women with previous uncomplicated pregnancies at least 3 months and at a median interval of 3 years postpartum. Flow-mediated dilatation, as a measure of endothelial function, was lower in women with previous preeclampsia compared with controls. The defect was more severe in women with recurrent preeclampsia compared with a single episode of preeclampsia [41]. In contrast, there were no significant differences in glyceryl trinitrate–induced, endothelium-independent dilatation between the three groups. Multivariable regression analysis showed that the relationship between previous preeclampsia and impaired flow-mediated dilatation was independent of age, BMI, blood pressure, family history of hypertension, fasting plasma glucose levels, and lipid profile. These results indicate that endothelial function is impaired in women with previous preeclampsia and cannot be explained by maternal risk factors [41]. Similarly, Germain et al. have also demonstrated significantly decreased endothelium-dependent vasodilatation among patients with previous preeclampsia compared with women with previous healthy pregnancies 11–27 months after pregnancy. Among the previously preeclamptic women, 40% exhibited endothelial dysfunction. Of note, diastolic and mean blood pressures as well as serum cholesterol were higher in women with previous preeclampsia and a trend to an inverse correlation was found between serum cholesterol levels and endothelial-mediated vasodilatation [43].

Arterial stiffness is a key determinant of central aortic pressure and is an independent predictor of adverse cardiovascular outcomes [44]. An augmentation index, which is expressed as a percentage of the aortic pulse pressure, is a measure of the stiffness of the arterial walls and can be determined non-invasively using applanation tonometry. Robb et al. evaluated the effect of normal pregnancy and pre-eclampsia on arterial stiffness and found that the augmentation index increased from 24 weeks over the third trimester. In women with preeclampsia, the augmentation index increased during pregnancy compared with gestationally matched women with uncomplicated pregnancies and remained elevated at 7 weeks postpartum [45]. The aforementioned studies did not differentiate between early- and late-onset preeclampsia and did not include patients with isolated intrauterine growth restriction (IUGR). Since early-onset preeclampsia and late-onset preeclampsia are considered by some to be different disease entities [46,47], women with a history of preeclampsia in their last pregnancy were studied 6–24 months postpartum but were divided into early-onset (diagnosed before 34 weeks of gestation) and late-onset preeclampsia (diagnosed after 34 weeks of gestation) [48]. In early-onset disease, underperfusion of the placenta is the predominant precipitating factor, whereas in late-onset preeclampsia, there is often minimal or no placental involvement [14,49]. In addition, this study also included an interesting group of patients with a history of IUGR without preeclampsia. All patients with IUGR included in this study had early-onset IUGR and delivered before 34 weeks of gestation. Flow-mediated vasodilatation was significantly reduced in women with previous early-onset preeclampsia and women with previous iso-lated IUGR compared with women with previous late-onset preeclampsia and control subjects (3.2% and 2.1% vs. 7.9% and 9.1%, respectively; $p < .0001$). In support of the concept that early- and late-onset preeclampsia represent different disease entities, flow-mediated vasodilatation in women with previous late-onset preeclampsia was comparable to that in the control group [48]. In addition, 93% and 89% of the early preeclampsia and IUGR women, respectively, exhibited endothelial dysfunction defined as flow-mediated dilatation <4.5%, whereas only 22% of late preeclamptic women and 12.5% of the control subjects met the criteria for endothelial dysfunction ($p = .0024$). Similarly, the radial arterial stiffness measured by the augmentation index was significantly increased only among women with pre-vious early-onset preeclampsia and women with previous isolated IUGR, but not among the late-onset preeclamptic women, whose augmentation index values were similar to those of the control subjects [48]. In accordance with these findings, Khalil et al. reported a significantly higher augmentation index in early- compared with late-onset preeclampsia and in severe compared with mild preeclampsia when patients were studied during pregnancy [50]. These interesting results suggest that early- but not late-onset preeclampsia is associated with endothelial dysfunction and increased arterial stiffness that extend beyond pregnancy and might contribute to adverse cardiovascular outcomes observed mainly in women with previous early-onset preeclampsia. Women with previous late-onset preeclampsia, however, exhibit normal physiological vascular profiles, which explains their relative low risk of future cardiovascular disease as shown by epidemiological studies [16,18]. Of interest, women who had isolated IUGR in their previous pregnancy also exhibited endothelial dysfunction, which was even more pronounced compared with early preeclamptic patients. Moreover, in the early preeclamptic women, those who also had fetal growth restriction had markedly reduced flow-mediated dilatation compared with those without fetal growth restriction [48]. Similarly, Khalil et al. have shown that the augmentation index during pregnancy was significantly elevated in women with preeclampsia who also had fetal growth restriction compared with those with preeclampsia without fetal growth restriction [50]. Therefore, in patients with previous preeclampsia, the degree of endothelial dysfunction seems to be more severe in the presence of IUGR, putting these women at higher risk of future cardiovascular disease.

The mechanism accounting for an increased risk of cardiovascular disease in women with a history of preeclampsia is probably related to endothelial dysfunction. However, it is still unanswered whether preeclamptic pregnancy results in damage to the endothelium leading to future cardiovascular disease or whether preexisting endothelial dysfunction underlies both the predisposition to preeclampsia and the later development of cardiovascular disease (Figure 1.2).

It is possible that shared risk factors may jointly predispose women to preeclampsia, endothelial dysfunction, and cardiovascular disease. Diabetes mellitus, chronic hypertension, renal disease, and

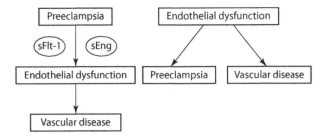

FIGURE 1.2　Mechanism accounting for the increased risk of cardiovascular diseases in women with a history of preeclampsia.

subclinical insulin resistance predispose women to preeclampsia and elevate the risk of cardiovascular disease [51–53]. Smith et al. assessed the physical and biochemical cardiovascular risk markers in women who had developed preeclampsia in their previous pregnancy at 1 year postpartum. Women with a history of preeclampsia had increased blood pressure, total cholesterol, higher LDL cholesterol, triglycerides, increased BMI, fasting insulin HOMA index, and microalbumin/creatinine ratio compared with women with previous normotensive pregnancies [54]. Of note, patients were not evaluated in this study before pregnancy, and the authors could not therefore determine whether cardiovascular risk factors play a role in the pathogenesis of preeclampsia or whether cardiovascular risk factors are being caused by preeclampsia. In order to answer this question, Romundstad et al. studied the cardiovascular risk factors before and after pregnancy in women who had experienced preeclampsia or gestational hypertension. They found that nearly half of the elevated cardiovascular risk factors after pregnancy could be explained by prepregnancy risk factors, rather than reflecting a direct influence of the hypertensive disorder in pregnancy [55]. Therefore, pregnancy may be viewed as a stress test that can reveal subclinical cardiovascular disease phenotypes long before overt disease [52].

Role of Antiangiogenic Factors in the Pathogenesis of Preeclampsia and Future Cardiovascular Disease

It has become clear in recent years that the circulating antiangiogenic factors sFlt-1 and sEng released from the placenta play a major role in the pathogenesis of preeclampsia. It has been proposed that in preeclampsia the placenta produces elevated levels of sFlt-1, which captures free vascular endothelial growth factor (VEGF) and placental growth factor (PLGF), inhibits their action, and causes endothelial dysfunction together with sEng, which inhibits transforming growth factorβ1 (TGF-β1) signaling [5,7,8]. Adenoviral-mediated overexpression of both sFlt-1 and sEng causes severe vascular damage, proteinuria, and severe hypertension in rats. Thus, sEng and sFlt-1, two antiangiogenic proteins operating through separate mechanisms, may combine to produce endothelial dysfunction and severe preeclampsia [6]. It has been hypothesized that endothelial damage resulting from maternal exposure to these angiogenic factors during pregnancy may be the cause of future maternal vascular disease. Although levels of sFlt-1 decline after the delivery of the placenta, a persistent and subtle antiangiogenic milieu may contribute to endothelial dysfunction and an elevated risk of cardiovascular disease in women with a history of preeclampsia [52]. It has been shown that monocytes in women with preeclampsia produce elevated levels of sFlt-1 compared with controls [56], and thus the source of sFlt-1 in nonpregnant women may be peripheral blood mononuclear cells. However, comparison of the circulatory levels of sFlt-1, sEng, VEGF, and PLGF 6–24 months after delivery between women with previous early-onset preeclampsia and women with previous normal pregnancy revealed no differences despite the presence of endothelial dysfunction in women with a history of preeclampsia [48]. Similarly, Germain et al. found similar circulatory levels of sFlt-1 and VEGF in women with previous severe preeclampsia and women with previous normal pregnancies 11–27 months after pregnancy [43]. In contrast, Wolf et al. found increased levels of sFlt-1 in women with prior preeclampsia 18 months postpartum, but instead of decreased levels of free

VEGF as expected, they found a trend toward increased free VEGF levels in the preeclamptic group [57]. Therefore, the basal levels of sFlt-1 appeared to be too low to influence circulating VEGF, suggesting that sFlt-1 is not likely to play a clinically significant role in the postpartum state. However, more studies are needed in order to determine whether antiangiogenic and proangiogenic molecules contribute to the development of cardiovascular disease in women. Of note, high sFlt-1 levels are also associated with carotid intima-media thickness and the progression of atherosclerosis in hypertensive patients [58]. Interestingly, Noori et al. have shown that in contrast to the observation during pregnancy, serum PLGF levels 12 weeks postpartum were higher in women who had a hypertensive pregnancy compared with women with a previous normotensive pregnancy [59]. PLGF has been shown to stimulate atherosclerotic intimal thickening [60], and elevated PLGF levels have been associated with an increased risk of coronary heart disease more than 10 years after a baseline test in asymptomatic women [61]. The authors speculate that the increased risk of cardiovascular disease after a pregnancy affected by preeclampsia may be partly mediated through PLGF, which increases atherosclerotic plaque formation [59].

Bytautiene et al. have evaluated the long-term effects of preeclampsia on vascular function in a mouse model of sFlt-1-induced preeclampsia. Mice at day 8 of gestation were injected with adenovirus carrying sFlt-1, and vascular function in the mothers was investigated 6–8 months after delivery [62]. At 6–8 months postpartum, blood sFlt-1 had returned to low levels and was comparable between the sFlt-1-injected mice and the controls injected with saline. Moreover, there was no difference in postpartum blood pressure or vascular reactivity between the groups. Hence, in a mouse model, overexpression of sFlt-1 does not lead to impaired vascular function after delivery [62]. These findings favor the hypothesis that the increased risk of cardiovascular disease in women with a history of preeclampsia is likely the result of preexisting risk factors common to preeclampsia and cardiovascular disease.

In order to determine whether endothelial function is a preexisting condition in preeclamptic patients, it is preferable to assess patients during or even before pregnancy. Savvidou et al. measured flow-mediated dilatation at 23–25 weeks of gestation in 86 women, and found that women who developed preeclampsia had significantly lower flow-mediated dilatation than did women who had normal outcomes (3.65% vs. 8.65%; $p < .0001$). Therefore, it appears that maternal endothelial function is impaired in women who eventually develop preeclampsia, and it occurs before the development of the clinical syndrome [63]. In accordance with these findings, Noori et al. have also demonstrated decreased flow-mediated dilatation at 10–17 weeks of gestation in women who later developed preeclampsia [59]. Therefore, the evidence in the literature appears to support the hypothesis that endothelial dysfunction is a preexisting condition, and pregnancy unmasks a woman preexisting risk of cardiovascular disease.

Large population-based prospective studies assessing endothelial function preconception are required in order to help in understanding the causality and whether endothelial dysfunction is a preexisting condition leading to both preeclampsia and future cardiovascular disease, or whether preeclampsia itself via antiangiogenic factors may injure the endothelium and thereby increase the risk of future cardiovascular disease.

Preeclampsia and Future Cardiovascular Disease: How Should We Manage Our Patients?

The consistent data showing that women with prior preeclampsia are at increased risk of cardiovascular disease have led the AHA to recommend that a history of preeclampsia be considered a major risk factor for coronary heart disease and cerebrovascular disease [9]. According to these guidelines, clinicians should obtain a pregnancy history for preeclampsia in all women to assess the risk of cardiovascular disease. A positive history of preeclampsia should be used to classify a woman as being at risk of cardiovascular disease, similar to a woman who is a cigarette smoker. Women with such a history should be counseled regarding preventive treatment and lifestyle modifications, including smoking cessation, physical activity, and weight reduction if overweight. However, there is no evidence that such interventions will decrease cardiovascular morbidity in this population of women. Nevertheless, the AHA recommends that women with a history of preeclampsia be screened for hypertension and other cardiovascular risk factors beginning at 6 months to 1 year postpartum [9]. In addition, the American

Congress of Obstetricians and Gynecologists (ACOG) has recently provided specific recommendations for cardiovascular disease risk factor screening for women with prior preeclampsia that was preterm (<37 weeks) or recurrent [64]. In this group of women, ACOG recommends yearly screening of blood pressure, lipids, fasting blood sugar, and BMI. This recommendation relates only to women with preterm or recurrent preeclampsia as they are at the highest risk of cardiovascular mortality, whereas the issue of screening for women with term preeclampsia is not addressed. Despite its recommendation, ACOG point out that the value of screening for cardiovascular risk factors in this group of women has not been established yet [64]. Veerbeek et al. have recently evaluated postpartum differences in cardiovascular risk factors 2–5 years after delivery in three subgroups of patients with a history of hypertensive pregnancy: early-onset preeclampsia, late-onset preeclampsia, and pregnancy-induced hypertension [65]. Women with previous early-onset preeclampsia had significantly higher fasting blood glucose, insulin, triglycerides, and total cholesterol compared with women with previous late-onset preeclampsia and women with previous pregnancy-induced hypertension. Almost half of the early-onset preeclampsia women had developed hypertension, compared with 39% and 25% of women in the pregnancy-induced hypertension and late-onset preeclampsia groups [65]. Therefore, preventive strategies should be stratified according to severity and the gestational age of onset of the hypertensive disease. Although the value of screening or intervention in previously preeclamptic women has not been established, a cost-effectiveness analysis has recently been done. A decision-analytic model was constructed to evaluate health-care costs and the potential effects of screening and treatment for hypertension in women with a history of early-onset preeclampsia [66]. Outcomes were measured in absolute costs, events, life-years, and quality-adjusted life-years (QALYs). Over a 20-year period, events occurred in 7.2% of the population after screening and in 8.5% of the population without screening. QALYs increased from 16.37 without screening to 16.4 with screening. Furthermore, screening was found to be less expensive than no screening, saving expenditures of €1071 per person over a 20-year period. Consequently, the authors concluded that annual hypertension screening and treatment for women with a history of preeclampsia may save costs for at least a similar quality of life and survival compared with standard care [66]. In order to initiate preventive health screening and intervention in women with prior preeclampsia, the clinician needs to be aware of the patient's history of preeclampsia. However, there is a wide range of variability in the validity of maternal self-recall of preeclampsia. A systematic review found that the sensitivity of recalling a diagnosis of preeclampsia ranged from 57% to 87% [67]. Furthermore, if the clinician does not actively ask the patient about a history of preeclampsia, the likelihood that a patient will spontaneously offer her history depends on the patient's awareness of the link between prior preeclampsia and future cardiovascular disease. Previous studies have shown that few women with prior preeclampsia know that it is associated with future health risks [68,69]. Nevertheless, even if a patient provides a history of preeclampsia, many clinicians are not aware of the link between prior preeclampsia and future cardiovascular disease, and will not therefore address the issue of cardiovascular risk reduction in these patients. In a Canadian study of obstetricians and midwives, only 54% were aware that women with prior preeclampsia have an increased long-term risk of hypertension [70]. In an online survey performed in the United States, only 9% of internists and 38% of obstetricians reported that they had provided cardiovascular risk reduction counseling to women with prior preeclampsia [71]. In addition, a study from the Netherlands indicted that only 50% of women with prior preeclampsia had had their blood pressure checked within 3 months of delivery [72]. Despite these obstacles, given the evidence to date, clinicians should make an effort to identify which of their patients has a history of preeclampsia and identify and treat known and modifiable cardiovascular risk factors in these women [73].

SUMMARY

Although the symptoms of preeclampsia resolve over a number of weeks after delivery, epidemiological data suggest that maternal vascular dysfunction may persist for years, manifested by an increased risk of future development of hypertension, stroke, coronary artery disease, and end-stage renal disease. Women with early-onset preeclampsia resulting in IUGR have the highest risk of future cardiovascular disease. Therefore, a woman's obstetric history becomes an important consideration toward her cardiovascular risk assessment. The evidence linking a history of preeclampsia with future cardiovascular disease is strong and has led the AHA and ACOG to recommend including a history of preeclampsia as a risk factor for cardiovascular disease. It is the role of the obstetrician to highlight the consequences of pregnancy outcomes to the primary care physician as well as the mother, as these middle-age women with previous preeclampsia, especially if early and severe, might benefit from lifestyle adaptation or prophylactic treatment. Monitoring and controlling weight, hypertension, and dyslipidemia may reduce long-term morbidity and mortality in this group of women.

The mechanism that accounts for an increased risk of cardiovascular disease in women with history of preeclampsia is thought to be endothelial dysfunction, which has been shown to persist in previously preeclamptic women many years after an affected pregnancy. It is still uncertain whether preeclampsia itself injures the endothelium, which leads to an increased risk of future cardiovascular disease, or whether preexisting endothelial dysfunction underlies both the predisposition to preeclampsia and the later development of cardiovascular disease. A growing body of literature in recent years indicates that endothelial dysfunction is a preexisting condition leading to both preeclampsia and cardiovascular disease later in life. Therefore, women who develop preeclampsia have greater underlying vascular risk. This manifests during pregnancy in the form of preeclampsia and later in life in the form of hypertension, stroke, and ischemic heart disease. However, it is still undetermined how women with prior preeclampsia should be screened for cardiovascular risk factors, and whether interventions to decrease cardiovascular risk factors will decrease cardiovascular morbidity and mortality in this population of women.

REFERENCES

1. ACOG. Diagnosis and management of preeclampsia and eclampsia. Practice bulletin no. 33, January 2002. *Obstet Gynecol*. 2002;99:159–67.
2. Berg CJ, Mackay AP, Qin C, Callaghan WM. Overview of maternal morbidity during hospitalization for labor and delivery in the United States: 1993–1997 and 2001–2005. *Obstet Gynecol*. 2009;113:1075–81.
3. MacKay AP, Berg CJ, Atrash HK. Pregnancy-related mortality from preeclampsia and eclampsia. *Obstet Gynecol*. 2001;97:533–8.
4. Roberts JM, Gammill HS. Preeclampsia: Recent insights. *Hypertension*. 2005;46:1243–9.
5. Maynard SE, Min JY, Merchan J, et al. Excess placental soluble fms-like tyrosine kinase 1 (sFlt1) may contribute to endothelial dysfunction, hypertension, and proteinuria in preeclampsia. *J Clin Invest*. 2003;111:649–58.
6. Venkatesha S, Toporsian M, Lam C, et al. Soluble endoglin contributes to the pathogenesis of preeclampsia. *Nat Med*. 2006;12:642–9.
7. Levine RJ, Lam C, Qian C, et al. Soluble endoglin and other circulating antiangiogenic factors in preeclampsia. *N Engl J Med*. 2006;355:992–1005.
8. Levine RJ, Maynard SE, Qian C, et al. Circulating angiogenic factors and the risk of preeclampsia. *N Engl J Med*. 2004;350:672–83.
9. Mosca L, Benjamin EJ, Berra K, et al. Effectiveness-based guidelines for the prevention of cardiovascular disease in women: 2011 update; A guideline from the American Heart Association. *Circulation*. 2011;123:1243–62.
10. Magnussen EB, Vatten LJ, Lund-Nilsen TI, et al. Prepregnancy cardiovascular risk factors as predictors of pre-eclampsia: Population based cohort study. *BMJ*. 2007;335:978.
11. Parretti E, Lapolla A, Dalfra M, et al. Preeclampsia in lean normotensive normotolerant pregnant women can be predicted by simple insulin sensitivity indexes. *Hypertension*. 2006;47:449–53.
12. Wolf M, Kettyle E, Sandler L, et al. Obesity and preeclampsia: The potential role of inflammation. *Obstet Gynecol*. 2001;98:757–62.
13. Agatisa PK, Ness RB, Roberts JM, et al. Impairment of endothelial function in women with a history of preeclampsia: An indicator of cardiovascular risk. *Am J Physiol Heart Circ Physiol*. 2004;286:H1389–93.
14. Lampinen KH, Ronnback M, Kaaja RJ, Groop PH. Impaired vascular dilatation in women with a history of pre-eclampsia. *J Hypertens*. 2006;24:751–6.
15. Poston L. Endothelial dysfunction in pre-eclampsia. *Pharmacol Rep*. 2006;58(Suppl):69–74.
16. Bellamy L, Casas JP, Hingorani AD, Williams DJ. Pre-eclampsia and risk of cardiovascular disease and cancer in later life: Systematic review and meta-analysis. *BMJ*. 2007;335:974.
17. Hannaford P, Ferry S, Hirsch S. Cardiovascular sequelae of toxaemia of pregnancy. *Heart*. 1997;77:154–8.

18. Irgens HU, Reisaeter L, Irgens LM, Lie RT. Long term mortality of mothers and fathers after pre-eclampsia: Population based cohort study. *BMJ*. 2001;323:1213–17.
19. Kestenbaum B, Seliger SL, Easterling TR, et al. Cardiovascular and thromboembolic events following hypertensive pregnancy. *Am J Kidney Dis*. 2003;42:982–9.
20. Ray JG, Vermeulen MJ, Schull MJ, Redelmeier DA. Cardiovascular health after maternal placental syndromes (CHAMPS): Population-based retrospective cohort study. *Lancet*. 2005;366:1797–803.
21. Vikse BE, Irgens LM, Leivestad T, et al. Preeclampsia and the risk of end-stage renal disease. *N Engl J Med*. 2008;359:800–9.
22. Williams D. Long-term complications of preeclampsia. *Semin Nephrol*. 2011;31:111–22.
23. Wilson BJ, Watson MS, Prescott GJ, et al. Hypertensive diseases of pregnancy and risk of hypertension and stroke in later life: Results from cohort study. *BMJ*. 2003;326:845.
24. Shalom G, Shoham-Vardi I, Sergienko R, et al. *Is preeclampsia a significant risk factor for long-term hospitalizations and morbidity? J Matern Fetal Neonatal Med*. 2013;26:13–15.
25. Mongraw-Chaffin ML, Cirillo PM, Cohn BA. Preeclampsia and cardiovascular disease death: Prospective evidence from the child health and development studies cohort. *Hypertension*. 2010;56:166–71.
26. Cirillo PM, Cohn BA. Pregnancy complications and cardiovascular disease death: 50-year follow-up of the child health and development studies pregnancy cohort. *Circulation*. 2015;12:1234–42.
27. Skjaerven R, Wilcox AJ, Klungsoyr K, et al. Cardiovascular mortality after pre-eclampsia in one child mothers: Prospective, population based cohort study. *BMJ*. 2012;345:e7677.
28. McDonald SD, Malinowski A, Zhou Q, et al. Cardiovascular sequelae of preeclampsia/eclampsia: A systematic review and meta-analyses. *Am Heart J*. 2008;156:918–30.
29. Kessous R, Shoham-Vardi I, Pariente G, et al. Long-term maternal atherosclerotic morbidity in women with pre-eclampsia. *Heart*. 2015;101:442–6.
30. Lykke JA, Langhoff-Roos J, Sibai BM, et al. Hypertensive pregnancy disorders and subsequent cardio-vascular mortality and type 2 diabetes mellitus in the mother. *Hypertension*. 2009;53:944–51.
31. Williams D, Davison J. Chronic kidney disease in pregnancy. *BMJ*. 2008;336:211–15.
32. Fisher KA, Luger A, Spargo BH, Lindheimer MD. Hypertension in pregnancy: Clinical-pathological correlations and remote prognosis. *Medicine (Baltimore)*. 1981;60:267–76.
33. Bar J, Kaplan B, Wittenberg C, et al. Microalbuminuria after pregnancy complicated by pre-eclampsia. *Nephrol Dial Transplant*. 1999;14:1129–32.
34. McDonald SD, Han Z, Walsh MW, et al. Kidney disease after preeclampsia: A systematic review and meta-analysis. *Am J Kidney Dis*. 2010;55:1026–39.
35. Joffe GM, Esterlitz JR, Levine RJ, et al. The relationship between abnormal glucose tolerance and hyper-tensive disorders of pregnancy in healthy nulliparous women: Calcium for Preeclampsia Prevention (CPEP) Study Group. *Am J Obstet Gynecol*. 1998;179:1032–7.
36. Sibai BM, Gordon T, Thom E, et al. Risk factors for preeclampsia in healthy nulliparous women: A prospective multicenter study; The National Institute of Child Health and Human Development Network of Maternal–Fetal Medicine Units. *Am J Obstet Gynecol*. 1995;172:642–8.
37. Smith GD, Harding S, Rosato M. Relation between infants' birth weight and mothers' mortality: Prospective observational study. *BMJ*. 2000;320:839–40.
38. Smith GD, Hart C, Blane D, et al. Lifetime socioeconomic position and mortality: Prospective observa-tional study. *BMJ*. 1997;314:547–52.
39. Smith GC, Pell JP, Walsh D. Pregnancy complications and maternal risk of ischaemic heart disease: A retrospective cohort study of 129,290 births. *Lancet*. 2001;357:2002–6.
40. DeRoo L, Skjaerven R, Wilcox A, et al. Placental abruption and long-term maternal cardiovascular disease mortality: A population-based registry study in Norway and Sweden. *Eur J Epidemiol*. 2016;31(5):501–11.
41. Chambers JC, Fusi L, Malik IS, et al. Association of maternal endothelial dysfunction with preeclamp-sia. *JAMA*. 2001;285:1607–12.
42. Evans CS, Gooch L, Flotta D, et al. Cardiovascular system during the postpartum state in women with a history of preeclampsia. *Hypertension*. 2011;58:57–62.
43. Germain AM, Romanik MC, Guerra I, et al. Endothelial dysfunction: A link among preeclampsia, recurrent pregnancy loss, and future cardiovascular events? *Hypertension*. 2007;49:90–95.
44. Laurent S, Boutouyrie P, Asmar R, et al. Aortic stiffness is an independent predictor of all-cause and cardiovascular mortality in hypertensive patients. *Hypertension*. 2001;37:1236–41.

45. Robb AO, Mills NL, Din JN, et al. Influence of the menstrual cycle, pregnancy, and preeclampsia on arterial stiffness. *Hypertension*. 2009;53(6):952–8.

46. Crispi F, Dominguez C, Llurba E, et al. Placental angiogenic growth factors and uterine artery Doppler findings for characterization of different subsets in preeclampsia and in isolated intrauterine growth restriction. *Am J Obstet Gynecol*. 2006;195:201–7.

47. Ness RB, Sibai BM. Shared and disparate components of the pathophysiologies of fetal growth restriction and preeclampsia. *Am J Obstet Gynecol*. 2006;195:40–49.

48. Yinon Y, Kingdom JC, Odutayo A, et al. Vascular dysfunction in women with a history of preeclampsia and intrauterine growth restriction: Insights into future vascular risk. *Circulation*. 2010;122:1846–53.

49. Redman CW, Sargent IL. Pre-eclampsia, the placenta and the maternal systemic inflammatory response: A review. *Placenta*. 2003;24(Suppl A):S21–7.

50. Khalil A, Jauniaux E, Harrington K. Antihypertensive therapy and central hemodynamics in women with hypertensive disorders in pregnancy. *Obstet Gynecol*. 2009;113:646–54.

51. Laivuori H, Tikkanen MJ, Ylikorkala O. Hyperinsulinemia 17 years after preeclamptic first pregnancy. *J Clin Endocrinol Metab*. 1996;81:2908–11.

52. Powe CE, Levine RJ, Karumanchi SA. Preeclampsia, a disease of the maternal endothelium: The role of antiangiogenic factors and implications for later cardiovascular disease. *Circulation*. 2011;123:2856–69.

53. Wolf M, Sandler L, Munoz K, et al. First trimester insulin resistance and subsequent preeclampsia: A prospective study. *J Clin Endocrinol Metab*. 2002;87:1563–8.

54. Smith GN, Walker MC, Liu A, et al. A history of preeclampsia identifies women who have underlying cardiovascular risk factors. *Am J Obstet Gynecol*. 2009;200:58.e51–8.

55. Romundstad PR, Magnussen EB, Smith GD, Vatten LJ. *Hypertension in pregnancy and later cardiovascular risk: Common antecedents? Circulation*. 2010;122:579–84.

56. Rajakumar A, Michael HM, Rajakumar PA, et al. Extra-placental expression of vascular endothelial growth factor receptor-1 (Flt-1) and soluble Flt-1 (sFlt-1), by peripheral blood mononuclear cells (PBMCs) in normotensive and preeclamptic pregnant women. *Placenta*. 2005;26:563–73.

57. Wolf M, Hubel CA, Lam C, et al. Preeclampsia and future cardiovascular disease: Potential role of altered angiogenesis and insulin resistance. *J Clin Endocrinol Metab*. 2004;89:6239–43.

58. Shin S, Lee SH, Park S, et al. Soluble fms-like tyrosine kinase-1 and the progression of carotid intima-media thickness: 24-month follow-up study. *Circ J*. 2010;74:2211–15.

59. Noori M, Donald AE, Angelakopoulou A, et al. Prospective study of placental angiogenic factors and maternal vascular function before and after preeclampsia and gestational hypertension. *Circulation*. 2010;122:478–87.

60. Khurana R, Moons L, Shafi S, et al. Placental growth factor promotes atherosclerotic intimal thickening and macrophage accumulation. *Circulation*. 2005;111:2828–36.

61. Cassidy A, Chiuve SE, Manson JE, et al. Potential role for plasma placental growth factor in predicting coronary heart disease risk in women. *Arterioscler Thromb Vasc Biol*. 2009;29:134–9.

62. Bytautiene E, Lu F, Tamayo EH, et al. Long-term maternal cardiovascular function in a mouse model of sFlt-1-induced preeclampsia. *Am J Physiol Heart Circ Physiol*. 2010;298:H189–93.

63. Savvidou MD, Hingorani AD, Tsikas D, et al. Endothelial dysfunction and raised plasma concentrations of asymmetric dimethylarginine in pregnant women who subsequently develop pre-eclampsia. *Lancet*. 2003;361:1511–17.

64. American College of Obstetricians and Gynecologists. Hypertension in pregnancy: Report of the American College of Obstetricians and Gynecologists' Task Force on Hypertension in Pregnancy. *Obstet Gynecol*. 2013;122:1122–31.

65. Veerbeek JH, Hermes W, Breimer AY, et al. Cardiovascular disease risk factors after early-onset preeclampsia, late-onset preeclampsia and pregnancy-induced hypertension. *Hypertension*. 2015;65:600–606.

66. Drost JT, Grutters JP, vab der Wilt GJ, et al. Yearly hypertension screening in women with a history of pre-eclampsia: A cost-effectiveness analysis. *Neth Heart J*. 2015;23:585–91.

67. Stuart JJ, Bairey Merz CN, Berga SL, et al. Maternal recall of hypertensive disorders in pregnancy: A systematic review. *J Women Health*. 2013;22:37–47.

68. Brown MC, Bell R, Collins C, et al. Women's perception of future risk following pregnancies complicated by preeclampsia. *Hypertens Pregnancy*. 2013;32:60–73.

69. Seely EW, Rich-Edwards J, Lui J, et al. Risk of future cardiovascular disease in women with prior pre-eclampsia: A focus group study. *BMC Pregnancy Childbirth*. 2013;13:240.

70. MacDonald SE, Walker M, Ramsha H, et al. Hypertensive disorders of pregnancy and long term risk of hypertension: What do Ontario prenatal care providers know, and what do they communicate? *J Obstet Gynaecol Can*. 2007;29:705–10.

71. Young B, Hacker MR, Rana S. Physicians' knowledge of future vascular disease in women with pre-eclampsia. *Hypertens Pregnancy*. 2012;31:50–58.

72. Nijdam ME, Timmerman M, Franx A, et al. Cardiovascular risk factor assessment after pre-eclampsia in primary care. *BMC Family Practice*. 2009;10:77.

73. Seely EW, Tsigas E, Rich-Edwards JW. Preeclampsia and future cardiovascular disease in women: How good are the data and how can we manage our patients? *Semin Perinatol*. 2015;39:276–83.

2

Gestational Diabetes Mellitus: Definition, Pregnancy Complications, and Long-Term Maternal Complications

Shelly Meshel and Yariv Yogev

Today, gestational diabetes mellitus (GDM) is defined as carbohydrate intolerance of variable severity with onset or first recognition during pregnancy. The definition is applicable regardless of whether insulin is used for treatment or the condition persists after pregnancy. It does not exclude the possibility that unrecognized glucose intolerance may have antedated the pregnancy [1].

GDM complicates 3%–15% of all pregnancies and is a major cause of perinatal morbidity and mortality as well as maternal long-term morbidity. Of all types of diabetes, GDM accounts for approximately 90%–95% of all cases of diabetes in pregnancy [2].

Introduction: Historical Milestones

The first reference to diabetes in pregnancy was made by Bennewitz in 1823. He considered diabetes to be a transient symptom of pregnancy and proved his theory when after two pregnancies all symptoms and glucosuria disappeared [3]. The next significant milestone in diabetic research during pregnancy was achieved by Priscilla White. Back in the early twentieth century, women with diabetes had a low chance of a successful pregnancy outcome. Pricilla was the first to believe that diabetes is not a contraindication to pregnancy. In 1949, White published the first version of her classification system, which would have an immense clinical value to practitioners all over the world [4]. In 1979, the White classification underwent its final revision [5].

In 1952, Jorgan Pedersen pointed out his (maternal) hyperglycemia–(fetal) hyperinsulinism hypothesis. According to his hypothesis, maternal hyperglycemia results in fetal hyperglycemia and, hence, in hypertrophy of fetal pancreatic islet tissue with insulin hypersecretion. Hyperinsulinism in the presence of more than adequate supplies of glucose, abruptly eliminated at birth, explains several of the characteristic features observed in the offspring [6]. This theory is still in use more than 20 years after Pedersen's death and is now called the *Pedersen theory*.

In 1989, representatives of government health departments and patient organizations from all European countries met with diabetes experts under the aegis of the regional offices of the World Health Organization (WHO) and the International Diabetes Federation in St. Vincent, Italy. They unanimously agreed on the need to search for the ways to prevent, treat, and cure diabetes. The St. Vincent Declaration highlights the importance of diabetes-related issues and the need to address them on a local, regional, and national level.

As for today, GDM is a cause of concern to both health providers and patients. In national audits that challenged the St. Vincent Declaration regarding both GDM and pre-GDM, poor pregnancy outcome was found in pregnancies complicated with diabetes [7,8]. The goal of this review is to summarize what is known today regarding GDM with points of interest for the future.

Epidemiology of Gestational Diabetes Mellitus

It is hard to relate to the epidemiology of GDM as it depends on the screening methods, the diagnostic criteria, and the clinical surveillance among different research studies.

The prevalence of GDM varies in direct proportion to the prevalence of type 2 diabetes in a given population or ethnic group [9]. The reported prevalence of GDM in the United States ranges from 3% to 20%, with 3%–5% being the most common rate [10]. In a study of the prevalence of diabetes and impaired glucose tolerance (IGT) in diverse populations in women between the ages of 20 and 39 years, the WHO Ad Hoc Diabetes Report Group [11] noted the lowest rate (<1%) of diabetes was in Bantu (Tanzania), while the highest rate was found in Pima/Papago and Nauruan Indians (14%–22%). King et al. [12] summarized the collected data on the prevalence of diabetes in pregnancy and showed that for a given population and ethnicity, the risk of diabetes in pregnancy reflects the underlying frequency of type 2 diabetes. The main reported risk factors for GDM are advanced maternal age, maternal obesity, high parity, previous delivery of a macrosomic infant, and a family history of type 2 diabetes (Box 2.1). Other reported risk factors are maternal short stature, polycystic ovary disease, a high intake of saturated fat, low birth weight, thalassemia trait, prior GDM, prior neonatal death, prior cesarean delivery, previous stillbirth or congenital malformations, high blood pressure during pregnancy, and multiple pregnancies [13–21].

The recurrence of GDM is observed in about 35%–70% of consecutives pregnancies and is associated with high prepregnancy maternal weight, a short interval between pregnancies (<24 months), and an early diagnosis of GDM [22–25].

There is an association between cumulative risk factors in a given pregnant woman and her risk of GDM.

What lies in the future? Studies show an increased prevalence of obesity and diabetes during the last few years [26]. Provided this trend is going to continue and given the similarity between the pathogenesis of GDM and type 2 diabetes, we can expect a rise in GDM in the upcoming years. Moreover, studies show that one of the adverse outcomes pregnancy in obese diabetic women is obese offspring with young-age metabolic syndrome. This shows the "vicious cycle" related to diabetes and emphasizes the need for health authorities to restrain it [27–29].

BOX 2.1   SELECTED RISK FACTORS FOR GDM

- Advanced maternal age
- Obesity
- High parity
- Previous macrosomic newborn
- A family history of type 2 diabetes
- Maternal short stature
- Polycystic ovary disease
- High intake of saturated fat
- Prior GDM
- Hypertensive disorders of pregnancy
- Multiple pregnancies

Short-Term and Long-Term Maternal and Fetal Complications

The adverse outcomes associated with GDM can be divided into both the short and long term, either maternal or fetal.

Maternal Adverse Outcomes

Short Term

Adverse maternal short-term outcomes can be divided into the exacerbation of GDM or prior diabetes first recognized during pregnancy or other complications with major contributions to maternal morbidity and mortality such as hydramnios, hypertension, preeclampsia, and an increased risk of cesarean section [30].

There is epidemiological and physical evidence that connects GDM with hypertensive disease during pregnancy. Epidemiological studies show higher rates of hypertensive complications in diabetic pregnancies compared with normal pregnancies [31,32] and a slightly increased risk of preeclampsia (15%–20% vs. 5%–7%) [33–35]. Physiological studies show that patients with the severest form of glucose intolerance are more likely to exhibit preeclampsia than patients with milder forms [36,37]. Yogev et al. [38] showed that the rate of preeclampsia is influenced by the severity of GDM and prepregnancy BMI. Optimizing glucose control during pregnancy may decrease the rate of preeclampsia, even in those with a greater severity of GDM.

Joffe et al. [39] reported that the level of plasma glucose at 1 hour after an oral glucose challenge was an important predictor of preeclampsia, even if it was within the normal range. This suggests that there is also a continuum of insulin resistance in women with normal glucose tolerance that may predispose them to hypertensive disease [40]. The relation is bidirectional: a long-term study reported persistent mild hyperinsulinemia in women 17 years after a preeclamptic pregnancy, despite their current normoglycemic rate [41].

The association between maternal diabetes and cesarean delivery is hard to prove because of many other confounders relevant to the decision regarding the mode of delivery. However, this association was suggested in a multivariate analysis that controlled for maternal demographics and obstetric complications [16,42–47].

Long Term

Long-term maternal adverse effects are mainly due to an increased risk of developing diabetes later in life, with the magnitude of the risk ranging from 20% to 80% [46,47]. The Copenhagen study [48] explored the predictors of subsequent diabetes after GDM. It found prepregnancy BMI, early diagnosis of GDM, high fasting blood glucose at GDM diagnosis, and postpartum IGT to be connected with future diabetes (mainly type 2). A family history of diabetes was associated with type 2 diabetes, whereas preterm delivery was associated with type 1 diabetes. A large-for-gestational-age (LGA) infant was not associated with future diabetes.

Moreover, insulin resistance is the cornerstone of GDM and type 2 diabetes and part of metabolic syndrome, which is defined by the American Heart Association as a combination of medical disorders that includes central obesity, high blood pressure, high serum triglyceride, low levels of high-density lipoprotein (HDL), and glucose intolerance. The presence of metabolic syndrome predicts a significantly increased risk of cardiovascular disease and long-term morbidity and mortality [49]. In the Copenhagen study, up to 40% of women with previous diet-treated GDM had metabolic syndrome, and this was three times higher than in the control group. Among glucose-tolerant women with prior GDM, the prevalence of the syndrome increased more than twofold compared with the control group [50].

Emerging data suggest an association between long-term maternal morbidity and pregnancy complicated by diabetes [51–53] (Box 2.2). Kessous et al. [51] studied a cohort of women with and without a diagnosis of GDM. Approximately 50,000 deliveries were studied, and the rate of GDM was 10.3%. During a follow-up period of more than 10 years, after adjustment for age and ethnicity,

---

BOX 2.2   SELECTED LONG-TERM COMPLICATIONS FOLLOWING GDM

- Type 2 diabetes
- Metabolic syndrome
- Vascular endothelial dysfunction
- Cardiac disease
- Renal disease

---

patients with GDM had higher rates of cardiovascular morbidity, including noninvasive cardiac diagnostic procedures (OR 1.8, 95% CI 1.4–2.2), simple cardiovascular events (OR 2.7, 95% CI 2.4–3.1), and total cardiovascular hospitalizations (OR 2.3, 95% CI 2.0–2.5). GDM was found to be an independent risk factor for long-term cardiovascular morbidity in a follow-up period of more than a decade.

An association between GDM and long-term and vascular endothelial dysfunction is supported in another study [52] proposing an association between GDM and a future risk of long-term maternal renal disease. In a population-based noninterventional study that compared the incidence of future renal morbidity in women with previous GDM, women with GDM had higher rates of total renal morbidity (0.1% vs. 0.2%; OR 2.3, 95% CI 1.4–3.7). In addition, a significant dose response association was found between the number of pregnancies with GDM and the future risk of renal morbidity (0.1%, 0.2%, and 0.4% for no GDM, one episode of GDM, and two episodes of GDM, respectively). It was suggested that the risk is more substantial for patients with recurrent episodes of GDM.

Another issue of interest was to examine the association between glucose level during pregnancy and the subsequent development of long-term maternal atherosclerotic morbidity. Charach et al. [53] in a retrospective case-control examined women who had at least one glucose measurement during their pregnancies. Cases were all women who delivered and subsequently developed atherosclerotic morbidity ($n = 815$). Controls were randomly matched by age and the year of delivery ($n = 6065$). The atherosclerotic morbidity group was further divided by severity: major events (cardiovascular, cerebrovascular disease, and chronic renal failure), minor events (hypertension, diabetes, and hyperlipidemia without target organ damage or complications), and cardiac evaluation tests (e.g., coronary angiography without records of atherosclerosis, cardiac scan, and stress test). The mean follow-up duration for the study group was 74 months. A significant linear association was found between glucose levels during pregnancy and long-term maternal atherosclerotic morbidity. Among the cases with severe atherosclerotic morbidity, the proportion of women with a high glucose level (>5.5 mmol/L) was the highest, whereas in controls it was the lowest. When adjustment was performed for atherosclerotic confounders such as GDM, preeclampsia, and obesity, a glucose level of >5.5 mmol/L was noted as an independent risk factor for hospitalizations later in nonpregnant life (hazard ratio 1.3, 95% CI 1.1–1.5; $p < .003$).

Fetal Adverse Outcomes

Short Term

The infants of GDM women are at increased risk of stillbirth and aberrant fetal growth (macrosomia and growth restriction) as well as metabolic (e.g., hypoglycemia and hypocalcemia), hematological (e.g., hyperbilirubinemia and polycythemia), and respiratory complications that increase neonatal intensivecare unit admission rates and birth trauma (e.g., shoulder dystocia) [54,55].

Congenital anomalies and spontaneous abortions are not as serious in GDM as they are in pregestational diabetes. However, due to the relatively high rate (10%) of undiagnosed type 2 diabetic women in the GDM population, there should be a concerted effort to rule out the presence of congenital malformations.

Early, albeit flawed, studies showed a fourfold increase in perinatal mortality in women with GDM. These studies did not control for variables affecting perinatal mortality such as fetal malformations or a maternal history of stillbirth, as well as advanced maternal age. Other studies also showed an increased risk of perinatal mortality up to a relative risk of 4.3 over control [56].

Being relatively common and easily documented, macrosomia is the perinatal outcome most investigators refer to when addressing GDM. Macrosomia has surrogate complications such as cesarean section, shoulder dystocia, and brachial plexus injury (BPI). The overall rate of macrosomia for the nondiabetic population is 7%–9% [57]. In contrast, the incidence reported for macrosomia in GDM is management dependent. It was shown that accelerated fetal growth is associated with the maternal glycemic profile. When good glycemic control is not achieved, the incidence of macrosomia can be as high as 20%–45% [58]. The macrosomic fetus is a result of diabetic fetopathy and is characterized by organomegaly [59,60]. Complications directly and indirectly associated with fetal macrosomia are neonatal hypoglycemia, hypocalcemia, hyperbilirubinemia, and polycythemia.

Neonatal hypoglycemia is defined clinically as a glucose level below 44 mg% [61]. The prevalence of early neonatal hypoglycemia is about 25% [62] and depends on maternal glycemic control, especially at the time of delivery. The most accepted explanation is based on the Pedersen theory: the fetus, in response to maternal hyperglycemia, develops a hyperinsulinemic state, which immediately after birth, as the hyperglycemic environment vanishes, causes neonatal hypoglycemia. The key to the treatment of neonatal hypoglycemia is to take preventive measures: adequate maternal glycemic control during delivery, early neonatal feeding, and screening for hypoglycemia.

Neonatal hypocalcemia was reported in up to 10%–20% of infants of GDM mothers and, as neonatal hypomagnesemia, is directly related to the severity of maternal diabetes [63]. Neonatal polycythemia is defined as hematocrit above 65% and has been reported in 5% of infants of GDM mothers [64]. The main explanation for it is intrauterine hypoxemia and erythropoietin elevation. Another explanation is a change in the placentofetal blood distribution in order to compensate for the hypoxemia. Polycythemia also gives a partial explanation for infant hyperbilirubinemia, which is more common in the infants of diabetic mothers.

Neonatal respiratory distress is more frequent in infants of diabetic mothers [65] and is caused mainly by respiratory distress syndrome (deficient surfactant production) but also by transient tachypnea of the newborn (TTN), meconium aspiration syndrome, polycythemia, and hypertrophic cardiomyopathy.

Long Term

Since Barker's primary epidemiologic studies in 1989 [66,67] showing an inverse relationship between birth weight and mortality due to adult ischemic heart disease, it has become increasingly clear over the past few decades that fetal stress may lead to fetal programming and the alteration of the normal developmental gene expression pattern. Research indicates that children of diabetic mothers remain at increased risk of a variety of developmental disturbances: obesity [68], impaired glucose tolerance or diabetes [69], and diminished neurobehavioral capacities [70]. It has not yet been proved for GDM; however, we can assume that fetal distress, which causes all the short-term neonatal complications in infants of GDM mothers, can also be associated with this risk.

Silverman et al. [71] demonstrated that the growth of the offspring of diabetic mothers is similar to that of nondiabetic populations after 12 months. However, after age 5, there was rapid weight gain to a point at which, at 8 years, almost half of the offspring of diabetic mothers had a weight at or above the 90th percentile. In addition, a slight upward trend in height was noted. Pettitt et al. [72], in a Pima Indian population, demonstrated that by 5–9 years of age, both macrosomic and normal birth weight infants of GDM mothers are more obese than the normal birth weight offspring of nondiabetic mothers. Adiposity in children is strongly correlated with childhood hypertension (both systolic and diastolic) and resembles metabolic syndrome, albeit at a younger age. Moreover, the presence of hypertension in LGA infants was suggested as a cause for this condition in children [73]. In another study, Vohr et al. [74] reported that LGA infants of GDM mothers had a higher BMI, waist circumference, and number of abdominal skin folds at 1 year compared with infants of nondiabetic mothers. The mean postprandial glucose value for the second and third trimester correlated with waist circumference ($r = .28$; $p < .04$) and the number of subscapular skin folds ($r = .37$; $p < .007$). They concluded that macrosomic infants of GDM mothers have unique patterns of adiposity that are present at birth and persist at 1 year of age.

Cognitive development in children of diabetic mothers has also been shown to be different relative to nondiabetic mothers: there is a relation between gestational ketonemia and a lower IQ in the child. There is also evidence of lower scores on behavioral assessment and psychomotor development scales. Also, exposure to maternal GDM was recently noted as an independent risk factor for long-term neuropsychiatric morbidity in the offspring [75].

Detection and Diagnostic Strategies for Gestational Diabetes Mellitus

For many years, health providers around the world debated whether GDM stands for the definition of a disease—i.e., whether it has maternal and/or fetal adverse outcomes that can be ameliorated by proper treatment.

First, when discussing the detection of GDM, there is a need to differentiate the screening methods from diagnosing GDM. The diagnostic lab test for GDM is the 100 g oral glucose tolerance test (OGTT). Screening can be based on risk stratification regarding anamnestic risk factors or by doing a 50 g glucose challenge test (GCT).

Risk stratification refers to the division of all pregnant women into three risk groups.

- *Low risk*: Fitting all of the following criteria: being a member of an ethnic group with a low prevalence of GDM; no known diabetes in first-degree relatives; age <25 years; weight normal at birth; weight normal before pregnancy; no history of abnormal glucose metabolism; no history of poor obstetric outcome
- *Average risk*: Not classified as low/high risk or detected as high risk at early pregnancy and did not have GDM early pregnancy
- *High risk*: Morbid obesity; first-degree family history of type 2 diabetes; previous history of GDM or glucose intolerance outside of pregnancy and/or glucosuria

Belonging to one of these risk groups will define the need for further evaluation and taking diagnostic measures for GDM.

Another option is to suggest universal screening for the entire pregnant population. Of course, as it is a screening test, pregnant women who have a positive GCT will still need to be diagnosed for GDM. The GCT was developed by O'Sullivan and coworkers in the 1950s [56] and involves the administration of a 50 g glucose load with phlebotomy 60 minutes later. At threshold values that achieve the desired degree of sensitivity, the GCT has relatively low specificity. Using a cutoff of 140 mg/dL will detect 80%–90% of women with GDM and will require that an OGTT be performed in 15% of patients. Lowering the cutoff to 130 mg/dL will increase the sensitivity to nearly 100% but will require OGTTs in nearly 25% of all patients [2].

Is abnormal GCT, without GDM, a predictor for fetal outcome?

Mello et al. found that abnormal GCT in early or late pregnancy, without GDM, is a predictor for LGA [76]. Yogev et al. [77] found a gradual increase in the rate of macrosomia, LGA, and cesarean section in relation to increasing GCT severity categories in women without GDM.

It is generally agreed that a value of 200 mg/dL in a GCT is likely to be associated with a diagnosis of GDM; thus, an OGTT need not be performed and treatment can be started [2]. However, Yogev et al. [78] showed that even in high GCT thresholds (more than 180 mg/dL), the predictive value for GDM was only 50%.

When choosing screening based on risk stratification, the Fourth and Fifth International Workshop–Conferences on GDM suggested that for women who are low risk there is no need for assessment for GDM. For women who are high risk, OGTT should be performed as soon as it is feasible; for the average-risk group, it is advisable to do GCT between 24 and 28 weeks of gestation.

This approach may be cost-effective under two circumstances: first, the diagnostic test that is used should not be complicated to administer—e.g., a single sample drawn 2 hours after a 75 g glucose load (approaching the standard GCT in simplicity). Second, in populations that have a very high prevalence of GDM, a high proportion will have a positive GCT and require a diagnostic OGTT [79]. In this circumstance, it is cost-effective to administer the full diagnostic test to all subjects.

After screening is done, based on either risk stratification or GCT there is still a need for diagnosis—as noted before, by OGTT. OGTT is the most accepted diagnostic test for GDM. There are two ways to interpret the OGTT: as a 100 g or 75 g glucose tolerance test. The tests should be performed in the morning after an overnight fast of at least 8 but not more than 14 hours and after at least 3 days of unrestricted diet (≥ 150 g carbohydrate per day) and physical activity. The subject should remain seated and should not smoke throughout. Two sets of cutoff values are currently in use: those proposed by the National Diabetes Data Group (NDDG) in 1979 and a modification of these values by Carpenter and Coustan in 1982. The latter criteria have been endorsed by the American Diabetes Association. Use of these lower values will increase the number of patients diagnosed with GDM from approximately 3% to 5%. However, studies have demonstrated that this approach will identify women who are at a comparable risk of perinatal morbidity, insulin treatment, and the subsequent development of type 2 diabetes to those detected by the NDDG criteria [74]. Infants of women who meet these lower Carpenter–Coustan criteria are at similar risk of perinatal morbidity, including macrosomia, to those identified using the NDDG criteria.

Is a single pathological value in the OGTT, also referred to as gestational impaired glucose tolerance (GIGT), predictive of an adverse perinatal outcome? In a recent retrospective cohort study [80] these women, compared with negative GCT women, had higher rates of cesarean section, preeclampsia, LGA infants, and neonatal admissions to neonatal intensivecare units. As to future implications, it was also shown that GIGT is associated with postpartum glycemia, insulin resistance, and beta cell dysfunction [81].

As to when it is best to evaluate pregnant women for GDM it is custom to do OGTT if the women are considered high risk at the first antenatal visit. However, for all other pregnant women, whether it is a one- or two-step approach, the proposed time is 24–28 weeks because up to then there is a rise in glucose insensitivity and from there to the end of the pregnancy there is hardly any change in the degree of insensitivity to insulin. Moreover, the early identification and treatment of GDM has not been proved to be associated with enhanced perinatal outcome.

Initial reports from the Hyperglycemia and Adverse Pregnancy Outcome (HAPO) study show a direct relationship between fasting glucose level and pregnancy outcomes such as neonatal birth weight, primary cesarean section, and neonatal hypoglycemia. The primary goal of the HAPO study is to determine the degree of glucose intolerance short of diabetes that conveys a clinically important risk of adverse perinatal outcome. The data that have been collected in the HAPO study should permit the selection of *outcome-based* criteria for the diagnosis of GDM. When a translation of this information is implemented, strategies for the detection and diagnosis of GDM may well be changed extensively from their current status [82].

Postpartum Maternal Management and Care

Women with GDM have an increased risk of developing type 2 diabetes after pregnancy. Approximately 10% of GDM women present clinical overt diabetes soon after pregnancy, and in the remaining population the incidence rate constantly increases over the years from delivery up to 70% at 10 years in specific groups [47].

Obesity and the need for insulin therapy during pregnancy are factors that promote insulin resistance and appear to enhance the risk of type 2 diabetes after GDM [83].

In all women with a history of GDM and particularly those presenting the aforementioned risk factors, the American Diabetes Association advises a reclassification of the maternal glycemia at 6 weeks after delivery with a 75 g OGTT [84]. If the blood glucose levels are normal, another evaluation should be done after 3 years. In the case of impaired fasting glucose (IFG) or impaired glucose tolerance (IGT), glucose testing is advised every year. These patients should be placed in intensive medical nutrition therapy and put on an individualized exercise regime due to their very high risk of developing diabetes

[85]. Medications that provoke insulin resistance should be avoided if possible. Patients should be educated on the symptoms of hyperglycemia and they should be advised to seek medical attention if they should develop such symptoms [86]. They should also be educated on the need for family planning to ensure optimal glycemia control from the start of any subsequent pregnancy. The offspring of women with GDM are at increased risk of obesity, glucose intolerance, and diabetes in late adolescence and young adulthood [87].

SUMMARY

GDM is defined as carbohydrate intolerance of variable severity with onset or first recognition during pregnancy. The prevalence of GDM is about 3%–15% of normal pregnancies and it depends of the prevalence in the same population of type 2 diabetes. The pathogenesis of GDM is a combination of insulin resistance (of normal pregnancy and a chronic form in GDM patients) and beta cell dysfunction of autoimmune origin and/or from genetic mutations, and is associated with chronic insulin resistance, genetic changes, and placental transport differences in GDM and nondiabetic pregnant women. The pathogenesis of GDM resembles that of type 2 diabetes. Indeed, a large percentage of GDM patients develop type 2 diabetes in the upcoming years after pregnancy.

GDM has both maternal and fetal complications. For the mother the risk is mainly long term: the progress to type 2 diabetes and metabolic syndrome, as well as long-term cardiovascular disease. For the fetus there are both short- and long-term complications: intrauterine fetal death (IUFD), aberrant fetal growth (mainly macrosomia, with its effect on delivery and the risk of shoulder dystocia), and metabolic hematologic changes (hypoglycemia, hypokalemia, hyperbilirubinemia, hypocalcemia, polycythemia, and respiratory distress syndrome). The long-term risks for the fetus are adverse neurological and cognitive outcomes and mainly early-onset metabolic syndrome.

For most women, glucose screening should be conducted at 24–28 weeks' gestation with the use of a 50 g oral glucose load. A value of 140 mg/dL or greater necessitates a full diagnostic 100 g OGTT. Testing at this time not only enables the obstetrician to assess glucose tolerance in the presence of the insulin-resistant state of pregnancy but, should GDM be diagnosed, it also permits treatment to begin before excessive fetal growth has occurred. Those women who seem to be at high risk of GDM should be tested by OGTT as soon as possible. If the initial screen is negative, they should be retested at 24–28 weeks' gestation.

Future research is needed regarding the prevention of GDM, treatment goals and the effectiveness of interventions, guidelines for pregnancy care, and the prevention of long-term metabolic sequelae for both the infant and the mother.

REFERENCES

1. Metzger BE, Coustan DR, and the Organizing Committee. Summary and recommendations of the 4th International Workshop Conference on gestational diabetes. *Diabetes Care*. 1998;21(Suppl 2): B161–7.
2. Gabbe SG, Graves CR. Management of diabetes mellitus complicating pregnancy. *Obstet Gynecol*. 2003;102(4):857–68.
3. Bennewitz HG. De diabete mellito, gravidatatis symptomate. MD thesis, University of Berlin, Germany, 1824. (Translated into English. Deposited at the Wellcome Museum of the History of Medicine, Euston Road, London, 1987.)
4. White P. Pregnancy complicating diabetes. *Am J Med*. 1949;5:609–16.
5. Hare JW, White P. Gestational diabetes and the White classification. *Diabetes Care*. 1980;3:394.
6. Pedersen J. *Diabetes and Pregnancy: Blood Sugar of Newborn Infants*. Copenhagen, Denmark: Danish Science Press; 1952 (thesis).
7. Bhattacharyya A, Brown S, Hughes SM, Vice PA. St Vincent declaration on diabetic pregnancies: How far are we? *Diabetes Res Clin Pract*. 50:215–16.
8. Steel JM. St Vincent's declaration 10 years on: Outcome of diabetic pregnancies. *Diabet Med*. 2003;20(1):82.

9. American College of Obstetricians and Gynecologists. Gestational diabetes. ACOG Practice Bulletin no. 30; 2001.
10. Coustan DR. Gestational diabetes. In: National Institute of Diabetes and Digestive and Kidney Diseases, *Diabetes in America*, 2nd edn. NIH publication no. 95-1468. Bethesda, MA: NIDDK; 1995, 703–17.
11. WHO Ad Hoc Diabetes Reporting Group. Diabetes and impaired glucose tolerance in women aged 20–39 years. *World Health Stat*. 1992;45:321–7.
12. King H. Epidemiology of glucose intolerance and gestational diabetes in women of childbearing age. *Diabetes Care* 1998;21(Suppl 2):B9–13.
13. Silva JK, Kaholokula JK, Ratner R, Mau M. Ethnic differences in perinatal outcome of gestational diabetes mellitus. *Diabetes Care*. 2006;29:2058–63.
14. Branchtein L, Schmidt MI, Matos MC, et al. Short stature and gestational diabetes in Brazil. Brazilian Gestational Diabetes Study Group. *Diabetologia*. 2000;43:848–51.
15. Egeland GM, Skjærven R, Irgens LM. Birth characteristics of women who develop gestational diabetes: Population based study. *Br Med J*. 2000;321:546–7.
16. Xiong X, Saunders LD, Wang FL, Demianczuk NN. Gestational diabetes mellitus: Prevalence, risk factors, maternal and infant outcomes. *Int J Gynaecol Obstet*. 2001;75:221–8.
17. Wijendran V, Bendel RB, Couch SC, et al. Fetal erythrocyte phospholipid polyunsaturated fatty acids are altered in pregnancy complicated with gestational diabetes mellitus. *Lipids*. 2000;35:927–31.
18. Bo S, Menato G, Lezo A, et al. Dietary fat and gestational hyperglycaemia. *Diabetologia*. 2001; 44:972–8.
19. Franks S, Gilling-Smith C, Waston H. Insulin action in the normal and polycystic ovary. *Metab Clin North Am*. 1999;28:361–78.
20. Hoskins RE. Zygosity as a risk factor for complications and outcomes of twin pregnancy. *Acta Genet Med Gemellol*. 1995;44:11–23.
21. Ferber KM, Keller E, Albert ED, Ziegler AG. Predictive value of human leukocyte antigen class II typing for the development of islet autoantibodies and insulin-dependent diabetes postpartum in women with gestational diabetes. *J Clin Endocrinol Metab*. 1999;84:2342–8.
22. MacNeill S, Dodds L, Hamilton DC, Armson BA, Vanden Hof M. Rates and risk factors for recurrence of gestational diabetes. *Diabetes Care*. 2001;24:659–62.
23. Major CA, deVeciana M, Weeks J, Morgan MA. Recurrence of gestational diabetes: Who is at risk? *Am J Obstet Gynecol*. 1998;179:1038–42.
24. Spong CY, Guillermo L, Kuboshige J, Cabalum T. Recurrence of gestational diabetes mellitus: Identification of risk factors. *Am J Perinatol*. 1998;15:29–33.
25. Nohira T, Kim S, Nakai H, et al. Recurrence of gestational diabetes mellitus: Rates and risk factors from initial GDM and one abnormal GTT value. *Diabetes Res Clin Pract*. 2006;71:75–81.
26. Mokdad AH, Bowman BA, Ford ES, Vinicor F, Marks JS, Koplan JP. The continuing epidemics of obesity and diabetes in the United States. *JAMA* 2001;286:1195–1200.
27. Abdul FB. Type 2 diabetes and rural India. *Lancet*. 2007;369(9558):273–4.
28. Albert Reece E. Perspectives on obesity, pregnancy and birth outcomes in the United States: The scope of the problem. *Am J Obstet Gynecol*. 2008;198(1):23–7.
29. Boney CM, Verma A, Tucker R, Vohr BR. Metabolic syndrome in childhood: Association with birth weight, maternal obesity, and gestational diabetes mellitus. *Pediatrics*. 2005;115(3):e290–6.
30. Setji T, Brown A, Feinglos M. Gestational diabetes mellitus. *Clin Diabetes*. 2005;23(1):17–24.
31. Rudge MV, Calderon IM, Ramos MD, et al. Hypertension disorders in pregnant women with diabetes mellitus. *Am J Perinatol*. 1997;44:11–5.
32. Greco P, Loverro G, Selvaggi L. Does gestational diabetes represent an obstetric risk factor? *Gynecol Obstet Invest*. 1994;37:242–5.
33. Sacks DA, Greenspoon JS, Abu-Fadil S, et al. Toward universal criteria for gestational diabetes: The 75 gram glucose tolerance test in pregnancy. *Am J Obstet Gynecol*. 1995;172:607–14.
34. Sermer M, et al. Impact of increasing carbohydrate intolerance on maternal fetal outcomes in 3637 women without gestational diabetes. *Am J Obstet Gynecol*. 1995;173:146–56.
35. Pennison EH, Egerman RS, et al. Perinatal outcomes in gestational diabetes: A comparison of criteria for diagnosis. *Am J Obstet Gynecol*. 2001;184:1118–21.
36. Cioffi FJ, Amorosa LF, Vintzileos AM, et al. Relationship of insulin resistance and hyperinsulinemia to blood pressure during pregnancy. *J Matern Fetal Med*. 1997;6:174–9.

37. Solomon CG, Graves SW, Greene MF, et al. Glucose intolerance as a predictor of hypertension of pregnancy. *Hypertention*. 1994;23(6 pt1):717–21.
38. Yogev Y, Xenakis EM, Langer O. The association between preeclampsia and the severity of gestational diabetes: The impact of glycemic control. *Am J Obstet Gynecol*. 2004;191(5):1655–60.
39. Joffe GM, et al. The relationship between abnormal glucose tolerance and hypertensive disorders of pregnancy in healthy nulliparous women. *Am J Obstet Gynecol*. 1998;179:1032–7.
40. Yogev Y, Langer O, Brustman L, Rosenn B. Pre-eclampsia and gestational diabetes mellitus: Does a correlation exist early in pregnancy? *J Matern Fetal Neonatal Med*. 2004;15(1):39–43.
41. Laivuori H. Hyperinsulinemia 17 years after pre-eclamptic first pregnancy. *J Clin Endocrinol Metab*. 1996;81:2908–11.
42. Kjos SL, Berkowitz K, Xiang A. Independent predictors of cesarean delivery in women with diabetes. *J Matern Fetal Neonatal Med*. 2004;15:61–7.
43. Ray JG, Vermeulen MJ, Shapiro JL, et al. Maternal and neonatal outcomes in pregestational and gestational diabetes mellitus, and the influence of maternal obesity and weight gain: The DEPOSIT study. *QJM*. 2001;94:147–56.
44. Ehrenberg HM, Durnwald CP, Catalano P, et al. The influence of obesity and diabetes on the risk of cesarean delivery. *Am J Obstet Gynecol*. 2004;191:969–74.
45. Patel RR, Peters TJ, Murphy DJ, et al. Prenatal risk factors for caesarean section: Analysis of the ALSPAC cohort of 12,944 women in England. *Int J Epidemiol*. 2005;34:355–67.
46. Peters RK, Kjos SL, Xiang A, et al. Long-term diabetogenic effect of single pregnancy in women with previous gestational diabetes mellitus. *Lancet*. 1996;347:227–30.
47. Kim C, Newton KM, Knopp RH. Gestational diabetes and the incidence of type 2 diabetes. *Diabetes Care*. 2002;25:1862–8.
48. Damm P, Kühl C, Bertelsen A, Mølsted-Pedersen L. Predictive factors for the development of diabetes in women with previous gestational diabetes mellitus. *Am J Obstet Gynecol*. 1992;167:607–16.
49. Lakka HM, Laaksonen DE, Lakka TA, et al. The metabolic syndrome and total and cardiovascular disease mortality in middle-aged men. *JAMA*. 2002;288:2709–16.
50. Lauenborg J, Mathiesen E, Hansen T, et al. The prevalence of the metabolic syndrome in a danish population of women with previous gestational diabetes mellitus is three-fold higher than in the general population. *J Clin Endocrinol Metab*. 2005;90:4004–10.
51. Kessous R, Shoham-Vardi I, Pariente G, Sherf M, Sheiner E. An association between gestational diabetes mellitus and long-term maternal cardiovascular morbidity. *Heart*. 2013;99(15):1118–21.
52. Beharier O, Shoham-Vardi I, Pariente G, Sergienko R, Kessous R, Baumfeld Y, Szaingurten-Solodkin I, Sheiner E. Gestational diabetes mellitus is a significant risk factor for long-term maternal renal disease. *J Clin Endocrinol Metab*. 2015;100(4):1412–6.
53. Charach R, Wolak T, Shoham-Vardi I, Sergienko R, Sheiner E. Can slight glucose intolerance during pregnancy predict future maternal atherosclerotic morbidity? *Diabet Med*. 2016;33(7):920–5.
54. Langer O, Yogev Y, Most O, Xenakis MJ. Gestational diabetes: The consequences of not treating. *Am J Obstet Gynecol*. 2005;192:989–97.
55. Crowther CA, Hiller JE, Moss JR, et al. Effect of treatment of gestational diabetes mellitus on pregnancy outcomes. *N Engl J Med*. 2005;352:2477–86.
56. O'Sullivan JB, Mahan CM, Charles D. Screening criteria for high-risk gestational diabetic patients. *Am J Obstet Gynecol*. 1973;116:895.
57. American College of Obstetricians and Gynecologists. Fetal macrosomia. Practice Bulletin no. 22; 2000.
58. Langer O, Rodriguez D, Xenakis EMJ, et al. Intensified versus conventional management of gestational diabetes. *Am J Obstet Gynecol*. 1994;170;1036–47.
59. Naeye RL. Infants of diabetic mothers: A quantitative, morphologic study. *Pediatrics*. 1965;35:980–88.
60. Langer O, Kagan-Hallet K. Diabetic vs. non-diabetic infants: A quantitative morphological study. In: *Proceedings of the 38th Annual Meeting of the Society for Gynecologic Investigation*. San Antonio, TX; 1992.
61. Koh THHG, Aynsley-Green A, Tarbit M, Eyre JA. Neural dysfunction during hypoglycemia. *Arch Dis Child*. 1998;63:1353–8.
62. Agrawal RK, Lui K, Gupta JM. Neonatal hypoglycemia in infants of diabetic mothers. *J Paediatr Child Health*. 2000;36:354–6.
63. Reece EA, Homko CJ. Infant of diabetic mother. *Semin Perinatol*. 1994;18:459–69.

64. Cordero L, Treuer SH, Landon M, Gabbe SG. Management of infants of diabetic mothers. *Arch Pediatr Adolesc Med*. 1998;152:249–54.

65. Robert MF, Neff RK, Hubbell JP, et al. Association between maternal diabetes and the respiratory distress syndrome in the newborn. *N Engl J Med*. 1976;294:357–60.

66. Barker D, Osmond C, Golding J, et al. Growth in utero, blood pressure in childhood and adult life, and mortality from cardiovascular disease. *Br Med J*. 1989;298:564–7.

67. Barker DJ. In utero programming of cardiovascular disease. *Theriogenology*. 2000;53:555–74.

68. Silverman B, Rizzo T, Green O, et al. Long-term prospective evaluation of offspring of diabetic mothers. *Diabetes*. 1991;40(Suppl 2):121–5.

69. Silverman B, Metzger B, Cho N, et al. Fetal hyperinsulinism and impaired glucose tolerance in adolescent offspring of diabetic mothers. *Diabetes Care*. 1995;18:611–7.

70. Rizzo T, Freinkel N, Metzger B, et al. Correlations between antepartum maternal metabolism and newborn behavior. *Am J Obstet Gynecol*. 1990;163:1458–64.

71. Silverman B, Landsberg L, Metzger B. Fetal hyperinsulinism in offspring of diabetic mothers. *Ann NY Acad Sci*. 1993;699:36–45.

72. Pettitt D, Knowler W, Bennett P, et al. Obesity in offspring of diabetic Pima Indian women despite normal birth weight. *Diabetes Care*. 1987;10:76–80.

73. Vohr B, McGarvey S, Coll C. Effects of maternal gestational diabetes and adiposity on neonatal adiposity and blood pressure. *Diabetes Care* 1995;18:467–75.

74. Vohr B, McGarvey S. Growth patterns of large-for-gestational age and appropriate-for-gestational age infants of gestational diabetic mothers and control mothers at age 1 year. *Diabetes Care*. 1997;20:1066–72.

75. Nahum Sacks K, Friger M, Shoham-Vardi I, Abokaf H, Speigel E, Sergienko R, Landau D, Sheiner E. Prenatal exposure to gestational diabetes mellitus as an independent risk factor for long-term neuropsychiatric morbidity of the offspring. *Am J Obstet Gynecol*. 2016;215(3):380.e1–7.

76. Mello G, Parretti E, Mecacci F, et al. Anthropometric characteristics of full-term infants: Effects of varying degrees of "normal" glucose metabolism. *J Perinat Med*. 1997;25:197–204.

77. Yogev Y, Langer O, Xenakis EM, Rosenn B. The association between glucose challenge test, obesity and pregnancy outcome in 6390 non-diabetic women. *J Matern Fetal Neonatal Med*. 2005;17(1):29–34.

78. Yogev Y, Langer O, Xenakis EM, Rosenn B. Glucose screening in Mexican-American women. *Obstet Gynecol*. 2004;103(6):1241–5.

79. Pettitt DJ, Knowler WC, Baird R, Bennett PH. Gestational diabetes: Infant and maternal complications of pregnancy in relation to third-trimester glucose tolerance in the Pima Indians. *Diabetes Care*. 1980;3:458–64.

80. McLaughlin GB, Cheng YW, Caughey AB. Women with one elevated 3-hour glucose tolerance test value: Are they at risk for adverse perinatal outcomes? *Am J Obstet Gynecol*. 2006;194:e16–9.

81. Retnakaran R, Qi Y, Sermer M, Connelly PW, Zinman B, Hanley AJ. Isolated hyperglycemia at 1-hour on oral glucose tolerance test in pregnancy resembles gestational diabetes in predicting postpartum metabolic dysfunction. *Diabetes Care*. 2008;31(7):1275–81.

82. HAPO Study Cooperative Research Group, Metzger BE, Lowe LP, et al. Hyperglycemia and adverse pregnancy outcomes. *N Engl J Med*. 2008;358(19):1991–2002.

83. Ben-Haroush A, Yogev Y, Hod M. Epidemiology of gestational diabetes mellitus and its association with type 2 diabetes. *Diabet Med* 2004;21:103–13.

84. American Diabetes Association. Report of the expert committee on the diagnosis and classification of diabetes mellitus. *Diabetes Care*. 2003;26(Suppl 1):S5–20.

85. American Diabetes Association. Report of the expert committee on the diagnosis and classification of diabetes mellitus. *Diabetes Care* 2002;25(Suppl 1):S5–20.

86. American Diabetes Association. Preconception care of women with diabetes. *Diabetes Care*. 2002;25(Suppl 1):S82–4.

87. Lapolla A, Botta RM, Vitacolonna E. Diabete in gravidanza. *Diabete*. 2001;13:269–83.

3

Placental Syndrome and Long-Term Maternal Complications

Gali Pariente, Tom Leibson, Howard Berger, and Eyal Sheiner

Introduction

In the past, we believed that pregnancy complications associated with placental disease resolved quickly and completely after the delivery of the placenta. Placental disease was thought primarily and solely to affect immediate perinatal outcome. In the last decade, it has slowly become apparent that placental disease has a long-lasting effect on maternal health as a result of subsequent vascular disease. Women who have suffered from placental complications during pregnancy experience a different health course than those who have had adequate placental function and normal pregnancy outcomes. The enigmatic association between placenta-related complications and long-term maternal morbidity is at the heart of this discussion. It is not yet clear whether future maternal vascular morbidity is a result of preexisting factors preceding placental complications or whether it is, in fact, the diseased placenta that paves the way for the secondary disseminated vascular endothelial insult, later manifesting as maternal vascular disease. Accumulated data from the last decade reveal that some seemingly healthy young women with complicated placental pathologies develop cardiovascular complications when followed long enough.

It is therefore possible that the pregnancy course and placenta-related morbidity will serve as screening tools, much like a "physiological stress test," allowing timely identification of the population at risk of subsequent vascular disease [1].

The Placenta

Normal Placentation

Normal pregnancy is dependent on the harmonization of three processes [2].

1. Decidualization of the maternal tissue
2. Placental formation
3. Embryonic development

Decidualization, the extent of which correlates with the degree of trophoblast invasion, starts in the late secretory phase of the menstrual cycle, continues during the pregnancy, and is believed to be one of the processes that control later trophoblast invasion and placental formation [3]. In normal pregnancies, the course of placentation starts when blastocyst cells adhere to the uterine endometrium, creating a line of epithelial cells termed the *cytotrophoblast*. Cytotrophoblast cells invade the uterine spiral arteries, replacing the endothelial layers of these vessels; the subsequent destruction of the medial elastic, muscular, and neural tissue results in the transformation of the spiral arteries into low-resistance, high-capacity uteroplacental vessels. This remodeling of the uterine spiral arteries results in the formation of a low-resistance arteriolar system and a dramatic increase in blood supply to the growing fetus. The endovascular invasion of the spiral arteries begins between 14 and 15 weeks of gestation, and by 18 weeks the endovascular trophoblast is incorporated into the vessel walls of one-third of the arteries [4,5].

Abnormal Placentation

Abnormal transformation of the spiral arteries was suggested to be a result of impaired trophoblast function [6]. Conversely, other studies have contradicted this by either demonstrating no differences in interstitial trophoblast invasion [7] or by showing no differences in integrin expression [8] in placentas from pregnancies with abnormal placentation compared with normal pregnancies. These studies imply that abnormal placentation results from impaired maternal decidualization rather than impaired trophoblast function.

Regardless of the cause of abnormal placentation, impaired development of the uteroplacental vasculature involves inadequate endovascular trophoblast invasion, resulting (and perhaps originating) in decidual vasculopathy with small, poorly developed spiral arteries that contain features of acute atherosis [9]. These poorly developed spiral arteries compromise blood flow to the maternal–fetal interface. As the pregnancy progresses, the fetus outgrows the placental reserve, creating placental insufficiency, which may result in placental ischemia and infarction as well as maternal placenta-associated syndrome.

Placenta-Associated Syndrome (Box 3.1)

Intrauterine growth restriction (IUGR), hypertensive disorders of pregnancy, stillbirth, and placental abruption may indicate chronic processes associated with vascular dysfunction and placental insufficiency [10]. A large number of studies regarding the association between these different placenta-related complications can be found in the literature. It has been well documented that preeclampsia is associated with placental abruption or placental infarction [11,12], necessitating preterm delivery [13], and can be further complicated by IUGR and intrauterine fetal death [2,14].

In their population-based cohort study, Rasmussen et al. [15] demonstrated that women who delivered infants below the 10th birth weight percentile had a relative risk of 3.0 of experiencing placental abruption compared with women who did not deliver small-for-gestational-age (SGA) infants. This finding was found to be consistent with other studies [16,17]. A prospective cohort study of 30,681 singleton pregnancies found a relationship between IUGR and placental abruption even after adjusting for smoking [18]. In this study, women with placental abruption were two to three times more likely to deliver an SGA neonate (below the 10th birth weight percentile) compared with women without placental abruption.

Hence, an underlying common factor may cause both fetal growth restriction and placental abruption—i.e., vascular dysfunction that results in an abnormal fetoplacental relationship and presents as growth restriction or placental abruption. Alternatively, one of these conditions may predispose to the other; IUGR may predispose to placental abruption via a common pathway of preeclampsia or, alternatively, placental abruption may result in partial placental separation before birth and thus impair fetal nourishment, resulting in IUGR.

Ananth et al. [19] suggested that there are acute and more commonly chronic disease mechanisms involved in the established risk factors for placental abruption. While the incidence of acute

---

BOX 3.1   PLACENTA-ASSOCIATED SYNDROME

Chronic processes associated with vascular dysfunction and placental insufficiency:

1. IUGR/SGA
2. Stillbirth
3. Hypertensive disorders of pregnancy
4. Placental abruption

inflammation-associated risk factors declines with advancing gestation in both women with or without placental abruption, the incidence of chronic processes such as IUGR or preeclampsia increases with gestational age among women with placental abruption, as opposed to women without placental abruption.

The clustering and shared predisposing factors of preeclampsia, IUGR, and placental abruption have led to the development of the concept of *placenta-associated syndrome*.

Intrauterine Growth Restriction and Long-Term Maternal Risk

Intrauterine Growth Restriction

IUGR is the term used to designate a fetus that has not met its growth potential; any fetus with an estimated fetal weight below the 10th percentile according to the week of pregnancy is considered growth restricted [20]. The extent of fetal growth can be approximated as birth weight standardized to gestational age, whereby SGA is the extreme [21]. SGA neonates are at significantly greater risk of mortality and morbidity. Associated neonatal complications include respiratory distress syndrome (RDS), necrotizing enterocolitis (NEC), chronic lung disease (CLD), impaired thermoregulation, and hypoglycemia [22–24].

In addition, IUGR is known to be associated with increased rates of cardiovascular disease (CVD) and type 2 diabetes in adult life via the concept known as *fetal programming* [25,26]. The long-term morbidity associated with being born SGA is beyond the scope of this chapter and is discussed comprehensively in another chapter.

Young age at first pregnancy, race, inflammation and infection, smoking, hypertension, and pregestational diabetes mellitus have all been associated with IUGR [27]. Being a part of placenta-associated syndrome, IUGR is obviously linked to placental insufficiency and chronic vascular dysfunction [10] and by sharing similar risk factors is believed to be associated with maternal metabolic syndrome and subsequent maternal morbidity and mortality.

Intrauterine Growth Restriction and Long-Term Maternal Risk

Smith et al. published one of the first studies reporting the association between birth weight and subsequent maternal mortality in 1997 [28] (Table 3.1). This was a prospective observational study that analyzed mortality in relation to the birth weight of offspring among members of married couples who participated in the Renfrew–Paisley study [40,41]. Participants in the Renfrew–Paisley study were residents aged 45–64 that were recruited during 1972–1976 by door-to-door census of all households in two towns in western Scotland, and were invited to attend a screening examination for CVDs. Participants completed a questionnaire regarding cardiovascular symptoms, smoking, and social class. Between 1993 and 1994, 794 married couples were identified and provided information regarding their offspring, and this information was used to search the hospital records and obtain the offspring's birth weight. The main outcome measured was mortality from all causes and from CVD over a 15-year follow-up. Mortality was inversely related to the offspring's birth weight for both mothers (relative risk [RR] for a 1 kg lower birth weight 1.82, 95% confidence interval [CI] 1.23–2.70) and fathers (RR 1.35, 95% CI 1.03–1.79). For mortality from CVD, inverse associations were seen for mothers (RR 2.00, 95% CI 1.18–3.33) and fathers (RR 1.52, 95% CI 1.03–2.17). Adjustment for confounding variables such as blood pressure, plasma cholesterol, body mass index (BMI), height, social class, and smoking had little effect on these risk estimates [28]. One of the weaknesses of this study is that it did not relate birth weight to the gestational age at the time of the delivery. Thus, it is uncertain whether the association was related to uterine growth restriction or to preterm delivery. Furthermore, both preterm delivery and growth restriction can be a result of preeclampsia, and this study did not adjust for its possible confounding effect.

Another early study, published in 2001, investigated the association between pregnancy complications related to low birth weight and later ischemic heart disease of the mother [42]. In this retrospective study, routine discharge data were used to identify all singleton first births in Scotland between 1981 and 1985. Linkage to the mothers' subsequent admissions and deaths provided 15–19 years of follow-up. The mothers' risks of death from any cause or from ischemic heart disease and admission for or death from ischemic heart disease were related to low birth weight, preterm delivery, and preeclampsia in the first pregnancy.

TABLE 3.1

Summary of Selected Studies on SGA/IUGR and Subsequent Maternal Morbidity and Mortality after Delivery of an SGA Neonate

Study (Author, Year, Country)	Cases	Comparison Group	Pregnancy Complication	Outcome Measured	Main Findings
Davey Smith et al. [28], 1997, Scotland, United Kingdom	159 deliveries	Mothers in same cohort, ($n = 794$)	Lower birth weight	Maternal and paternal mortality	Mortality was inversely related to offspring's birth weight for both mothers and fathers.
Lawlor et al. [33], 2002, United Kingdom	Not provided	Mothers in the same cohort ($n = 3265$)	Lower birth rate	Maternal insulin resistance	Birth weight of offspring was inversely related to the mother's insulin resistance.
Gordon et al. [32], 2004, Scotland, United Kingdom	Lower birth weight quartile ($n = 24,143$)	Mothers in the same cohort, with normal birth infant ($n = 119,668$)	LBW (preterm delivery and spontaneous abortion also investigated)	Maternal cerebrovascular event	Compared with women who delivered babies ≥3500 g, women who delivered LBW (<2500 g) infants were at increased risk of CVE with a consistent trend across birth weight categories. The lowest birth weight quintile was predictive of subsequent maternal CVE. Additive effect; women who experienced all three complications had a sevenfold risk of cerebrovascular disease.
Catov et al. [36], 2007, United States	56 women with LBW infant	Mothers in the same cohort ($n = 446$)	LBW	Maternal cardiovascular risk factors and body composition	Women who had delivered a LBW infant had a larger abdominal circumference for BMI. After adjustment for BMI, race, and age, women with a history of an LBW neonate had elevations in systolic BP, greater IL-6 levels, and were more insulin resistant compared with women with a normal-weight infant.
Kanagalingam et al. [37], 2008, Scotland, United Kingdom	Mothers with SGA neonates ($n = 28$)	Matched controls ($n = 29$)	SGA	Maternal cardiovascular risk factors and markers of vascular dysfunction	Delivery of an SGA infant was associated with altered lipids, higher systolic BP subclinical inflammation, and endothelial activation with differences robust to confounder adjustment. Endothelium-dependent and -independent microvascular functions were also impaired in mothers of SGA offspring.
Lykke et al. [33], 2010, Denmark	Mothers with SGA neonate ($n = 43,109$)	Mothers in the same cohort ($n = 796,806$)	SGA (preterm delivery, hypertensive disorders of pregnancy, placental abruption, and stillbirth also investigated)	Maternal cardiovascular and noncardiovascular mortality	Previous delivery of SGA neonate was associated with subsequent death of mothers from cardiovascular and noncardiovascular causes.

Study	Exposed	Comparison	Exposure	Outcome	Findings
Li et al. [34], 2010, Taiwan	Parents with LBW neonate (n = 85,285)	Parents with Non LBW neonate (n = 1,315,098)	LBW	Maternal and paternal cardiovascular mortality	Significant association between bearing LBW offspring (<2500 g) and CVD mortality for mothers. On standardizing the birth weight for gestational age, the observed associations persisted, although these associations were relatively weak.
Bonamy et al. [35], 2011, Sweden	Women with LBW neonate (n = 239,903)	Women from the same cohort (n = 923,686)	SGA (preterm delivery was also investigated)	Maternal CVD	The risk of maternal CVD increased relative to fetal growth but was restricted to very SGA infants. There was a significant interaction between preterm birth and fetal growth with respect to mothers' risk of CVD. Among mothers to very SGA infants, the hazard ratio of CVD ranged from 1.38 to 3.40 in mothers to term and very preterm infants, respectively.
Bukowski et al. [36], 2012, United States	Women with SGA neonate (n = 309)	Women from the same cohort (n = 6608)	SGA	Maternal ischemic heart disease	Delivery of an SGA infant was strongly associated with greater maternal risk of IHD. The association was independent of the family history of IHD, stroke, hypertension diabetes, and other risk factors for IHD. Delivery of an SGA infant was associated with earlier onset of IHD and preceded it by a median of 30 years.
Dietz et al. [37], 2013, United States	Women who delivered a term LBW neonate (n = 150)	Women from the same cohort (n = 4820)	LBW	Maternal CVD	Women with a history of LBW neonate had an OR of 2.07 for CVD compared with women without a history of LBW neonate. After adjustment for hypertension and high cholesterol, the association did not remain statistically significant.
Pariente et al. [38], 2013, Israel	Women who delivered SGA neonate (n = 4411)	Women from the same cohort (n = 47,612)	SGA	Maternal simple and complex cardiovascular events; maternal cardiovascular mortality	Delivery of an SGA neonate was a risk factor for long-term complex cardiovascular events. Women who delivered an SGA neonate had a significantly higher risk of cardiovascular mortality during the follow-up period. Delivery of an SGA neonate remained an independent risk factor for long-term maternal cardiovascular mortality after controlling for confounders such as GDM, hypertensive disorders of pregnancy, and obesity.
Almasi et al. [39], 2015, Israel	Women with SGA (n = 10,701)	Women from the same cohort (n = 99,342)	SGA	Maternal chronic kidney disease	Women with a delivery of an SGA neonate had higher rates of renal-related morbidity such as kidney transplantation, chronic renal failure, and hypertensive renal disease. After adjusting for confounders, previous delivery of an SGA neonate was independently associated with subsequent maternal renal disease.

Abbreviations: LBW: low birth weight; SGA: small for gestational age; GDM: gestational diabetes mellitus; CVE: cerebrovascular event; CVD: cardiovascular disease; IHD: ischemic heart disease; BMI: body mass index; BP: blood pressure; HR: hazard ratio; OR: odds ratio.

Hazard ratios were adjusted for socioeconomic deprivation, maternal age and height, and essential maternal hypertension. Complete data were available on 129,920 deliveries. Maternal risk of ischemic heart disease admission or death was associated with delivering a baby in the lowest birth weight quintile for gestational age (adjusted hazard ratio [HR] 1.9, 95% CI 1.5–2.4). The effect was synergistic; women with all three complications (i.e., low birth weight, preeclampsia, and preterm birth) had a risk of ischemic heart disease admission or death seven times greater (95% CI 3.3–14.5) than the control group [42].

Another retrospective study used the same Scottish databases to assess subsequent maternal cerebrovascular events among women with a history of delivering a low–birth weight infant [30]. The authors identified all first singleton live births in Scotland (1981–1985) and found that 342 of the 119,668 mothers suffered cerebrovascular events over 14–19 years' follow-up. Compared with women who delivered babies ≥3500 g, women who delivered low–birth weight (<2500 g) infants were at increased risk of cerebrovascular disease (adjusted HR 2.51, 95% CI 1.71–3.70), with a consistent trend across birth weight categories. The lowest birth weight quintile (adjusted HR 1.29, 95% CI 1.01–1.65), preterm delivery (adjusted HR 1.91, 95% CI 1.35–2.70), and previous spontaneous abortion (adjusted HR 1.49, 95% CI 1.09–2.03) were all predictive of subsequent maternal cerebrovascular events. The effects were additive. Women who experienced all three complications had a sevenfold increased risk of cerebrovascular disease (adjusted HR 7.03, 95% CI 2.24–22.06) [30].

As evidence regarding the association between the delivery of a low–birth weight infant and the risk of subsequent vascular complications emerged, questions regarding the mechanisms underlying this association began to be addressed, primarily by unifying theories, such as pointing to a common vascular and metabolic maladaptation to pregnancy and senescence as an underlying factor. One of the studies that highlighted this association was published by Lawlor et al. in 2002 [29]. In this cross-sectional survey, the association between the birth weight of the offspring and the mother's insulin resistance in late adulthood was investigated. The authors used information from the British Women's Heart and Health Study, which sampled women 60–79 years old, randomly selected from general practitioners' lists in 23 towns in the United Kingdom [43]. Participants (4286) were asked how many pregnancies and live births they had experienced and women with at least one live birth were asked to provide the sex and birth weight of their firstborn child. Fasting blood samples were taken and insulin resistance was estimated with the homeostasis model assessment. Women with clinical diabetes at the time of the interview were excluded from the analysis. The birth weight of the offspring was inversely related to maternal insulin resistance in late adulthood. For each 1 kg higher birth weight of the offspring, women had a 15% reduction in the odds of being in the quartile with highest insulin resistance compared with other quartiles (odds ratio [OR] 0.85, 95% CI 0.71–1.00). This increased to 27% (OR 0.73, 95% CI 0.60–0.90) after adjusting data for potential confounders such as age, BMI, blood pressure, cholesterol, and triglyceride levels [29]. One major limitation of this study derived from the fact that exposure (delivering an SGA neonate) was based on the maternal recall of an event that may have occurred 40 or 50 years before (recall bias).

Other studies have assessed the association between delivering an SGA infant and cardiovascular risk factors [31,32,44]. Older women (mean age of 80 years) who delivered low–birth weight infants were demonstrated to have a larger abdominal circumference for BMI. After adjusting for BMI, race, and age, they were found to have elevations in systolic blood pressure, had greater IL-6 levels, and were more likely to be insulin resistant compared with women who had delivered a normal-weight infant [31]. Evidence of elevated classic and new cardiovascular risk factors was also demonstrated among younger women who delivered a low–birth weight infant. One study reported impaired glucose metabolism among younger women (on average, 39 years old, 8 years postpartum) with a history of delivering a low–birth weight infant [44], while other studies were able to demonstrate alterations in triglycerides and cholesterol, elevated systolic blood pressure, and increased levels of subclinical inflammation markers (CRP, IL-6, and ICAM) among women who delivered a low–birth weight infant only 4 years prior to the analysis [32].

During the last decade, robust supporting evidence regarding the association between maternal mortality from cardiovascular and noncardiovascular causes following the delivery of an SGA infant has accumulated. Studies with large sample sizes from the United Kingdom [45], Sweden [46], Taiwan [34], and Denmark [33] have all demonstrated associations between the delivery of an SGA infant and the subsequent elevation of maternal mortality from cardiovascular and noncardiovascular causes.

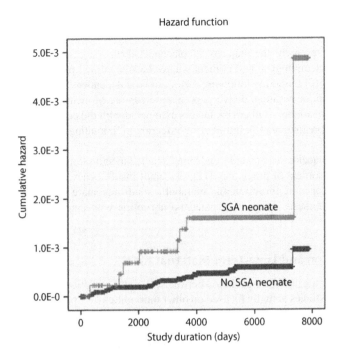

FIGURE 3.1　Kaplan–Meier curve for cardiovascular-associated mortality of women with and without a history of delivering an SGA neonate. Survival analysis (presenting hazard function) showed that women who delivered an SGA neonate had a significantly higher risk of cardiovascular mortality during the follow-up period.

Recently, alongside mortality reports, other studies have also described an association between the birth of an SGA infant and later maternal CVD [35,36,47]. One study, published by our group, compared long-term cardiovascular morbidity between women with and without SGA infants [38]. Cardiovascular morbidity was divided into four categories according to severity and type. During the study period, 47,612 deliveries met the inclusion criteria and 4411 (9.3%) women delivered an SGA neonate. Women who delivered an SGA neonate had a significantly higher risk of cardiovascular mortality during the follow-up period (Kaplan–Meier survival analysis, log-rank test 0.002; Figure 3.1). The delivery of an SGA neonate was a risk factor for long-term complex cardiovascular events, including congestive heart failure, hypertensive heart disease, and acute cor pulmonale (OR 2.3, 95% CI 1.3–4.4; $p = .006$), and long-term cardiovascular mortality (OR 3.4, 95% CI 1.5–7.6; $p = .006$). The delivery of an SGA neonate remained an independent risk factor for long-term maternal cardiovascular mortality after controlling for confounders such as maternal age and ethnicity (Cox multivariable regression: adjusted HR 3.5, 95% CI 1.5–8.2; $p = .004$) [38]. Another recent study published by our group assessed the association between the delivery of an SGA neonate and long-term maternal chronic kidney disease [39]. In this retrospective study, with a mean follow-up duration of 11.2 years, the previous delivery of an SGA neonate was independently associated with subsequent renal morbidity such as chronic renal failure, kidney transplantation, and hypertensive renal disease (adjusted HR 1.7, 95% CI 1.1–2.8).

Placental Abruption and Long-Term Maternal Risk

Placental Abruption

Placental abruption complicates roughly 1 in 100–200 (0.5%–1%) pregnancies [48,49] and is associated with a substantial risk of significant maternal and perinatal morbidity and mortality [11–13]. Evidence from the United States [50], Norway [15], and Israel [12] indicates that the frequency of placental abruption is increasing.

Despite extensive research, the majority of placental abruption cases are of unknown cause [51]. However, several epidemiological and clinical studies have identified predisposing risk factors for this disorder. Our group [12] found the following factors to be independently linked with the occurrence of placental abruption: prior cesarean delivery, premature rupture of membranes, habitual abortions, and a history of fertility treatments. Other risk factors associated with the occurrence of placental abruption are smoking during pregnancy [48], intrauterine infection [52], multiparity [53], and gestational hypertension [11].

Being a part of placenta-associated syndrome, placental abruption is obviously linked to IUGR [11], hypertensive disorders of pregnancy [12], placental insufficiency, and chronic vascular dysfunction. The fact that placental abruption and metabolic syndrome share several risk factors have led to the formation of hypotheses associating placental abruption with long-term maternal morbidity and mortality.

Placental Abruption and Long-Term Maternal Risk

Few studies have investigated the association between placental abruption and subsequent cardiovascular morbidity, and these studies actually focused on other morbidities (i.e., preeclampsia) [33,54] (Table 3.2). Ray and colleagues [54] examined the risk of early CVD in women with a history of pregnancy affected by maternal placental syndromes (gestational hypertension, preeclampsia, placental abruption, and placental infarction). In their study, patients with a history of placental abruption or infarction had an adjusted HR of 1.7 (95% CI 1.3–2.2) for CVDs.

Lykke et al. [33] studied the association between pregnancy complications and premature maternal death in a registry-based retrospective cohort study in Denmark. Women ($n = 782,287$) with a first single-ton delivery between 1978 and 2007 were followed for a median of 14.8 years. While placental abruption was associated with death from noncardiovascular causes (HR 1.4; $p < .001$), placental abruption was not found to be associated with death from cardiovascular causes, unless it was combined with preeclampsia (HR 1.23; $p = .37$). The authors concluded that these findings imply that placental abruption might act as an indicator of severity in preeclamptic pregnancies.

Rather than focusing on disease outcomes, Veerbeek et al. [58] assessed common risk factors for CVD 6–9 months after delivery in 75 women with a history of placental abruption and in 79 controls with uncomplicated pregnancies. Women with a history of placental abruption had significantly higher BMI, mean systolic blood pressure, fasting blood glucose, C-reactive protein, total cholesterol, high-density lipoprotein cholesterol, and low-density lipoprotein cholesterol. The author concluded that these finding suggest a higher risk of CVD among women with previous placental abruption.

One of the first studies that focused on the association between placental abruption per se and long-term maternal outcomes was published by our group in 2013 [55]. The aim of this retrospective population-based study was to investigate the risk of subsequent cardiovascular events in women with a history of placental abruption. The incidence of cardiovascular events was compared between women with and without placental abruption during 1988–1999 with a follow-up period of more than a decade. During the study period, there were 47,585 deliveries meeting the inclusion criteria; of these, 653 occurred in patients with placental abruption. No significant association was noted between placental abruption and subsequent long-term hospitalizations because of cardiovascular causes. However, placental abruption was associated with long-term cardiovascular mortality (OR 6.6, 95% CI 2.3–18.3). The cardiovascular case fatality rate for the placental abruption group was 13.0% versus 2.5% in the comparison group ($p < .001$). Using Cox multivariable regression models, placental abruption remained an independent risk factor for long-term maternal cardiovascular mortality after adjusting for multiple factors such as BMI, hypertension, maternal age, and gestational diabetes mellitus (adjusted HR 4.3, 95% CI 1.1–18.6). Figure 3.2 presents a Kaplan–Meier hazard function curve for the cumulative incidence of cardiovascular mortality following an event of placental abruption. Patients with a history of placental abruption had a significantly higher risk of mortality during a hospitalization for CVD for the whole follow-up period ($p = .017$) [55].

TABLE 3.2

Summary of Selected Studies on Placental Abruption and Subsequent Maternal Morbidity and Mortality

Study (Author, Year, Country)	Cases	Comparison Group	Pregnancy Complication	Outcome Measured	Main Findings
Ray et al. [54], 2005, Canada	Women with placental abruption (*n* = 11,156) or placental infarction (*n* = 9,303)	Women from the same cohort (*n* = 1,033,559)	Placental abruption (placental syndrome; preeclampsia and gestational hypertension also investigated)	Maternal composite CVD; hospital admission for revascularization for coronary artery; cerebrovascular disease; peripheral artery disease	The incidence of CVD was 500 per million person years in women who had had maternal placental syndrome compared with 200 per million in women who did not. This risk was higher in the combined presence of maternal placental syndrome and poor fetal growth or maternal placental syndrome and intrauterine fetal death relative to neither.
Pariente et al. [55], 2013, Israel	Women with placental abruption (*n* = 653)	Women from the same cohort (*n* = 47,585)	Placental abruption	Maternal simple and complex cardiovascular events; maternal cardiovascular mortality	No significant association was noted between placental abruption and subsequent long-term cardiovascular hospitalizations. Placental abruption was associated with long-term cardiovascular mortality. The cardiovascular case fatality rate for the placental abruption group was 13.0% vs. 2.5% in the comparison group.
Arazi et al. [56], 2015, Israel	Women with placental abruption (*n* = 1,807)	Women from the same cohort (*n* = 99,354)	Placental abruption	Maternal renal-related hospitalizations	During the follow-up period patients with a history of placental abruption did not have a higher rate of renal morbidity.
DeRoo et al. [57], 2015, Norway, Sweden	Women with placental abruption in first pregnancy (*n* = 10,981); fathers with a history of placental abruption in first pregnancy (*n* = 821,156); women with placental abruption in any pregnancy (*n* = 23,529)	Women from the same cohort (*n* = 2,117,797); men from the same cohort (*n* not provided)	Placental abruption	Maternal cardiovascular mortality; paternal cardiovascular mortality	Women with placental abruption in first pregnancy had an increased risk of CVD death. Results were unchanged by excluding women with pregestational hypertension, preeclampsia, or diabetes. Women with placental abruption in any pregnancy also had a 1.8-fold increased risk of CVD mortality compared with women who never experienced the condition. No significant difference in mortality between fathers with and without placental abruption in first delivery.

Note: CVD: cardiovascular disease.

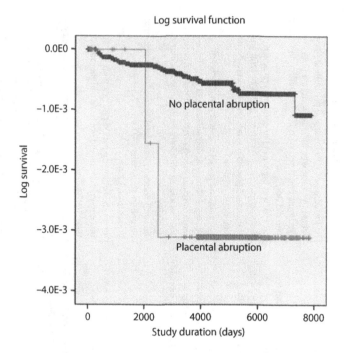

FIGURE 3.2   Kaplan–Meier curve for cardiovascular-associated mortality of patients with and without a history of placental abruption. Survival analysis (presenting the log survival function) showed that women with a history of placental abruption had a significantly higher risk of cardiovascular mortality during the follow-up period.

A recent study focused on the association between maternal placental abruption and subsequent maternal renal complications [56]. In this retrospective analysis of a prospectively collected database, delivery data ($n = 99,354$) were collected over a 25-year period, with a mean follow-up duration of 11.2 years. Renal morbidity included kidney transplantation, chronic renal failure, hypertensive renal disease, and so on. A history of placental abruption ($n = 1807$) was not found to be associated with subsequent renal morbidity (0.2% vs. 0.1%; OR 1.8, 95% CI 0.6–4.8; $p = .261$) [56]. Patients with placental abruption did not have higher cumulative incidence of renal-related hospitalizations using a Kaplan–Meier survival curve (Figure 3.3).

Recently, a population-based registry study from Scandinavia (Norway and Sweden) assessed the association between long-term maternal cardiovascular mortality and placental abruption [57]. The authors used linked Medical Birth Registry and Death Registry data to study CVD-related mortality among over two million women with a first singleton birth between 1967 and 2002 in Norway and 1973 and 2003 in Sweden. Women were followed through 2009 and 2010, respectively, to ascertain subsequent pregnancies and mortality. There were 49,944 deaths after an average follow-up of 23 years, of which 5453 were due to CVD. Women with placental abruption in first pregnancy ($n = 10,981$) had an increased risk of CVD death (HR 1.8, 95% CI 1.3–2.4). Results were essentially unchanged by excluding women with pregestational hypertension, preeclampsia, or diabetes. Women with placental abruption in any pregnancy ($n = 23,529$) also had a 1.8-fold increased risk of CVD mortality (95% CI 1.5–2.2) compared with those who had never experienced the condition [57].

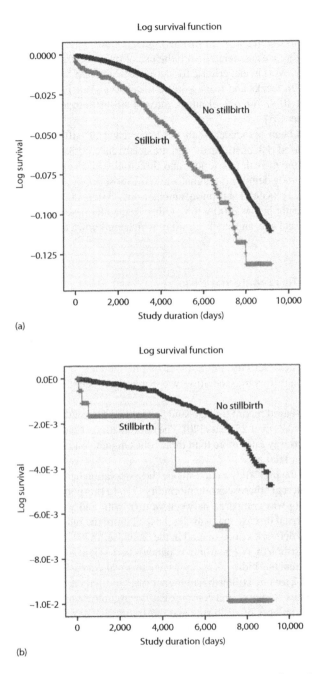

FIGURE 3.3   Kaplan–Meier curve for (a) cardiovascular-associated morbidity and (b) renal-associated morbidity of patients with and without a history of stillbirth. Survival analysis (presenting the log survival function) showed that women with a history of stillbirth had a significantly higher risk of cardiovascular and renal morbidity during the follow-up period.

Stillbirth and Long-Term Maternal Risk

Stillbirth

The World Health Organization (WHO) defines stillbirth as a baby born dead at 28 weeks of gestation or more, with a birth weight of ≥ 1000 g or a body length of ≥ 35 cm.

A universal research- and registry-oriented definition of stillbirth is impossible to establish due to differences in the definitions of fetal death in various countries, differences in norms and criteria for reporting fetal death, and differences associated with the use of birth weight versus gestational-age criteria to define fetal nonviability. Worldwide, criteria for defining fetal death or stillbirth vary from a gestational age of ≥16 weeks to ≥26 weeks and from ≥400 g to ≥500 g [59]. The reported incidence of stillbirth varies from 3.0–7.4 per 1000 [60–62], although rates of stillbirth in low-income countries are believed to be substantially higher [63].

Several factors have been associated with the occurrence of stillbirth. Al Kadri and Tamim [64] showed a 25-fold increased risk of stillbirth with the occurrence of placental abruption, 10-fold with the occurrence of intrauterine growth restriction, and threefold with the presence of hypertensive disorder in pregnancy. Another study demonstrated that while the most important factor associated with stillbirth among white women was placental abruption, among South Asian and black women the most significant risk factor was birth weight below 2000 g [65]. Other frequently described risk factors for stillbirth are obesity, advanced maternal age, and smoking, all of which are known to be risk factors of atherosclerosis [66–68].

Stillbirth and Long-Term Maternal Risk

Few studies have assessed the association between a history of stillbirth and long-term maternal morbidity and mortality (Table 3.3). Kharazmi et al. [69] examined the association between stillbirth and the subsequent maternal risk of MI or stroke. A history of stillbirth was associated with a risk of MI more than 3.4 times higher (95% CI 1.53–7.72) after adjusting for several confounders such as smoking, BMI, physical activity, the number of pregnancies, hypertension, hyperlipidemia, and diabetes mellitus. No significant association was found between a history of stillbirth and the risk of stroke.

A Danish population-based record linkage study examined associations between pregnancy outcomes and maternal mortality rates over 25 years [70]. The combination of induced abortions and natural losses was associated with mortality rates more than three times higher compared with parturients who had not experienced abortions or fetal loss.

Our group published the first study to investigate the association between a previous diagnosis of stillbirth and long-term maternal atherosclerotic morbidity [71]. In this population-based retrospective study, atherosclerotic morbidity was compared between women with and without previous stillbirth. Women with cardiovascular or renal disease that was diagnosed before the index pregnancy were excluded from the study. Of the 99,280 deliveries documented in the database, 1879 (1.9%) occurred in patients who had a history of at least one stillbirth. After stillbirth, patients had a significantly higher cumulative incidence of cardiovascular and renal morbidity (Kaplan–Meier survival curve; Figure 3a,b). During the follow-up period, patients with at least one stillbirth had higher rates of total cardiovascular and renal hospitalizations and had higher rates of simple and complex cardiovascular events. A significant stepwise increase was found between the number of stillbirths and the future risk of cardiovascular morbidity. In a Cox proportional hazards model that was adjusted for confounders, previous stillbirth was associated independently with atherosclerotic morbidity.

Mechanisms for Placental Syndrome

This chapter strengthens the hypothesis that IUGR and placental abruption are associated with a higher risk of long-term maternal morbidity and mortality. Although these studies are relatively consistent in their findings, the underlying mechanisms are not fully understood.

It is uncertain whether the metabolic, inflammatory, and hemodynamic loads of pregnancy unmask underlying phenotypic vulnerability to CVD that is subsequently expressed as pregnancy complications, or whether the complicated pregnancy itself prompts vascular damage and/or inflammatory responses that predispose to future cardiovascular morbidity and mortality [72].

TABLE 3.3

Summary of Selected Studies on Stillbirth and Subsequent Maternal Morbidity and Mortality

Study (Author, Year, Country)	Cases	Comparison Group	Pregnancy Complication	Outcome Measured	Main Findings
Kharazmi et al. [69], 2011, Germany	Women with at least one stillbirth ($n = 209$)	Women from the same cohort ($n = 11,518$)	Stillbirth (miscarriage and abortion also investigated)	Maternal myocardial infarction or stroke	A history of stillbirth was significantly associated with an increased the risk of MI compared with the general population. After adjusting for confounders such as age, smoking, BMI, physical activity, number of pregnancies, hypertension, hyperlipidemia, and diabetes mellitus the association remained significant. No significant association was found between a history of stillbirth and stroke.
Coleman et al. [70], 2012, United States	Women with stillbirth ($n = 64,625$)	Women from the same cohort ($n = 1,001,266$)	Stillbirth (miscarriage and abortion also investigated)	Maternal mortality rate	The combination of induced abortions and natural losses was associated with mortality rates more than three times higher compared with parturients who had not experienced abortions or fetal loss.
Pariente et al. [71], 2014, Israel	Women with stillbirth ($n = 1879$)	Women from the same cohort ($n = 99,280$)	Stillbirth	Atherosclerotic morbidity; simple and complex cardiovascular events; renal-related morbidity	Patients with at least one stillbirth had higher rates of total cardiovascular and renal hospitalizations and had higher rates of simple and complex cardiovascular events. A significant stepwise increase was found between the number of stillbirths and future risk of cardiovascular morbidity. After adjusting for confounders such as maternal age, pregestational diabetes, chronic hypertension, preeclampsia, obesity, and placental abruption, previous stillbirth was associated independently with atherosclerotic morbidity.

Several mechanisms have been suggested to explain the association between placenta-associated syndrome and subsequent maternal morbidity and mortality.

Shared Risk Factors

Placenta-associated syndrome and its components IUGR and placental abruption share several risk factors with CVD. Among them are early maternal age [73], black race [73,74], inflammation and infection [21], cigarette smoking [73,75], hypertension [76,77], and pregestational diabetes [78]. It was proposed that failed adaptation to the intense biologic demands of pregnancy may result in abnormal placentation that in turn will be manifested as growth restriction or placental abruption, and the reasons for maladaptation to pregnancy could involve metabolic and vascular disease pathways [27].

These indicators of abnormal metabolism not only pave the way to a pregnancy affected by maternal placental syndrome, but might also appear afterward. For example, Kanagalingam and colleagues [37] have demonstrated substantial metabolic abnormalities among women who delivered an SGA infant only 4 years after the delivery. Hence, metabolic syndrome and its components could be one mediating factor between maternal placental syndrome and premature CVD.

Shared Genetic Pathways

The genetic theory states that delivering a low–birth weight baby is, in a proportion of cases, a perinatal manifestation of genotypes that also predispose to cardiovascular morbidity. Thus, common genetic risk factors for CVD and uterine growth restriction may explain the relation between an individual's birth weight and her risk of CVD in later life. This effect is often referred to as the *intergenerational association*.

According to the intergenerational association hypothesis, women who were born SGA will more likely parent an SGA infant. Delivering their SGA neonate, rather than the personal history of SGA, has been shown to place these women at increased susceptibility for cardiovascular morbidity [25,26].

Since the intergenerational association of birth weight has been seen for mothers [79] this may contribute to associations between the offspring's birth weight and maternal mortality.

Moreover, factors related to both insulin resistance and birth weight explain at least part of the relationship between birth weight and the risk of adult CVD and diabetes of the offspring in adulthood [80] and the mother later on in life.

The association between the birth weight of offspring and insulin resistance in older age, rather than during the mothers' reproductive years, is more supportive of a genetic mechanism than a temporary hormonal effect of pregnancy on metabolic risk factors for CVD [81].

Intergenerational effects may also be a result of epigenetic processes where methylation imprinting in one generation influences gene expression in the next one. In a historical Swedish cohort, grandparents' food supply in childhood was associated with cardiovascular and diabetic mortality in their grandchildren [82]. Additionally, data from the Avon Longitudinal Study of Parents and Children (ALSPAC) showed that early paternal smoking initiation was linked with greater BMI in sons [83].

In addition, other genetic pathways may explain these associations; mutations that are associated with both an increased risk of ischemic heart disease and restricted growth have been identified in genes encoding G proteins [84], glucokinase [85], and clotting factors [86].

Shared Physiological Processes

Inflammation

The levels of inflammatory markers such as CRP and IL-6 were shown to be elevated in women with low–birth weight neonates [36], suggesting that these women may be exposed to upregulation of inflammation, a process that has been linked to both IUGR [87,88] and an increased risk of CVD [89,90].

Coagulation Cascade

Recent publications have demonstrated that thrombophilic mutations act synergistically with other risk factors to increase the risk of ischemic heart disease in young women [91]. Some studies have shown an association between inherited and acquired forms of thrombophilia and pregnancies complicated with IUGR [92]. However, other studies have demonstrated no association between thrombophilia polymorphism and IUGR [93]; the link between the observed association and causality has not been strongly established, and screening for thrombophilia in the context of uterine growth restriction is currently not a standard practice [10] and has not been associated with improved perinatal outcome.

Endothelial Dysfunction

Endothelial progenitor cells play a role in repairing damaged endothelium. Mothers with SGA infants have demonstrated a reduction in the number and function of circulating endothelial progenitor cells (20% decline in number in mothers delivering an SGA infant compared with mothers of appropriate-for-gestational-age babies) [94]. A decrease in the number and function of endothelial progenitor cells has been linked to cardiovascular risk in the nonpregnant population. It is not clear, however, whether the reduced availability of functioning endothelial progenitor cells in pregnancy is a cause of ischemic placental disease, a result of ischemic placental disease, or represents the link of ischemic placental disease with its clinical manifestations.

CONCLUSION

The present chapter presents robust evidence regarding the association of placenta-associated syndrome and long-term maternal morbidity and mortality. As pregnancy outcomes are progressively being recognized as predictors of subsequent maternal health, a formal definition of placenta-associated syndrome as a pregnancy outcome could contribute to individual risk assessment and improvements in health maintenance.

The American Heart Association recently incorporated a history of preeclampsia, gestational diabetes, and pregnancy-induced hypertension into its cardiovascular risk-assessment guidelines for women [1]. We suggest that the delivery of an SGA infant and/or placental abruption should also be considered additional risk factors for long-term maternal CVD.

REFERENCES

1. Mosca L, Benjamin EJ, Berra K, et al., Effectiveness-based guidelines for the prevention of cardiovascular disease in women: 2011 update; A guideline from the American Heart Association. *Circulation.* 2011; 123(11):1243–62.
2. Brosens JJ, Pijnenborg R, Brosens IA. The myometrial junctional zone spiral arteries in normal and abnormal pregnancies: A review of the literature. *Am J Obstet Gynecol.* 2002;187(5):1416–23.
3. Christensen S, Verhage HG, Nowak G, et al. Smooth muscle myosin II and alpha smooth muscle actin expression in the baboon (*Papio anubis*) uterus is associated with glandular secretory activity and stromal cell transformation. *Biol Reprod.* 1995;53(3):598–608.
4. Pijnenborg R, Bland JM, Robertson WB, et al. Uteroplacental arterial changes related to interstitial trophoblast migration in early human pregnancy. *Placenta.* 1983;4(4):397–413.
5. Kam EP, Gardner L, Loke YW, et al. The role of trophoblast in the physiological change in decidual spiral arteries. *Hum Reprod.* 1999;14(8):2131–8.
6. Lim KH, Zhou Y, Janatpour M, et al. Human cytotrophoblast differentiation/invasion is abnormal in pre-eclampsia. *Am J Pathol.* 1997;151(6):1809–18.
7. Pijnenborg R, Anthony J, Davey DA, et al. Placental bed spiral arteries in the hypertensive disorders of pregnancy. *Br J Obstet Gynaecol.* 1991;98(7):648–55.

8. Lyall F, Bulmer JN, Duffie E, et al. Human trophoblast invasion and spiral artery transformation: The role of PECAM-1 in normal pregnancy, preeclampsia, and fetal growth restriction. *Am J Pathol*. 2001;158(5):1713–21.

9. Meekins JW, Pijnenborg R, Hanssens M, et al. A study of placental bed spiral arteries and trophoblast invasion in normal and severe pre-eclamptic pregnancies. *Br J Obstet Gynaecol*. 1994;101(8):669–74.

10. Lausman A, Kingdom J, Gagnon R, Basso M, et al. Intrauterine growth restriction: Screening, diagnosis, and management. *J Obstet Gynaecol Can*. 2013;35(8):741–57.

11. Sheiner E, Shoham-Vardi I, Hallak M, et al. Placental abruption in term pregnancies: Clinical significance and obstetric risk factors. *J Matern Fetal Neonatal Med*. 2003;13(1):45–9.

12. Pariente G, Wiznitzer A, Sergienko R, et al. Placental abruption: Critical analysis of risk factors and perinatal outcomes. *J Matern Fetal Neonatal Med* 2011;24(5):698–702.

13. Sheiner E, Shoham-Vardi I, Hadar A, et al. Incidence, obstetric risk factors and pregnancy outcome of preterm placental abruption: A retrospective analysis. *J Matern Fetal Neonatal Med*. 2002;11(1):34–9.

14. Granger JP, Alexander BT, Llinas MT, et al. Pathophysiology of hypertension during preeclampsia linking placental ischemia with endothelial dysfunction. *Hypertension*. 2001; 38 (3 Pt 2): 718–22.

15. Rasmussen S, Irgens LM, Bergsjo P, et al. The occurrence of placental abruption in Norway 1967–1991. *Acta Obstet Gynecol Scand*. 1996;75(3):222–8.

16. Krohn M, Voigt L, McKnight B, et al. Correlates of placental abruption. *Br J Obstet Gynaecol*. 1987;94(4):333–40.

17. Voigt LF, Hollenbach KA, Krohn MA, et al. The relationship of abruptio placentae with maternal smoking and small for gestational age infants. *Obstet Gynecol*. 1990;75(5):771–4.

18. Raymond EG, Mills JL. Placental abruption: Maternal risk factors and associated fetal conditions. *Acta Obstet Gynecol Scand*. 1993;72(8):633–9.

19. Ananth CV, Getahun D, Peltier MR, et al. Placental abruption in term and preterm gestations: Evidence for heterogeneity in clinical pathways. *Obstet Gynecol*. 2006;107(4):785–92.

20. Mikolajczyk RT, Zhang J, Betran AP, et al. A global reference for fetal-weight and birthweight percentiles. *Lancet*. 2011;377(9780):1855–61.

21. Goldenberg RL, Cliver SP. Small for gestational age and intrauterine growth restriction: Definitions and standards. *Clin Obstet Gynecol*. 1997;40(4):704–14.

22. Zeitlin J, El Ayoubi M, Jarreau PH, et al. Impact of fetal growth restriction on mortality and morbidity in a very preterm birth cohort. *J Pediatr*. 2010;157(5):733–9.e1.

23. Peacock JL, Lo JW, D'Costa W, et al. Respiratory morbidity at follow-up of small-for-gestational-age infants born very prematurely. *Pediatr Res*. 2013; 73 (4 Pt 1): 457–63.

24. Doctor BA, O'Riordan MA, Kirchner HL, et al. Perinatal correlates and neonatal outcomes of small for gestational age infants born at term gestation. *Am J Obstet Gynecol*. 2001;185(3):652–9.

25. Barker DJ. The developmental origins of well-being. *Philos Trans R Soc Lond B Biol Sci*. 2004;359(1449):1359–66.

26. Barker DJ, Winter PD, Osmond C, et al. Weight in infancy and death from ischaemic heart disease. *Lancet*. 1989;2(8663):577–80.

27. Sattar N, Greer IA. Pregnancy complications and maternal cardiovascular risk: Opportunities for intervention and screening? *BMJ*. 2002;325(7356):157–60.

28. Davey Smith G, Hart C, Ferrell C, et al. Birth weight of offspring and mortality in the Renfrew and Paisley study: Prospective observational study. *BMJ*. 1997;315(7117):1189–93.

29. Hawthorne VM, Watt GC, Hart CL, et al. Cardiorespiratory disease in men and women in urban Scotland: Baseline characteristics of the Renfrew/Paisley (midspan) study population. *Scott Med J*. 1995;40(4):102–7.

30. Watt GC, Hart CL, Hole DJ, et al. Risk factors for cardiorespiratory and all cause mortality in men and women in urban Scotland: 15 year follow up. *Scott Med J*. 1995;40(4):108–12.

31. Smith GC, Pell JP, Walsh D. Pregnancy complications and maternal risk of ischaemic heart disease: A retrospective cohort study of 129,290 births. *Lancet*. 2001;357(9273):2002–6.

32. Pell JP, Smith GC, Walsh D. Pregnancy complications and subsequent maternal cerebrovascular events: A retrospective cohort study of 119,668 births. *Am J Epidemiol*. 2004;159(4):336–42.

33. Lawlor DA, Davey Smith G, Ebrahim S. Birth weight of offspring and insulin resistance in late adulthood: Cross sectional survey. *BMJ*. 2002;325(7360):359.

34. Lawlor DA, Bedford C, Taylor M, et al. Geographical variation in cardiovascular disease, risk factors, and their control in older women: British Women's Heart and Health Study. *J Epidemiol Community Health*. 2003;57(2):134–40.
35. Catov JM, Dodge R, Yamal JM, et al. Prior preterm or small-for-gestational-age birth related to maternal metabolic syndrome. *Obstet Gynecol*. 2011; 117 (2 Pt 1): 225–32.
36. Catov JM, Newman AB, Roberts JM, et al. Association between infant birth weight and maternal cardiovascular risk factors in the health, aging, and body composition study. *Ann Epidemiol*. 2007;17(1):36–43.
37. Kanagalingam MG, Nelson SM, Freeman DJ, et al. Vascular dysfunction and alteration of novel and classic cardiovascular risk factors in mothers of growth restricted offspring. *Atherosclerosis*. 2009;205(1):244–50.
38. Davey Smith G, Hyppönen E, Power C, et al. Offspring birth weight and parental mortality: Prospective observational study and meta-analysis. *Am J Epidemiol*. 2007;166(2):160–69.
39. Manor O, Koupil I. Birth weight of infants and mortality in their parents and grandparents: The Uppsala Birth Cohort Study. *Int J Epidemiol*. 2010;39(5):1264–76.
40. Li CY, Chen HF, Sung FC, et al. Offspring birth weight and parental cardiovascular mortality. *Int J Epidemiol*. 2010;39(4):1082–90.
41. Lykke JA, Langhoff-Roos J, Lockwood CJ, et al. Mortality of mothers from cardiovascular and non-cardiovascular causes following pregnancy complications in first delivery. *Paediatr Perinat Epidemiol*. 2010;24(4):323–30.
42. Bonamy AK, Parikh NI, Cnattingius S, et al. Birth characteristics and subsequent risks of maternal cardiovascular disease: Effects of gestational age and fetal growth. *Circulation*. 2011;124(25):2839–46.
43. Lykke JA, Paidas MJ, Triche EW, et al. Fetal growth and later maternal death, cardiovascular disease and diabetes. *Acta Obstet Gynecol Scand*. 2012;91(4):503–10.
44. 44. Bukowski R, Davis KE, Wilson PW. Delivery of a small for gestational age infant and greater maternal risk of ischemic heart disease. *PLoS One*. 2012;7(3):e33047.
45. Pariente G, Sheiner E, Kessous R, et al. Association between delivery of a small-for-gestational-age neonate and long-term maternal cardiovascular morbidity. *Int J Gynaecol Obstet*. 2013;123(1):68–71.
46. Almasi O, Pariente G, Kessous R, et al. Association between delivery of small-for-gestational-age neonate and long-term maternal chronic kidney disease. *J Matern Fetal Neonatal Med*. 2016;29(17):2861–4.
47. Ananth CV, Savitz DA, Bowes WA Jr, et al. Influence of hypertensive disorders and cigarette smoking on placental abruption and uterine bleeding during pregnancy. *Br J Obstet Gynaecol*. 1997;104(5):572–8.
48. Ananth CV, Savitz DA, Williams MA. Placental abruption and its association with hypertension and prolonged rupture of membranes: A methodologic review and meta-analysis. *Obstet Gynecol*. 1996;88(2):309–18.
49. Ananth CV, Oyelese Y, Yeo L, et al. Placental abruption in the United States, 1979 through 2001: Temporal trends and potential determinants. *Am J Obstet Gynecol*. 2005;192(1):191–8.
50. Ananth, CV, Mulian JC, Demissie K, et al. Placental abruption among singleton and twin births in the United States: Risk factor profiles. *Am J Epidemiol*. 2001;153(8):771–8.
51. Saftlas, AF, Ison DR, Atrash HK, et al. National trends in the incidence of abruptio placentae, 1979–1987. *Obstet Gynecol*. 1991;78(6):1081–6.
52. Abu-Heija A, al-Chalabi H, el-Iloubani N. Abruptio placentae: Risk factors and perinatal outcome. *J Obstet Gynaecol Res*. 1998;24(2):141–4.
53. Ray JG, Vermeulen MJ, Schull MJ, et al. Cardiovascular health after maternal placental syndromes (CHAMPS): Population-based retrospective cohort study. *Lancet*. 2005;366(9499):1797–803.
54. Veerbeek JH, Smit JG, Koster MP, et al. Maternal cardiovascular risk profile after maternal placental abruption. *Hypertension*. 2013;61(6):1297–301.
55. Pariente G, Shoham-Vardi I, Kessous R, et al. Placental abruption as a significant risk factor for long-term cardiovascular mortality in a follow-up period of more than a decade. *Paediatr Perinat Epidemiol*. 2014;28(1):32–8.
56. Arazi ES, Kessous R, Shoham-Vardi I, et al. Is there an association between a history of placental abruption and long-term maternal renal complications? *J Matern Fetal Neonatal Med*. 2015;28(14):1641–6.
57. DeRoo L, Skjærven R, Wilcox A, et al. Placental abruption and long-term maternal cardiovascular disease mortality: A population-based registry study in Norway and Sweden. *Eur J Epidemiol*. 2015;31(5):501–11.

58. Joseph KS, et al. Rationalizing definitions and procedures for optimizing clinical care and public health in fetal death and stillbirth. *Obstet Gynecol.* 2015;125(4):784–8.

59. Helgadottir LB, Skjeldestad FE, Jacobsen AF, et al. Incidence and risk factors of fetal death in Norway: A case-control study. *Acta Obstet Gynecol Scand.* 2011;90(4):390–97.

60. Stanton C, Lawn JE, Rahman H, et al. Stillbirth rates: Delivering estimates in 190 countries. *Lancet.* 2006;367(9521):1487–94.

61. Ohana O, Holcberg G, Sergienko R, et al. Risk factors for intrauterine fetal death (1988–2009). *J Matern Fetal Neonatal Med.* 2011;24(9):1079–83.

62. Cousens S, Blencowe H, Stanton C, et al. National, regional, and worldwide estimates of stillbirth rates in 2009 with trends since 1995: A systematic analysis. *Lancet.* 2011;377(9774):1319–30.

63. Al-Kadri HM, Tamim HM. Factors contributing to intra-uterine fetal death. *Arch Gynecol Obstet.* 2012;286(5):1109–16.

64. Balchin I, Whittaker JC, Patel RR, et al. Racial variation in the association between gestational age and perinatal mortality: Prospective study. *BMJ.* 2007;334(7598):833.

65. Fretts RC. Etiology and prevention of stillbirth. *Am J Obstet Gynecol.* 2005;193(6):1923–35.

66. Goldenberg RL, Kirby R, Culhane JF. Stillbirth: A review. *J Matern Fetal Neonatal Med.* 2004;16(2):79–94.

67. Silver RM. Fetal death. *Obstet Gynecol.* 2007;109(1):153–67.

68. Kharazmi E, Dossus L, Rohrmann S, et al. Pregnancy loss and risk of cardiovascular disease: A prospective population-based cohort study (EPIC-Heidelberg). *Heart.* 2011;97(1):49–54.

69. Coleman PK, Reardon DC, Calhoun BC. Reproductive history patterns and long-term mortality rates: A Danish, population-based record linkage study. *Eur J Public Health.* 2013;23(4):569–74.

70. Pariente G, Shoham-Vardi I, Kessous R, et al. Is stillbirth associated with long-term atherosclerotic morbidity? *Am J Obstet Gynecol.* 2014;211(4):416.e1–12.

71. Wenger NK. Recognizing pregnancy-associated cardiovascular risk factors. *Am J Cardiol.* 2014;113(2):406–9.

72. Shiono PH, Klebanoff MA. Ethnic differences in preterm and very preterm delivery. *Am J Public Health.* 1986;76(11):1317–21.

73. David RJ, Collins JW, Jr. Differing birth weight among infants of U.S.-born blacks, African-born blacks, and U.S.-born whites. *N Engl J Med.* 1997;337(17):1209–14.

74. Fox SH, Koepsell TD, Daling JR. Birth weight and smoking during pregnancy: Effect modification by maternal age. *Am J Epidemiol.* 1994;139(10):1008–15.

75. Abrams B, Newman V. Small-for-gestational-age birth: Maternal predictors and comparison with risk factors of spontaneous preterm delivery in the same cohort. *Am J Obstet Gynecol.* 1991;164(3):785–90.

76. Fang J, Madhavan S, Alderman MH. The influence of maternal hypertension on low birth weight: Differences among ethnic populations. *Ethn Dis.* 1999;9(3):369–76.

77. Zeitlin JA, Ancel PY, Saurel-Cubizolles MJ, et al. Are risk factors the same for small for gestational age versus other preterm births? *Am J Obstet Gynecol.* 2001;185(1):208–15.

78. Ounsted M. Transmission through the female line of fetal growth constraint. *Early Hum Dev.* 1986;13(3):339–41.

79. Hattersley AT, Tooke JE. The fetal insulin hypothesis: An alternative explanation of the association of low birthweight with diabetes and vascular disease. *Lancet.* 1999;353(9166):1789–92.

80. Ness RB, Schotland HM, Flegal KM, et al. Reproductive history and coronary heart disease risk in women. *Epidemiol Rev.* 1994;16(2):298–314.

81. Bygren LO, Kaati G, Edvinsson S. Longevity determined by paternal ancestors' nutrition during their slow growth period. *Acta Biotheor.* 2001;49(1):53–9.

82. Pembrey ME, ME, Bygren LO, Kaati G, et al. Sex-specific, male-line transgenerational responses in humans. *Eur J Hum Genet.* 2006;14(2):159–66.

83. Hocher B, Slowinski T, Stolze T, et al. Association of maternal G protein beta3 subunit 825T allele with low birthweight. *Lancet.* 2000;355(9211):1241–2.

84. Hattersley AT, et al. Mutations in the glucokinase gene of the fetus result in reduced birth weight. *Nature genetics.* 1998;19(3):268–70.

85. Kupferminc MJ, Eldor A, Steinman N, et al. Increased frequency of genetic thrombophilia in women with complications of pregnancy. *New Engl J Med.* 1999;340(1):9–13.

86. Bartha JL, Romero-Carmona R, Comino-Delgado R. Inflammatory cytokines in intrauterine growth retardation. *Acta Obstet Gynecol Scand.* 2003;82(12):1099–102.
87. Silver RM, Schwinzer B, McGregor JA. Interleukin-6 levels in amniotic fluid in normal and abnormal pregnancies: Preeclampsia, small-for-gestational-age fetus, and premature labor. *Am J Obstet Gynecol.* 1993;169(5):1101–5.
88. Ridker PM, Hennekens CH, Buring JE, et al. C-reactive protein and other markers of inflammation in the prediction of cardiovascular disease in women. *N Engl J Med.* 2000;342(12):836–43.
89. Tracy RP, Lemaitre RN, Psaty BM, et al. Relationship of C-reactive protein to risk of cardiovascular disease in the elderly: Results from the Cardiovascular Health Study and the Rural Health Promotion Project. *Arterioscler Thromb Vasc Biol.* 1997;17(6):1121–7.
90. Rosendaal FR, Siscovick DS, Schwartz SM, et al. A common prothrombin variant (20210 G to A) increases the risk of myocardial infarction in young women. *Blood.* 1997;90(5):1747–50.
91. Alfirevic Z, Roberts D, Martlew V. How strong is the association between maternal thrombophilia and adverse pregnancy outcome? A systematic review. *Eur J Obstet Gynecol Reprod Biol.* 2002;101(1):6–14.
92. Infante-Rivard C, , Rivard GE, Yotov WV, et al. Absence of association of thrombophilia polymorphisms with intrauterine growth restriction. *New Engl J Med.* 2002;347(1):19–25.
93. King TF, Bergin DA, Kent EM, et al. Endothelial progenitor cells in mothers of low-birthweight infants: A link between defective placental vascularization and increased cardiovascular risk? *J Clin Endocrinol Metab.* 2013;98(1):E33–9.
94. Dietz PM, , Kuklina EV, Bateman BT, et al. Assessing cardiovascular disease risk among young women with a history of delivering a low-birth-weight infant. *Am J Perinatol.* 2013;30(4):267–73.

4

Pregnancy Complications and Impact on Long-Term Oncological Morbidity of the Mother

Roy Kessous and Walter H. Gotlieb

Introduction

A Window of Opportunity

In recent years there has been growing interest based on accumulating evidence concerning a link between common pregnancy complications and future maternal cardiovascular, renal, ophthalmic, and other morbidities [1–3] (Figure 4.1). Studies provide evidence to support the hypothesis that pregnancy can be considered a window of opportunity in order to better evaluate a woman's future lifetime risk of certain morbidities.

Female Cancers

Cancer represents a wide array of diseases resulting from various factors including genetic predisposition, lifestyle characteristics, and environmental exposures [5]. With the turn of the millennium, cancer has become the leading cause of death in developed countries, with an estimated 12.7 million cases and 7.6 million deaths yearly worldwide [6]. Currently, cancer-related death under the age of 85 years is outranking death related to cardiovascular disease [7].

Worldwide, breast cancer is the most commonly diagnosed cancer in women [8–10], with most cases occurring after the age of 50 [8]. Cervical cancer is the most common gynecologic (i.e., from the woman's reproductive organs) cancer, and accounted for an estimated 528,000 new cancer cases worldwide and 266,000 deaths in 2012 [10]. This is followed by uterine cancer, with over 300,000 new cases diagnosed in 2012 [10]. Most cases of endometrial cancer are diagnosed after menopause, with the highest incidence after the age of 60 years [11]. Ovarian cancer, although less common, has the highest fatality rate of all gynecologic cancers, with a mortality rate of 7.5 per 100,000 women per year [12,13].

Pregnancy and Cancer

Throughout this chapter it is important to remember that pregnancy as a whole is associated with a reduced risk of developing ovarian, endometrial, and breast cancer later in life [14].

The underlining mechanisms that link pregnancy complications and the risk of cancer are likely associated with hormonal or epithelial/vascular changes. Several previous studies have investigated the carcinogenic effect of estrogen [15,16] and the influence of human chorionic gonadotropin on genes regulating cell proliferation, apoptosis, cell trafficking, and DNA repair [17]. Vascular endothelial growth factor (VEGF) is known to be an important mediator in the formation of blood vessels, which is essential for the development and progression of tumors [18,19]. Matrix metalloproteinases (MMPs) are also important angiogenic factors that are known to be associated with the development of cancer as well as the metastatic potential and overall survival [20,21].

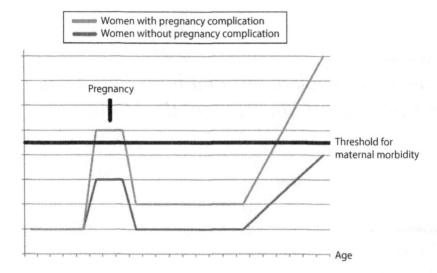

FIGURE 4.1 Theoretical increased risk of future maternal morbidities in women with common pregnancy complications. (Adapted from Sattar N, and Greer IA, *BMJ*, 325, 157–60, 2002.)

This chapter attempts to review the most recent available data on the link between common pregnancy complications and the future maternal risk of malignancies, and the possible pathophysiology. A better understanding of these associations may lead to clinical guidelines such as screening and recommendations about the information that should be provided to patients.

Pregnancy as a Checkpoint for Women

Young women rarely undergo routine examinations, and pregnancy gives an opportunity for health-care professionals to examine them and provide them with counseling and recommendations concerning lifestyle changes.

Young Age Obesity

Diagnosis of obesity and intervention strategies to reduce obesity represent some of the most important opportunities.

The prevalence of obesity has increased dramatically in the last few decades and has become a worldwide health problem. In the United States it is estimated that one-third of women are obese [22]. Literature is abundant on adult obesity and its association with the future risk of morbidities such as cardiovascular disease and thromboembolism [23]. Furthermore, adult obesity has also been recognized as a potential risk factor for cancer-related morbidity and mortality [24–27]. High levels of endogenous estrogen associated with obesity together with hyperinsulinemia, an increased level of insulin-like growth factor 1 (IGF-1), a proinflammatory state, and genetic susceptibility [24,28,29] might explain the link between obesity and cancer. Only a limited number of studies have tried to evaluate the association between young age obesity and future risk for female malignancies.

Endometrial Cancer

Young adult obesity is associated with earlier age at diagnosis of uterine cancer, and mortality from this cancer is linearly correlated with body mass index (BMI) [26]. Both BMI at age 25 and a 5% weight gain were significantly correlated with endometrial cancer incidence [30]. Using data from the Cancer Prevention Study II, in which 33,027 women were enrolled in 1992–1993 and were followed until 2009,

TABLE 4.1

Summary of Selected Studies on Young Age Obesity and Future Risk of Specific Female Malignancies

Study (Author, Year)	No. of Cases	Type of Study	Type of Data Collected	Main Findings
Ovarian Cancer				
Olsen et al., 2008, [34]	1269	Case control	Self-administered questionnaires; BMI at age 20	OR 0.7 (95% CI 0.4–1.3)
Leitzmann et al., 2009, [37]	303	Retrospective	Self-administered questionnaires; BMI at age 18	Overweight: OR 1.29 (95% CI 0.82–2.04) Obese: OR 1.74 (95% CI 0.86–3.53)
Kessous et al., 2015, [41]	57	Retrospective	Prepregnancy medical records	OR 3.3 (95% CI 1.1–9.1)
Breast Cancer				
Zhu et al., 2005, [38]	304	Case control	Telephone interview; BMI at age 18	OR 1.6 (95% CI 0.35–3.22)
Sangaramoorthy et al., 2011, [39]	931	Case control	Body figure image questionnaire at ages 10, 15, 20 (lighter, same, heavier)	Premenopausal OR 0.38 (95% CI 0.21–0.68) Postmenopausal OR 1.04 (95% CI 0.59–1.82)
Berstad et al., 2010, [40]	3,997	Case control	Self-reported BMI at age 18	OR (BMI > or = 25 kg/m^2 vs. < 20 kg/m^2) = 0.76 (95% CI 0.63–0.90)
Han et al., 2014, [30]	372	Retrospective	Self-administered questionnaires; BMI at age 25	OR 1.28 (95% CI 1.13–1.46)
Kessous et al., 2015, [41]	529	Retrospective	Prepregnancy medical records	OR 1.8 (95% CI 1.2–2.8)
Uterine Cancer				
Han et al., 2014, [30]	78	Retrospective	Self-administered questionnaires; BMI at age 25	OR 1.83 (95% CI 1.47–2.26)
Stevens et al., 2014, [31]	447	Retrospective	Self-administered questionnaires; BMI at age 18	RR 1.29 (95% CI 1.12–1.49 per 5 BMI units)
Lu et al., 2011, [32]	668	Case control	In-person interview regarding anthropometric features in each decade	BMI at age 20s: BMI 25–30: OR 2.21 (95% CI 1.42–3.44). BMI >30: OR 1.96 (95% CI 1.16–3.29)
Hosono et al., 2011, [33]	222	Case control	Self-administered questionnaires; BMI at age 20	OR 1.3 (95% CI 1.29–4.11)
Kessous et al., 2015, [41]	61	Retrospective	Prepregnancy medical records	OR 1.5 (95% CI 0.4–6.1)

the authors found a significant correlation between BMI at age 18 and risk of endometrial cancer (RR 1.29, 95% CI 1.12–1.49 per 5 BMI units) [31]. This association was further confirmed in other studies [32,33] (Table 4.1).

Ovarian Cancer

Links between adult obesity and ovarian cancer remain controversial. However, in their meta-analysis, Poorolajal et al. showed that adult obesity increases the risk of ovarian cancer by 8%–27% [25]. Data is even less convulsive with regard to the association of young age obesity and ovarian cancer. In a case-control study that included 1269 patients with a diagnosis of invasive ovarian cancer, patients filled self-administered questionnaires concerning risk factors that included height and weight at the age of 20, and no association was found between BMI at age 20 and future risk of ovarian cancer [34]. Another prospective study with 7 years follow-up on 94,525 women, of whom 303 developed ovarian cancer, could not detect an association between self-reported BMI >25 at the age of 18 and ovarian cancer. Methodological concerns limit the validity of these studies since it is well known that a significant

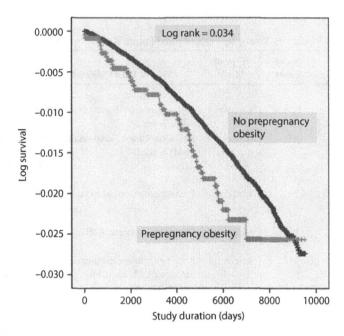

FIGURE 4.2   Kaplan–Meier log survival function for cumulative incidence of hospitalizations for female malignancies, in patients with and without a history of prepregnancy obesity. (Adapted from Kessous R, et al., *AJOG*, 212(Suppl 1), S268, 2015.)

underreporting bias exists when using self-report methods to retrospectively establish young adult obesity [35,36]. Nevertheless, when combining obesity at the age of 18 and obesity at the time of diagnosis, patients had a significantly increased risk of ovarian cancer [37].

Breast Cancer

A weak but significant association has been shown between obesity at a young age and postmenopausal, but not premenopausal, breast cancer [27]. In a case-control study, recollection of the BMI at age 18 during a telephone interview of 304 patients with breast cancer did not show an increased risk of breast cancer [38]; two similar studies surprisingly showed obesity at a young age to be protective [39,40]; and yet another cohort study indicated that a 5% increase in weight from the age of 25 was related to a higher risk of postmenopausal breast cancer [30]. In a study from our group, women with a history of high prepregnancy BMI (>30) were at higher risk of developing breast cancer (Figure 4.2) [41].

Fertility Treatments

Infertility, defined as the inability to conceive within one year of regular sexual activity, is not considered a disease, but rather the consequence of many possible disorders including anatomical malformations and endocrine and autoimmune diseases [42,43]. Infertility is diagnosed in approximately 5%–15% of couples, and female causes are identified in approximately 40% of cases [42–44]. In the past three decades there has been a significant increase in the use of assisted reproductive technology (ART) [45], and there is a growing concern regarding the long-term implications of these treatments.

The etiological role of hormones in the development of cancer has long been studied, particularly in female cancers such as those of the breast, uterus, and ovary [46].

Endometrial Cancer

Although hormones are directly implicated in the development of endometrial cancer, the association between hormonal use in fertility treatments and the development of uterine cancer is unclear. Early retrospective studies on 9832 women with infertility in the 1960s, 1970s, and 1980s did not find an association between clomiphene citrate or gonadotropins and endometrial cancer [48]. The incidence of endometrial cancer in 9165 women who purchased IVF drugs was similar to age-matched controls [49]. On the other hand, in Denmark, the use of gonadotropins and more than six cycles of fertility drugs was found to increase the risk of uterine cancer [50]. A follow-up study of 2431 infertile woman reported the occurrence of 31 cases of uterine cancer over a 30-year period. This rate was significantly higher than expected with a SIR of 1.69 (95% CI 1.14–2.41) [51]. In the cohort study reported by our group, 61 cases of uterine cancer were diagnosed, with an increased risk only in patients with a history of IVF treatments [47]. Overall there seems to be a slight increase in the risk of endometrial cancer than needs to be weighed against the benefits of childbearing (Table 4.2).

Ovarian Cancer

Since the publication of Atlas et al. [52] in 1982 linking fertility drugs to ovarian cancer, controversy has remained whether fertility treatments as such are associated with an increased risk of ovarian cancer. There are several reasons for this difficulty, including the low incidence of ovarian cancer, the short follow-up times, the small cohorts, and differentiating between the contribution of the fertility drugs and infertility as a risk factor on its own. There is good evidence that infertility in itself increases the risk of ovarian cancer. Indeed, subfertile women that have not been treated with fertility drugs are at increased risk of ovarian cancer, compared with women that are not diagnosed with subfertility [53]. Another important difficulty lies in the variety of fertility treatments and protocols, which leads to inconsistency in results and difficulty in reaching conclusions.

When looking at ovulation induction treatments separately, clomiphene citrate or gonadotropins increased the risk of ovarian cancer (SIR 5.89, 95% CI 1.91–13.75) in one study [54], but in our cohort of 106,031 patients, out of whom 3214 patients underwent ovulation induction and 1124 patients in vitro fertilization (IVF), we found no increased risk of the development of ovarian cancer [47]. Similarly, in a cohort of 12,193 infertile patients, 45 ovarian cancers were diagnosed during prolonged follow-up, and no increased risk was associated with clomiphene citrate or gonadotropins (RR 0.82, 95% CI 0.4–1.5) [55,56]. The same results were found in another large European study of 156 cases of ovarian cancer. Results from this study showed no increased risk of ovarian cancer in any of the ovulation induction drugs that were evaluated [57]. Although the jury is still out, the majority of the data regarding ovulation induction are reassuring.

When searching the literature for an association between IVF treatment and ovarian cancer the results are even less conclusive. Some found no association [49], but a meta-analysis of eight studies including 746,455 patients following IVF treatment showed an increased relative risk of 1.59 (95% CI 1.24–2.03) [58]. The risk becomes apparent when extending the surveillance time to 15 years from first IVF [59]. This increased risk appears only when comparing IVF patients with the general population, and seems to disappear when compared with subfertile women [60]. Overall, it appears that there is a possible link between IVF treatments and the future risk of ovarian cancer (Figure 4.3).

Breast Cancer

Neither a large Danish cohort study (54,362 women with infertility problems between 1963 and 1998) [61] nor our single-center cohort study found a significant correlation between fertility treatments and the future risk of breast cancer [47]. A large meta-analysis published by Sergentanis et al. included eight cohort studies with a total of 14,961 cases of breast cancer. According to the results from this meta-analysis, no significant association was found between IVF and breast cancer both when compared with the general population and to infertile women [62]. When considering this current available data, it seems that there is no link between a history of fertility treatments and the future risk of developing breast cancer.

TABLE 4.2

Summary of Selected Studies on Fertility Treatment and Future Risk of Specific Female Malignancies

Study (Author, Year)	No. of Cancer Cases	Type of Study	Type of Fertility Treatment	Main Findings
Ovarian Cancer: Ovulation Induction				
Sanner et al., 2009, [54]	17	Historical cohort study	Gonadotropin	SIR 5.89 (95% CI 1.91–13.75)
Kessous et al., 2015, [47]	58	Retrospective	Gondotropins/ clomiphen	No association
Brinton et al., 2004, [55]	45	Retrospective	Gondotropins/ clomiphen	RR 0.82 (95% CI 0.4–1.5)
Jensen et al., 2009, [57]	156	Retrospective	Gondotropins/ clomiphen/GnRH	No association
Ovarian Cancer: In Vitro Fertilization				
Yli-kuha et al., 2012, [49]	11	Retrospective	IVF drugs	OR 2.25 (95% CI 0.59–8.68)
Li et al., 2013, [58]		Meta-analysis	IVF	OR 1.59 (95% CI 1.24–2.03)
Van Leeuwen et al., 2011, [59]	30	Retrospective	IVF	OR 1.35 (95% CI 0.91–1.92)
Siristatidis et al., 2013, [60]	75	Meta-analysis	IVF	RR 1.50 (95% CI 1.17–1.92)
Kessous et al., 2015, [47]	58	Retrospective	IVF	HR 4.0 (95% CI 1.2–12.6)
Breast Cancer				
Yli-kuha et al., 2012, [49]	108	Retrospective	IVF drugs	RR 0.86 (95% CI 0.57–1.30)
Li et al., 2013, [55]		Meta-analysis		RR 0.89 (95% CI 0.79–1.01)
Jensen et al., 2007, [61]	331	Retrospective	All types of treatments	No association
Kessous et al., 2015, [47]	528	Retrospective	OI/IVF	No association
Sergentanis et al., 2014, [62]	14,961	Meta-analysis	IVF	RR 0.91 (95% CI 0.74–1.11)
Uterine Cancer				
Brinton et al., 2013, [48]	118	Retrospective	Gondotropins/ clomiphen	Clomiphene: HR 1.39 (95% CI 0.96–2.01) Gonadotropins: HR 1.34 (95% CI 0.76–2.37)
Yli-kuha et al., 2012, [49]	6	Retrospective	IVF drugs	OR 2.0 (95% CI 0.37–10.9)
Jensen et al., 2009, [50]	83	Case control	Fertility drugs	All: RR 1.10 (95% CI 0.69–1.76)Gonadotropins: RR 2.21 (95% CI 1.08–4.50)
Lerner-Geva et al., 2012, [51]	30	Retrospective	Fertility treatments	SIR 1.69 (95% CI 1.14–2.41)
Kessous et al., 2015, [47]	61	Retrospective	IVF	HR 4.6 (95% CI 1.4–15.0)

Cervical Cancer

A relatively small number of studies have been published regarding the link between fertility treatments and the future risk of cervical cancer. In these studies, patients with a history of fertility treatments were found to have either a significantly lower risk of developing cervical cancer [49,63] or no increased risk of cervical cancer [47,64]. This lower incidence of cervical cancer may be explained by a more meticulous surveillance of IVF patients that are used to perform gynecological exams and thus screening tests. These data allow us to reassure our patients regarding the lack of future risk of cervical cancer due to fertility treatments.

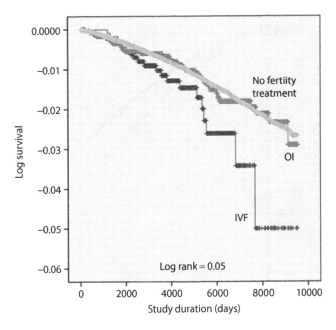

FIGURE 4.3   Kaplan–Meier log survival function for cumulative incidence of hospitalizations due to female malignancies in patients with and without a history of fertility treatments. (Adapted from Kessous R, et al., *J Cancer Res Clin Oncol*, 2015.)

Gestational Diabetes Mellitus

Gestational diabetes mellitus (GDM) is a worldwide public health problem. It is defined as carbohydrate intolerance that begins or is first recognized during pregnancy, and complicates about 7% of all pregnancies [65]. In the last few decades, there has been a rising incidence of GDM, with health consequences for the mothers as well as the offspring during the antepartum, intrapartum, and postpartum periods [66,67]. GDM is one of the most significant risk factors of the development of type 2 diabetes mellitus (T2DM), with 50% of women with a history of GDM in one of their pregnancies developing T2DM, representing a sevenfold increase in the risk of T2DM over time compared with women without a history of GDM. Furthermore, it is also a well-known risk factor of the development of metabolic syndromes and cardiovascular diseases [68–70].

Gestational diabetes mellitus is characterized by hyperinsulinemia and an increase in the IGF-1 cascade, leading to the possible unsupervised growth of cells and cancer [71,72] .

One retrospective population-based study, in which 104,715 patients (out of whom 9893 had a history of GDM) were followed for up to 26 years (mean of 11.2 years), revealed that patients with a history of GDM had an increased risk of female malignancies, including uterine and ovarian cancer, after adjusting for confounders such as parity, maternal age, and fertility treatments (adjusted HR 1.3, 95% CI 1.2–1.6; $p = .001$) [73] (Figure 4.4). Further studies are needed to confirm these findings.

In a cohort of 11,264 women with GDM diagnosed between 1995 and 2009, the authors found an increased risk of pancreatic cancer and hematological malignancies, but not any other cancers (including gynecological malignancies or breast cancer) [74]. This was also observed in a study on breast cancer [75] and other gynecologic cancers [76]. The low prevalence of cancer in young adults and the long time lag between GDM and observable malignancies has led others to reach different conclusions, with stronger associations in postmenopausal breast cancer (RR 1.5, 95% CI 1.0–2.1) [77]. One study found glucose intolerance during pregnancy to be associated with a dose-related increase in the risk of malignant neoplasm, particularly of the breast [78], and another showed a significantly increased risk of breast cancer (OR 2, CI 1.59–2.51; $p = .001$) in patients with a history of GDM [74].

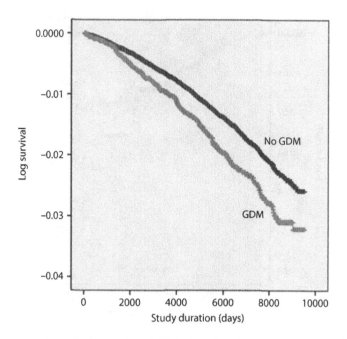

FIGURE 4.4 Kaplan–Meier log survival function for the cumulative incidence of female malignancies hospitalizations with or without a history of gestational diabetes mellitus. (Adapted from Kessous R, et al., *AJOG*, 214(Suppl 1), S240–S241, 2016.)

In summary, despite a good rational pathophysiological hypothesis linking GDM to cancer, clinical studies have shown contradicting results. In view of the rise of GDM, studies are needed to further establish the association of GDM to the long-term risk of cancer, especially breast cancer.

Preeclampsia

The incidence of hypertensive disorders such as preeclampsia and eclampsia in pregnancy is relatively high worldwide. These disorders are considered among the main obstetrical causes of maternal death during pregnancy [79,80]. Although the pathophysiology of preeclampsia is not determined, several potential mechanisms have been suggested. Clinical manifestations are thought to result from micro-angiopathy in different target organs [81]. This process leads to the release of antiangiogenic factors into the maternal circulation, thereby altering maternal systemic endothelial function [82,83]. This may also explain why women who develop preeclampsia have consistently been shown to carry a higher risk of later cardiovascular disease, end-stage renal disease, and hypothyroidism [84–87]. In addition, preeclampsia may also induce permanent endothelial and arterial changes that could lead to the future development of cancer [88,89].

Early studies suggested that immune, hormonal, or genetic mechanisms that induce preeclampsia during pregnancy may reduce the risk of breast cancer both in the mother and daughter [90–92]. Linking a perinatal registry to the Cancer Registry in Israel revealed an increased risk of cancer, including breast and ovarian cancer, in women with a history of preeclampsia [93,94]. A systematic review published in 2007 by Bellamy et al. found no increase or decrease in the risk of any cancer, including breast cancer, following pregnancies with preeclampsia [95]. Similarly, a cohort of 103,180 women, including 8328 with a history of preeclampsia, did not reveal an association between preeclampsia and gynecological malignancies, including breast cancer [96].

Taken together, it is hard to demonstrate a link between preeclampsia and the future risk of malignancy.

Recurrent Pregnancy Loss

Recurrent pregnancy loss (RPL) is defined as more than two or three spontaneous abortions occurring prior to 20 weeks gestation [97]. More than 15% of clinical pregnancies will end in spontaneous abortion, about 2% of pregnant women will suffer two consecutive abortions, and only 0.4%–1% will have three or more consecutive abortions [98]. Etiologies include thrombophilia, immunologic and genetic factors, vascular/placental changes, uterine malformations, and environmental factors [99]. This topic is covered thoroughly in the next chapter.

Pregnancy by itself is associated with decreased risks of ovarian, endometrial, and breast cancers [14], but it is not clear whether only full-term pregnancies have this protective effect or if abortions also confer some protection. Multiple hypotheses might support the lack of protection and even the increased risk conferred by recurrent pregnancy losses on future oncologic outcome. One such lack of a protection mechanism is related to the low levels of progesterone that characterize early pregnancy loss [100–102]. Another mechanism is related to the high levels of estrogen that are seen in early pregnancy and might increase the vulnerability of the breast tissues to different carcinogenesis later in life [103]. Finally, histocompatibility complex–linked genes that have been associated with recurrent pregnancy losses could be related to future susceptibility to cancer [104,105].

Several studies have analyzed the association between abortions and oncologic outcome, but methodological differences, including different definitions of RPL, and the mix of data from spontaneous and induced abortions make it challenging to reach solid conclusions.

Breast Cancer

A review of more than 50 studies and 83,000 patients that included all types of abortions did not show an association between RPL and the future risk of breast cancer [106]. When RPL is analyzed separately from induced or nonrecurring miscarriages, there is a higher incidence of breast cancer (HR 1.7, 95% CI 1.3–2.2; $p = .001$) [107].

Ovarian Cancer

Patients with a history of multiple spontaneous abortions were at higher risk of ovarian cancer, in contrast to patients with a history of multiple induced abortions who did not have a higher incidence of this cancer [108]. Other studies did not find patients with a history of RPL to be at higher risk of ovarian cancer [107,109].

Uterine Cancer

While several studies have reported the protective effect of RPL on the future risk of uterine cancer [110,111]; others have reported these patients to have increased risk [112,113] or no influence at all [107,113].

Cervical Cancer

Only one study evaluated the link between a history of RPL and cervical cancer. This study included data on 106,265 patients, out of whom 7052 had a history of RPL and 229 cases developed cervical cancer. Patients with a history of RPL had a higher incidence of cervical cancer [107]. More studies are needed in order to confirm this possible link.

SUMMARY OF KEY POINTS

1. Results need to be interpreted in the context of the established protective effect of pregnancy on the future development of ovarian, endometrial, and breast cancer.
2. Methodological limitations and inconclusive, often contradictory, results are creating difficulties in evaluating the link between pregnancy-associated complications and the future risk of female malignancies.
3. The link between young-age obesity and the future risk of endometrial cancer seems established, and possible but not conclusive evidence exists regarding the link between young-age obesity and the future risk of breast and ovarian cancer.
4. Based on the published studies available in 2016, it seems that data regarding ovulation-inducing drugs and the future risk of ovarian cancer are relatively reassuring, similar to fertility treatments and the future risk of breast and cervical cancers. However, it appears that there is a possible link between IVF treatments and the future risk of developing uterine and ovarian cancers. More studies are required to provide health-care professionals and patients with clear recommendations.
5. The link between gestational diabetes mellitus and the future development of ovarian and endometrial cancer has not been extensively studied, and despite possible implications suggested by published studies, more studies should be performed in order to support these preliminary results. More literature is available regarding GDM and breast cancer. These studies report contradicting results; nevertheless, a significant number of studies have found a positive association, which may compel physicians to inform patients regarding this possible risk.
6. It seems that for now it is hard to establish a link between preeclampsia and the future risk of malignancies. Therefore, no clear recommendations are available to physicians or patients.
7. For recurrent pregnancy loss, the situation is more complex in view of the mixed types of abortions included in the published series. Nevertheless, given the possible link in the literature, more studies should be done to provide patients with the proper counseling.
8. Given the tendency of young patients to underutilize medical services, pregnancy serves as a highly valuable unavoidable checkpoint in a women's life. When common complications are encountered by a physician, counseling and possible interventions such as surveillance and lifestyle changes might impact on the development of future diseases such as cancer.

REFERENCES

1. Mangos GJ, Spaan JJ, Pirabhahar S, Brown MA. Markers of cardiovascular disease risk after hypertension in pregnancy. *J Hypertens*. 2012;30:351–8.
2. McDonald SD, Han Z, Walsh MW, Gerstein HC, Devereaux PJ. Kidney disease after preeclampsia: A systematic review and meta-analysis. *Am J Kidney Dis*. 2010;55:1026–39.
3. Gordin D, Kaaja R, Forsblom C, Hiilesmaa V, Teramo K, Groop PH. Pre-eclampsia and pregnancy-induced hypertension are associated with severe diabetic retinopathy in type 1 diabetes later in life. *Acta Diabetol*. 2013;50:781–7.
4. Sattar N, Greer IA. Pregnancy complications and maternal cardiovascular risk: Opportunities for intervention and screening? *BMJ*. 2002;325:157–60.
5. Cogliano VJ, Baan R, Straif K, et al. Preventable exposures associated with human cancers. *J Natl Cancer Inst*. 2011;103:1827–39.
6. Jemal A, Bray F, Center MM, Ferlay J, Ward E, Forman D. Global cancer statistics. *CA Cancer J Clin*. 2011;61:69–90.
7. Siegel R, Ward E, Brawley O, Jemal A. Cancer statistics, 2011: The impact of eliminating socioeconomic and racial disparities on premature cancer deaths. *CA Cancer J Clin*. 2011;61:212–36.
8. DeSantis C, Ma J, Bryan L, Jemal A. Breast cancer statistics, 2013. *CA Cancer J Clin*. 2014;64:52–62.
9. McPherson K, Steel CM, Dixon JM. ABC of breast diseases: Breast cancer-epidemiology, risk factors, and genetics. *BMJ*. 2000;321:624–8.

10. Torre LA, Bray F, Siegel RL, Ferlay J, Lortet-Tieulent J, Jemal A. Global cancer statistics, 2012. *CA Cancer J Clin*. 2015;65:87–108.
11. Amant F, Moerman P, Neven P, Timmerman D, Van Limbergen E, Vergote I. Endometrial cancer. *Lancet*. 2005;366:491–505.
12. Sopik V, Iqbal J, Rosen B, Narod SA. Why have ovarian cancer mortality rates declined? Part I: Incidence. *Gynecol Oncol*. 2015;138(3):741–9.
13. Siegel RL, Miller KD, Jemal A. Cancer statistics, 2015. *CA Cancer J Clin*. 2015;65:5–29.
14. Beral V. Long term effects of childbearing on health. *J Epidemiol Community Health* 1985;39:343–6.
15. Fishman J, Osborne MP, Telang NT. The role of estrogen in mammary carcinogenesis. *Ann NY Acad Sci*. 1995;768:91–100.
16. Britton JA, Gammon MD, Schoenberg JB, et al. Risk of breast cancer classified by joint estrogen receptor and progesterone receptor status among women 20–44 years of age. *Am J Epidemiol*. 2002;156:507–16.
17. Guo S, Russo IH, Lareef MH, Russo J. Effect of human chorionic gonadotropin in the gene expression profile of MCF-7 cells. *Int J Oncol*. 2004;24:399–407.
18. Koochekpour S, Bullock P, Dean A, Pilkington G, Merzak A. Expression of vascular endothelial growth-factor in the cyst fluid of human cerebral gliomas. *Oncol Rep*. 1995;2:1147–9.
19. Cohen T, Nahari D, Cerem LW, Neufeld G, Levi BZ. Interleukin 6 induces the expression of vascular endothelial growth factor. *J Biol Chem*. 1996;271:736–41.
20. Nelson AR, Fingleton B, Rothenberg ML, Matrisian LM. Matrix metalloproteinases: Biologic activity and clinical implications. *J Clin Oncol*. 2000;18:1135–49.
21. Roomi MW, Kalinovsky T, Rath M, Niedzwiecki A. Modulation of u-PA, MMPs and their inhibitors by a novel nutrient mixture in human female cancer cell lines. *Oncol Rep*. 2012;28:768–76.
22. Gynecologists ACoOa. Obesity in pregnancy. ACOG Committee Opinion no. 549. *Obstet Gynecol*. 2013;121:213–7.
23. Ebbert JO, Elrashidi MY, Jensen MD. Managing overweight and obesity in adults to reduce cardiovascular disease risk. *Curr Atheroscler Rep*. 2014;16:445.
24. Burza MA, Spagnuolo R, Montalcini T, Doldo P, Pujia A, Romeo S. Effect of excess body weight on the genetic susceptibility to cancer. *J Clin Gastroenterol*. 2014;48(Suppl 1):S78–9.
25. Poorolajal J, Jenabi E, Masoumi SZ. Body mass index effects on risk of ovarian cancer: A meta-analysis. *Asian Pac J Cancer Prev*. 2014;15:7665–71.
26. Nevadunsky NS, Van Arsdale A, Strickler HD, et al. Obesity and age at diagnosis of endometrial cancer. *Obstet Gynecol*. 2014;124:300–306.
27. Cheraghi Z, Poorolajal J, Hashem T, Esmailnasab N, Doosti Irani A. Effect of body mass index on breast cancer during premenopausal and postmenopausal periods: A meta-analysis. *PLoS One*. 2012;7:e51446.
28. Vona-Davis L, Rose DP. Angiogenesis, adipokines and breast cancer. *Cytokine Growth Factor Rev*. 2009;20:193–201.
29. Bertolini F, Orecchioni S, Petit JY, Kolonin MG. Obesity, proinflammatory mediators, adipose tissue progenitors, and breast cancer. *Curr Opin Oncol*. 2014;26:545–50.
30. Han X, Stevens J, Truesdale KP, et al. Body mass index at early adulthood, subsequent weight change and cancer incidence and mortality. *Int J Cancer*. 2014;135:2900–909.
31. Stevens VL, Jacobs EJ, Patel AV, Sun J, Gapstur SM, McCullough ML. Body weight in early adulthood, adult weight gain, and risk of endometrial cancer in women not using postmenopausal hormones. *Cancer Causes Control*. 2014;25:321–8.
32. Lu L, Risch H, Irwin ML, et al. Long-term overweight and weight gain in early adulthood in association with risk of endometrial cancer. *Int J Cancer*. 2011;129:1237–43.
33. Hosono S, Matsuo K, Hirose K, et al. Weight gain during adulthood and body weight at age 20 are associated with the risk of endometrial cancer in Japanese women. *J Epidemiol*. 2011;21:466–73.
34. Olsen CM, Nagle CM, Whiteman DC, et al. Body size and risk of epithelial ovarian and related cancers: A population-based case-control study. *Int J Cancer*. 2008;123:450–56.
35. Shields M, Connor Gorber S, Janssen I, Tremblay MS. Bias in self-reported estimates of obesity in Canadian health surveys: An update on correction equations for adults. *Health Rep*. 2011;22:35–45.
36. Scribani M, Shelton J, Chapel D, Krupa N, Wyckoff L, Jenkins P. Comparison of bias resulting from two methods of self-reporting height and weight: A validation study. *JRSM Open*. 2014;5(6):2042533313514048.

37. Leitzmann MF, Koebnick C, Danforth KN, et al. Body mass index and risk of ovarian cancer. *Cancer.* 2009;115:812–22.
38. Zhu K, Caulfield J, Hunter S, Roland CL, Payne-Wilks K, Texter L. Body mass index and breast cancer risk in African American women. *Ann Epidemiol.* 2005;15:123–8.
39. Sangaramoorthy M, Phipps AI, Horn-Ross PL, Koo J, John EM. Early-life factors and breast cancer risk in Hispanic women: The role of adolescent body size. *Cancer Epidemiol Biomarkers Prev* 2011;20:2572–82.
40. Berstad P, Coates RJ, Bernstein L, et al. A case-control study of body mass index and breast cancer risk in white and African-American women. *Cancer Epidemiol Biomarkers Prev.* 2010;19:1532–44.
41. Kessous R, Davidson E, Meirovitz M, Sergienko R, Sheiner E. Prepregnancy obesity: A risk factor for future development of ovarian and breast cancer. *Eur J Cancer Prev.* 2016 Feb 22.
42. Mascarenhas MN, Flaxman SR, Boerma T, Vanderpoel S, Stevens GA. National, regional, and global trends in infertility prevalence since 1990: A systematic analysis of 277 health surveys. *PLoS Med.* 2012;9:e1001356.
43. Evers JL. Female subfertility. *Lancet.* 2002;360:151–9.
44. Boivin J, Bunting L, Collins JA, Nygren KG. International estimates of infertility prevalence and treatment-seeking: Potential need and demand for infertility medical care. *Hum Reprod.* 2007;22:1506–12.
45. Wysowski DK. Use of fertility drugs in the United States, 1973 through 1991. *Fertil Steril.* 1993;60:1096–8.
46. Bernstein L. Epidemiology of endocrine-related risk factors for breast cancer. *J Mammary Gland Biol Neoplasia.* 2002;7:3–15.
47. Kessous R, Davidson E, Meirovitz M, Sergienko R, Sheiner E. The risk of female malignancies after fertility treatments: A cohort study with 25-year follow-up. *J Cancer Res Clin Oncol.* 2016 Jan;142(1):287–93.
48. Brinton LA, Westhoff CL, Scoccia B, et al. Fertility drugs and endometrial cancer risk: Results from an extended follow-up of a large infertility cohort. *Hum Reprod.* 2013;28:2813–21.
49. Yli-Kuha AN, Gissler M, Klemetti R, Luoto R, Hemminki E. Cancer morbidity in a cohort of 9175 Finnish women treated for infertility. *Hum Reprod.* 2012;27:1149–55.
50. Jensen A, Sharif H, Kjaer SK. Use of fertility drugs and risk of uterine cancer: Results from a large Danish population-based cohort study. *Am J Epidemiol.* 2009;170:1408–14.
51. Lerner-Geva L, Liat LG, Rabinovici J, et al. Are infertility treatments a potential risk factor for cancer development? Perspective of 30 years of follow-up. *Gynecol Endocrinol.* 2012;28:809–14.
52. Atlas M, Menczer J. Massive hyperstimulation and borderline carcinoma of the ovary: A possible association. *Acta Obstet Gynecol Scand.* 1982;61:261–3.
53. Whittemore AS, Harris R, Itnyre J, Collaborative Ovarian Cancer Group. Characteristics relating to ovarian cancer risk: Collaborative analysis of 12 US case-control studies; II. Invasive epithelial ovarian cancers in white women. *Am J Epidemiol.* 1992;136:1184–203.
54. Sanner K, Conner P, Bergfeldt K, et al. Ovarian epithelial neoplasia after hormonal infertility treatment: Long-term follow-up of a historical cohort in Sweden. *Fertil Steril.* 2009;91:1152–8.
55. Brinton LA, Lamb EJ, Moghissi KS, et al. Ovarian cancer risk associated with varying causes of infertility. *Fertil Steril.* 2004;82:405–14.
56. Trabert B, Lamb EJ, Scoccia B, et al. Ovulation-inducing drugs and ovarian cancer risk: Results from an extended follow-up of a large United States infertility cohort. *Fertil Steril.* 2013;100:1660–66.
57. Jensen A, Sharif H, Frederiksen K, Kjaer SK. Use of fertility drugs and risk of ovarian cancer: Danish population based cohort study. *BMJ.* 2009;338:b249.
58. Li LL, Zhou J, Qian XJ, Chen YD. Meta-analysis on the possible association between in vitro fertilization and cancer risk. *Int J Gynecol Cancer.* 2013;23:16–24.
59. van Leeuwen FE, Klip H, Mooij TM, et al. Risk of borderline and invasive ovarian tumours after ovarian stimulation for in vitro fertilization in a large Dutch cohort. *Hum Reprod.* 2011;26:3456–65.
60. Siristatidis C, Sergentanis TN, Kanavidis P, et al. Controlled ovarian hyperstimulation for IVF: Impact on ovarian, endometrial and cervical cancer; a systematic review and meta-analysis. *Hum Reprod Update.* 2013;19:105–23.
61. Jensen A, Sharif H, Svare EI, Frederiksen K, Kjaer SK. Risk of breast cancer after exposure to fertility drugs: Results from a large Danish cohort study. *Cancer Epidemiol Biomarkers Prev.* 2007;16:1400–407.

62. Sergentanis TN, Diamantaras AA, Perlepe C, Kanavidis P, Skalkidou A, Petridou ET. IVF and breast cancer: A systematic review and meta-analysis. *Hum Reprod Update*. 2014;20:106–23.

63. Silva Idos S, Wark PA, McCormack VA, et al. Ovulation-stimulation drugs and cancer risks: A long-term follow-up of a British cohort. *Br J Cancer*. 2009;100:1824–31.

64. Dor J, Lerner-Geva L, Rabinovici J, et al. Cancer incidence in a cohort of infertile women who underwent in vitro fertilization. *Fertil Steril*. 2002;77:324–7.

65. Association AD. Gestational diabetes mellitus. *Diabetes Care*. 2004;27(Suppl 1):S88–90.

66. Malcolm J. Through the looking glass: Gestational diabetes as a predictor of maternal and offspring long-term health. *Diabetes Metab Res Rev*. 2012;28:307–11.

67. Kjos SL, Buchanan TA. Gestational diabetes mellitus. *N Engl J Med*. 1999;341:1749–56.

68. Bellamy L, Casas JP, Hingorani AD, Williams D. Type 2 diabetes mellitus after gestational diabetes: A systematic review and meta-analysis. *Lancet*. 2009;373:1773–9.

69. Xu Y, Shen S, Sun L, Yang H, Jin B, Cao X. Metabolic syndrome risk after gestational diabetes: A systematic review and meta-analysis. *PLoS One*. 2014;9:e87863.

70. Kessous R, Shoham-Vardi I, Pariente G, Sherf M, Sheiner E. An association between gestational diabetes mellitus and long-term maternal cardiovascular morbidity. *Heart*. 2013;99:1118–21.

71. Chodick G, Zucker I. Diabetes, gestational diabetes and the risk of cancer in women: Epidemiologic evidence and possible biologic mechanisms. *Womens Health (Lond)* 2011;7:227–37.

72. Giovannucci E, Harlan DM, Archer MC, et al. Diabetes and cancer: A consensus report. *Diabetes Care*. 2010;33:1674–85.

73. Kessous R, Fuchs O, Davidson E, Sergienko R, Sheiner E. A history of gestational diabetes mellitus: Is it a marker for future long-term female malignancies? *AJOG*. 2016;214(Suppl 1):S240–41.

74. Sella T, Chodick G, Barchana M, et al. Gestational diabetes and risk of incident primary cancer: A large historical cohort study in Israel. *Cancer Causes Control* 2011;22:1513–20.

75. Bejaimal SA, Wu CF, Lowe J, Feig DS, Shah BR, Lipscombe LL. Short-term risk of cancer among women with previous gestational diabetes: A population-based study. *Diabet Med*. 2015;39(6):445–50.

76. Tong GX, Cheng J, Chai J, et al. Association between gestational diabetes mellitus and subsequent risk of cancer: A systematic review of epidemiological studies. *Asian Pac J Cancer Prev*. 2014;15:4265–9.

77. Perrin MC, Terry MB, Kleinhaus K, et al. Gestational diabetes and the risk of breast cancer among women in the Jerusalem Perinatal Study. *Breast Cancer Res Treat*. 2008;108:129–35.

78. Dawson SI. Long-term risk of malignant neoplasm associated with gestational glucose intolerance. *Cancer*. 2004;100:149–55.

79. Abalos E, Cuesta C, Grosso AL, Chou D, Say L. Global and regional estimates of preeclampsia and eclampsia: A systematic review. *Eur J Obstet Gynecol Reprod Biol*. 2013;170:1–7.

80. Khan KS, Wojdyla D, Say L, Gülmezoglu AM, Van Look PF. WHO analysis of causes of maternal death: A systematic review. *Lancet*. 2006;367:1066–74.

81. Lain KY, Roberts JM. Contemporary concepts of the pathogenesis and management of preeclampsia. *JAMA*. 2002;287:3183–6.

82. Redman CW, Sacks GP, Sargent IL. Preeclampsia: An excessive maternal inflammatory response to pregnancy. *Am J Obstet Gynecol*. 1999;180:499–506.

83. Roberts JM, Taylor RN, Goldfien A. Clinical and biochemical evidence of endothelial cell dysfunction in the pregnancy syndrome preeclampsia. *Am J Hypertens*. 1991;4:700–708.

84. Harskamp RE, Zeeman GG. Preeclampsia: At risk for remote cardiovascular disease. *Am J Med Sci*. 2007;334:291–5.

85. McDonald SD, Malinowski A, Zhou Q, Yusuf S, Devereaux PJ. Cardiovascular sequelae of preeclampsia/eclampsia: A systematic review and meta-analyses. *Am Heart J*. 2008;156:918–30.

86. Vikse BE, Irgens LM, Leivestad T, Skjaerven R, Iversen BM. Preeclampsia and the risk of end-stage renal disease. *N Engl J Med*. 2008;359:800–809.

87. Levine RJ, Vatten LJ, Horowitz GL, et al. Pre-eclampsia, soluble fms-like tyrosine kinase 1, and the risk of reduced thyroid function: Nested case-control and population based study. *BMJ*. 2009;339:b4336.

88. Romundstad PR, Magnussen EB, Smith GD, Vatten LJ. Hypertension in pregnancy and later cardiovascular risk: Common antecedents? *Circulation*. 2010;122:579–84.

89. Bytautiene E, Bulayeva N, Bhat G, Li L, Rosenblatt KP, Saade GR. Long-term alterations in maternal plasma proteome after sFlt1-induced preeclampsia in mice. *Am J Obstet Gynecol*. 2013;208:388.e1–88. e10.

90. Polednak AP, Janerich DT. Characteristics of first pregnancy in relation to early breast cancer: A case-control study. *J Reprod Med*. 1983;28:314–18.

91. Troisi R, Weiss HA, Hoover RN, et al. Pregnancy characteristics and maternal risk of breast cancer. *Epidemiology*. 1998;9:641–7.

92. Ekbom A, Trichopoulos D, Adami HO, Hsieh CC, Lan SJ. Evidence of prenatal influences on breast cancer risk. *Lancet*. 1992;340:1015–18.

93. Paltiel O, Friedlander Y, Tiram E, Barchana M, Xue X, Harlap S. Cancer after pre-eclampsia: Follow up of the Jerusalem perinatal study cohort. *BMJ*. 2004;328:919.

94. Calderon-Margalit R, Friedlander Y, Yanetz R, et al. Preeclampsia and subsequent risk of cancer: Update from the Jerusalem Perinatal Study. *Am J Obstet Gynecol*. 2009;200:63.e1–5.

95. Bellamy L, Casas JP, Hingorani AD, Williams DJ. Pre-eclampsia and risk of cardiovascular disease and cancer in later life: Systematic review and meta-analysis. *BMJ*. 2007;335:974.

96. Walfisch A, Kessous R, Davidson E, Sergienko R, Sheiner E. Pre-eclampsia and future female malignancy. *Hypertens Pregnancy*. 2015;34(4):456–63.

97. Gynecologists ACoOa. Management of recurrent pregnancy loss. ACOG Practice Bulletin no. 24, February 2001. (Replaces Technical Bulletin no. 212, September 1995.) *Int J Gynaecol Obstet*. 2002;78:179–90.

98. Salat-Baroux J. Recurrent spontaneous abortions. *Reprod Nutr Dev*. 1988;28:1555–68.

99. Medicine PCotASfR. Evaluation and treatment of recurrent pregnancy loss: A committee opinion. *Fertil Steril*. 2012;98:1103–11.

100. Lukanova A, Kaaks R. Endogenous hormones and ovarian cancer: Epidemiology and current hypotheses. *Cancer Epidemiol Biomarkers Prev*. 2005;14:98–107.

101. Dai D, Wolf DM, Litman ES, White MJ, Leslie KK. Progesterone inhibits human endometrial cancer cell growth and invasiveness: Down-regulation of cellular adhesion molecules through progesterone B receptors. *Cancer Res*. 2002;62:881–6.

102. Brisken C. Reply to: Is progesterone a neutral or protective factor for breast cancer? *Nat Rev Cancer*. 2014;14:146.

103. Davidson T. Abortion and breast cancer: A hard decision made harder. *Lancet Oncol*. 2001;2:756–8.

104. Gill TJ. Influence of MHC and MHC-linked genes on reproduction. *Am J Hum Genet*. 1992;50:1–5.

105. Gill TJ. The borderland of embryogenesis and carcinogenesis: Major histocompatibility complex-linked genes affecting development and their possible relationship to the development of cancer. *Biochim Biophys Acta*. 1984;738:93–102.

106. Beral V, Bull D, Doll R, Peto R, Reeves G, Cancer CGoHFiB. Breast cancer and abortion: Collaborative reanalysis of data from 53 epidemiological studies, including 83,000 women with breast cancer from 16 countries. *Lancet*. 2004;363:1007–16.

107. Charach R, Kessous R, Beharier O, Sheiner E, Davidson E. Is there an association between recurrent pregnancy loss and future risk for famale malignancies? *AJOG*. 2016;214(1 Suppl).

108. Braem MG, Onland-Moret NC, Schouten LJ, et al. Multiple miscarriages are associated with the risk of ovarian cancer: Results from the European Prospective Investigation into Cancer and Nutrition. *PLoS One*. 2012;7:e37141.

109. Dick ML, Siskind V, Purdie DM, Green AC, Cancer ACSGO, Group AOCS. Incomplete pregnancy and risk of ovarian cancer: Results from two Australian case-control studies and systematic review. *Cancer Causes Control*. 2009;20:1571–85.

110. Xu WH, Xiang YB, Ruan ZX, et al. Menstrual and reproductive factors and endometrial cancer risk: Results from a population-based case-control study in urban Shanghai. *Int J Cancer*. 2004;108:613–19.

111. Parslov M, Lidegaard O, Klintorp S, et al. Risk factors among young women with endometrial cancer: A Danish case-control study. *Am J Obstet Gynecol*. 2000;182:23–9.

112. Brinton LA, Sakoda LC, Lissowska J, et al. Reproductive risk factors for endometrial cancer among Polish women. *Br J Cancer*. 2007;96:1450–56.

113. McPherson CP, Sellers TA, Potter JD, Bostick RM, Folsom AR. Reproductive factors and risk of endometrial cancer: The Iowa Women's Health Study. *Am J Epidemiol*. 1996;143:1195–202.

5

Recurrent Pregnancy Loss: Overview and Impact on Future Maternal Health

Oren Barak and Edi Vaisbuch

Introduction

Spontaneous pregnancy loss is a well-defined situation in which an established intrauterine pregnancy is involuntarily terminated before the fetus has reached viability [1] and is most commonly the consequence of a chromosomal abnormality.

Recurrent pregnancy loss (RPL) on the other hand is a situation of many different names (e.g., *habitual abortion, recurrent miscarriage*), many definitions, and many possible etiologies. The two most acceptable definitions nowadays are set by the European Society of Human Reproduction and Embryology (ESHRE), which defines RPL as three or more consecutive miscarriages occurring before 20 weeks postmenstruation [2], and by the American Society for Reproductive Medicine (ASRM), which defines RPL as two or more first-trimester pregnancy losses [3]. Depending on the specific definition chosen, the incidence of RPL is 1%–5% [1].

The possible etiologies causing RPL are divided into six major categories: endocrine, immunologic, anatomic, genetic, infectious, and unexplained [4]. The evaluation of RPL, as guided by those proposed etiologies, includes hormonal evaluation (progesterone, thyroid stimulating hormone, prolactin, hemoglobin A1C) for endocrine, antibody screening (lupus anticoagulant, antiphospholipid, anti-beta-2 glycoprotein 1 [a-β2gp1]) for autoimmune, uterine imaging (hysterosalpingography, hysteroscopy, sonohysterography, transvaginal ultrasonography) for anatomic, and karyotyping for genetic etiology. Noteworthy is the fact that even after a comprehensive evaluation, the etiology remains unexplained in the majority of the cases [2,5].

Deciding when and what to evaluate is almost as hard as finding the reason for RPL. Factors that must be taken into consideration when timing the evaluation of RPL include, among others, the number of prior losses, the age of the patient, and the period length the couple is trying to conceive [6]. In couples without a history of a successful pregnancy, the risk of a miscarriage in the subsequent pregnancy after two losses is 30% compared with 45% after three losses. Therefore, in order to spare couples from dealing with another "failure," it appears reasonable to start evaluation after two losses [7–9].

As for today, there is a paucity of knowledge regarding the management of couples with RPL. Most management strategies are based on clinical experience and observational studies rather than on randomized controlled trials. Therefore, the most important issue while addressing a couple with RPL is the couple itself. Indeed, several studies have shown that psychological support has a significant positive influence on the management and outcome in patients with RPL [10–12].

In recent years, evidence has built up about the association between RPL and an increased risk of future maternal morbidities. Some studies have shown a higher prevalence of cardiac, renal, and endothelial complications in later life in women with a history of RPL [13–16]. This chapter will present an overview of RPL and the possible impact on future maternal health.

Epidemiology

The incidence of RPL is dependent on the definition used, maternal age, and obstetrical history. If defined as two or more consecutive losses, RPL may be diagnosed in 5% of the population, compared with only 1% if a definition of three or more consecutive losses is selected [17].

The patient age has a negative influence on the miscarriage rate; for example, an 11% risk is found in patients aged 20–24 years compared with 24% at 40–44 years of age [18]. Thus, in patients diagnosed with RPL, the outcome of the subsequent pregnancy is strongly influenced by the patient age; for example, a 20-year-old patient with a history of two spontaneous losses has a 92% success rate in her subsequent pregnancy compared with only 69% for a 40-year-old woman with the same history [19]. The paternal age may also pose a risk of miscarriage, with the strongest influence being paternal age over 40 years combined with a spouse older than 35 years [20].

Etiology, Management, and Future Implications

There are several major etiologies to be taken into consideration when assessing couples with RPL. In almost half of the cases the etiology is related to immunologic factors, followed by endocrine, anatomic, genetic, and infectious etiologies. Yet, in up to 50% of cases the etiology remains obscure even after comprehensive evaluation (Figure 5.1) [4].

Genetic Factors

Parental genetic factors account for 2%–5% of RPL cases. The most common abnormality is a balanced translocation, either reciprocal or Robertsonian [4,21,22]. Carriers of a balanced translocation are phenotypically normal but have a one-half to two-thirds chance of having an unbalanced embryo, dependent on the type of translocation.

Other chromosomal abnormalities that may be associated with RPL are inversions, insertions, mosaicism, and (rarely) single-gene defects.

Karyotyping all couples suffering RPL is suggested by the American College of Obstetricians and Gynecologists [23]; however, more recent publications question the need and efficacy of routine parental karyotyping [24]. Chromosomal analysis of the conceptus itself is much more important and has a stronger influence on future pregnancies [25,26]. It has been shown in some studies that the frequency of abnormal embryonic karyotypes decreases with the number of recurrent losses and that the pregnancy outcome may be better after an aneuploid miscarriage [27–29].

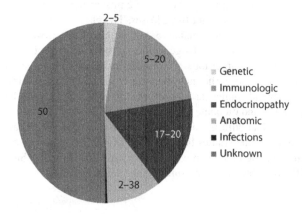

FIGURE 5.1   Etiology and prevalence (%) of RPL.

Due to those findings some experts suggest selective parental karyotyping in cases where no fetal products of conception (POC) can be achieved [6] or when an unbalanced chromosome abnormality is found in the POC [30].

If an abnormal parental karyotype is found, the couple should be referred to genetic counseling. Possible interventions include preimplantation genetic testing (PGD/PGS), egg or sperm donation and adoption [30]. Using PGD in couples known to carry a translocation reduced the miscarriage rate and increased the pregnancy rate [31].

Immunologic Factors

Alloimmunity (an immune response against a foreign object) and autoimmunity (an immune response against any part of the host) have both been suggested as possible etiologies for RPL. The alloimmune theories involve maternal cytotoxic antibody production, inadequate maternal blocking antibody production, and dysregulation in the natural killer (NK) cells response. As for today, no clear evidence has been found to support the relationship between those theories and RPL or the effectiveness of treatment; thus, routine evaluation of alloimmunity is not recommended [1,23,30].

Antiphospholipid syndrome (APLS) is probably the most important autoimmune disorder related to RPL. The syndrome is associated with the production of antiphospholipid antibodies (aPLs—e.g., lupus anticoagulant [LAC] and anticardiolipin antibodies [aCL]), acquired antibodies known to cause implantation failures through several mechanisms [7], and placental thrombosis and infarction [32]. The latter is the reason APLS is also categorized as a thrombotic factor causing RPL. Another important antibody that may be responsible for the syndrome is antibody against beta-2-glycoprotein-1 (β 2gp1; a-β 2gp1). This molecule is present on the surface of trophoblastic cell membranes and is another binding site for aPLs. β2gp1 is related to the coagulation cascade; it may inhibit thromboses by reducing the conversion of prothrombin to thrombin and by inhibiting the intrinsic coagulation pathway [7]. APLS is also known as a cause of other obstetrical complications such as preeclampsia and fetal growth restriction.

APLS may be regarded as *primary* when no evidence of an underlying condition is known or *secondary* if an underlying condition, most commonly systemic lupus erythematosus (SLE), is present [7]. APLS may be found in 5%–20% of patients with RPL [4,33,34]. Each antibody found in the syndrome may independently cause RPL, but it seems that the presence of a-β2gp1 increases the risk of RPL more than the presence of LAC or aCL [8,35]. The diagnosis of APLS requires both clinical and laboratory criteria. The criteria currently in use was set in 2006 in the International Consensus Definition for the Diagnosis of Antiphospholipid Syndrome (Table 5.1) [36].

If untreated, patients diagnosed with APLS have only a 20%–30% chance of a successful delivery in their next pregnancy [7]. Several treatment protocols have been investigated, including aspirin, prednisone, intravenous immunoglobulin (IVIG), heparin, and low-molecular-weight heparin (LMWH), alone or in various combinations. A Cochrane review [37] published in 2005 found that the most efficacious treatment to reduce the rate of pregnancy loss was the combination of unfractionated heparin and low-dose aspirin, with a reduction of 54% compared with aspirin alone. The suggested treatment protocol is a low dose of aspirin (81 mg) once a day started before conception and 5000 units of unfractionated heparin twice a day added after intrauterine pregnancy is confirmed. Due to the negative influence heparin may have on bone density, it is recommended to add calcium carbonate (1200–1500 mg) and vitamin D (800–1000 IU) to treatment. The use of LMWH may be as good as unfractionated heparin [38], and although this protocol has not been studied enough and the results of the studies evaluating this protocol are controversial [37,39], common practice nowadays includes the combination of LMWH and low-dose aspirin.

Inherited Thrombophilia

Inherited (congenital) thrombophilia, as well as acquired thrombophilia (e.g., APLS), is an established cause of thrombosis [30] and most commonly is the result of a genetic deletion/mutation in one of the proteins related to the coagulation cascade [40].

TABLE 5.1

Clinical and Laboratory Criteria for the Diagnosis of APLS (Based on the International Consensus Definition for the Diagnosis of Antiphospholipid Syndrome)

A. Clinical Criteria	Definition
1. Vascular thrombosis	One or more clinical episodes of arterial, venous, or small vessel thrombosis, in any tissue or organ.
	• Thrombosis must be confirmed by objective validated criteria (i.e., unequivocal findings of appropriate imaging studies or histopathology).
	• For histopathologic confirmation, thrombosis should be present without significant evidence of inflammation in the vessel wall.
2. Pregnancy morbidity	A. One or more losses after the 10th week of a morphologically normal fetus.
	B. One or more premature births of a normal neonate before the 34th week.
	C. Three or more unexplained consecutive early miscarriages.
B. Laboratory Criteria	Found in at least two tests more than 12 weeks apart.
1. Lupus anticoagulant	
2. Anticardiolipin antibody of IgG or IgM isotype in medium to high titer	
3. A-β2gp1 antibody of IgG or IgM isotype in 99th percentile titer	

Source: Miyakis S, et al., *J Thromb Haemost*, 4(2), 295–306, 2006.

The most common inherited thrombophilia include factor V Leiden (FVL), prothrombin gene mutation, protein C deficiency (PCD), protein S deficiency (PSD), methyltetrahydrofolate reductase (MTHFR) mutation, and antithrombin III (AT III) deficiency [23,30,40]. Due to its ability to induce thrombosis and clots, thrombophilia is suggested to be a risk factor for several pregnancy adverse outcomes (e.g., fetal loss, intrauterine growth retardation, placental abruption, and preeclampsia) [30,41].

The association between thrombophilia and pregnancy loss is not fully established, and while many studies and clinical guidelines agree that inherited thrombophilia does not cause early RPL and do not recommend routine laboratory assessment for inherited thrombophilia in these cases [2,9,23,40,42], some agree that inherited thrombophilia may be related to late pregnancy loss [23,30].

Endocrine Factors

A few maternal endocrine disorders have been associated with RPL, including diabetes mellitus (DM), thyroid diseases, hyperprolactinemia, polycystic ovary syndrome (PCOS), and luteal phase defects (LPD) [1,4,9,30,43]. These disorders may account for 17%–20% of RPL [4].

Insulin-dependent DM is a well-established etiology for pregnancy loss, but only when poorly controlled (e.g., glycosylated hemoglobin higher than 9%–10%) [44–46]. In addition, the rate of pregnancy loss has also been found to be higher in uncontrolled type 2 DM [47].

Thyroid disease has also been associated with pregnancy loss and RPL; however, as for DM, only uncontrolled disease may influence the rate of pregnancy loss [48,49].

The presence of antithyroid antibodies is more prevalent in cases of RPL, and in some studies the prevalence was higher even in euthyroid patients [50,51], but not in others [52–54]. The mechanism by which antithyroid antibodies induce pregnancy loss is not fully understood [55].

PCOS is another possible etiology for RPL. PCOS may be found in up to 40% of patients diagnosed with RPL, almost two times more prevalent than in the general population. It is important to note, however, that the various markers of PCOS (ovarian morphology, elevated luteinizing hormone, and elevated testosterone) are not predictive of future pregnancy loss or live birth in ovulating PCOS women with RPL [56].

Insulin resistance, either related to DM or PCOS, has been correlated with RPL [57]. This relationship was born through studies that showed a reduction in pregnancy loss in PCOS patients treated with metformin [58–60]. However, the mechanism was challenged by a study published in 2007 that showed similar abortion rates (as well as ovulation and pregnancy rates) in PCOS patients treated with either metformin or clomiphene citrate [61].

LPD has been described as a condition in which endogenous progesterone is not sufficient to maintain a functional secretory endometrium and allow normal embryo implantation and growth. A committee opinion published by the ASRM in 2015 concluded, "Although progesterone is important for the process of implantation and early embryonic development, LPD as an independent entity causing infertility has not been proven" [62]. Furthermore, the committee noted that diagnostic tests for LPD cannot be recommended and adding progesterone after pregnancy has been achieved is not an established treatment.

Anatomic Factors

Uterine anomalies, including congenital uterine malformations, intrauterine adhesions, and uterine masses (e.g., leiomyoma and polyps) are thought to cause RPL by interrupting the endometrial vasculature and placentation [4]. Cervical incompetence can also be regarded as a uterine anomaly causing RPL but through a different mechanism and mostly in the second trimester [6].

The reported prevalence of uterine malformations in RPL ranges from 2% to 38%. This wide range probably reflects differences in the diagnosis criteria of RPL, the imaging method used, and uterine anomalies included in the studies [4,63,64]. Although the real prevalence of RPL related to uterine anomalies is unknown, it is clear that it is higher than in the general population, in which it is about 4% [64]. Furthermore, uterine anomalies are more common in second-trimester pregnancy loss than in first-trimester losses.

Of all mullerian duct anomalies, the most relevant to RPL is the septate uterus, for two reasons: first, it is the most common anomaly found in RPL patients and endorsed the highest risk of pregnancy loss [63–65]; second, it is the only anomaly in which benefit was reported following treatment by hysteroscopic metroplasty [66–70].

Trauma to the uterine cavity (e.g., endometrial curettage and infection) may result in the formation of intrauterine adhesions. Those adhesions interfere with normal placentation and are a potential cause of RPL through three possible mechanisms: (1) constriction of the uterine cavity; (2) an insufficient amount of normal endometrium to support implantation; (3) defective endometrial vascularization [71].

An intrauterine mass can be found in 20%–50% of reproductive-aged women. Depending on the size and location, these benign tumors can also cause RPL. Masses that obliterate or alter the endometrial cavity have the strongest influence on pregnancy loss, especially submucous leiomyomas. In this setting, Simpson [72] suggested three possible explanations for pregnancy loss: thin endometrial surface, increased cytokine production due to rapid growth and necrosis of the mass during pregnancy, and occupying space required by the developing fetus. Whether removal of the leiomyoma will prevent the next loss is controversial, but some studies advocate removal of submucous or large fibroids in order to improve fertility [73,74].

Infectious Factors

Many infective pathogens have been related to spontaneous pregnancy loss, including, among others, *Lisreria monocytogens*, *Toxoplasma gondii*, rubella, herpes simplex virus, cytomegalovirus, Coxsackie viruses, and *Ureaplasma urealyticum*. As for today, no correlation has been found between infection and RPL; therefore, it is not recommended to routinely evaluate patients for infectious etiology [4,9,30].

Unexplained RPL

Although many factors have been found to be associated with RPL, still no specific cause can be found in approximately half of the patients [4,9]. In such cases, the prognosis of a future successful pregnancy is good, about 75%, with supportive care [19]. As previously mentioned, the two most important factors when consulting such women regarding their chance of a successful future pregnancy are maternal age and the number of previous losses [75].

The issue of treatment in cases of unexplained RPL was recently addressed by two randomized controlled trials. In the first, Clark et al. [76] compared combined treatment with aspirin and LMWH with no treatment, and in the second, by Kaandorp et al. [77], aspirin alone or in combination with LMWH was compared with placebo. Both trials found no improvements in the live birth rate or reduction in pregnancy loss rate with treatment.

Future Maternal Implications of Recurrent Pregnancy Loss

In the last few years, a possible link between RPL and future maternal complications has been suggested. Regardless of the diagnosis of RPL, the association between uncontrolled DM or thyroid diseases and long-term morbidities later in life is well established. Poorly controlled DM is an important risk factor for the development of micro- and macrovascular complications such as retinopathy, nephropathy, and cardiovascular disease [78–81], while patients with thyroid hormone imbalance may suffer, among other things, from hypercholesterolemia [82], cognitive dysfunction [83], and obstructive sleep apnea [84]. Similarly, patients diagnosed with APLS may develop future complications and long-term morbidities, primarily from vascular thrombosis and the possible side effects of long-term anticoagulant treatment. Thus, women with RPL diagnosed to have DM, thyroid hormone imbalance, or APLS are prone to similar future morbidities.

Other causes of RPL such as uterine malformations, genetic aberrations, and infections have less clear or direct implications on long-term maternal health, although it is important to remember that these patients may have related interventions, such as repeated medical or instrumental curettage, that may cause complications affecting their quality of life (e.g., chronic pain, pelvic inflammatory disease, and anemia).

More interesting is whether women with RPL of an unexplained etiology are also prone to an increased risk of future maternal morbidities. The first to address this issue were Pell et al., who reported in 2004 that patients with RPL, as well as patients with preterm deliveries, have an increased risk of future maternal cardiovascular events [15]. A possible pathophysiologic explanation for this relationship is endothelial dysfunction, which may be the link between several obstetric complications and may be found in some patients with RPL [16].

This observation was further supported by two recent studies demonstrating that patients experiencing RPL have a higher risk of future cardiovascular disease [13,14]. Kharazmi et al., in a prospective population-based cohort study, found a nine-times-higher risk of myocardial infarction later in life for patients with a history of three or more recurrent miscarriages, and this risk further increased with each additional pregnancy loss [13].

In a large population-based epidemiological study including almost 100,000 patients over a 15-year period, of whom 6.7% had a history of RPL, Sheiner et al. assessed the association between RPL and long-term maternal morbidities [14]. Compared with women without, those with RPL had a significantly higher rate of long-term cardiovascular morbidities and significantly higher rates of cardiovascular-related hospitalizations (5.8% vs. 3.1%; OR 1.9, 95% CI 1.7–22; $p = .001$) (Figure 5.2). The incidence of cardiac procedures (either invasive or noninvasive) and that of cardiovascular events (angina pectoris and congestive heart disease) was doubled in the RPL group. Furthermore, patients with a history of three recurrent abortions were at higher risk (adjusted HR 1.6, 95% CI 1.4–16) than women with two abortions (adjusted HR 1.3, 95% CI 1.1–1.5). Notably, RPL remained independently associated with a higher risk of cardiovascular morbidities even after controlling for possible confounders related to the metabolic syndrome such as diabetes, preeclampsia, and obesity as well as APLS and thrombophilia.

In the same study [14], the authors also examined a possible association between RPL and future renal-related hospitalizations; however, after controlling for other known risk factors for renal morbidities, RPL was not found to be an independent risk factor for such morbidities (adjusted HR 1.3, 95% CI 0.8–2.3; $p = .3$) (Figure 5.3).

Recently, Charach et al. reported an association between RPL and a higher incidence of future female malignancies (adjusted HR 1.4, 95% CI 1.1–1.6; $p = .003$): specifically, breast (OR 1.7, 95% CI 1.3–2.2; $p = .001$) and cervical cancer (OR 1.6, 95% CI 1.05–2.42; $p = .038$) [85].

In another report, a higher rate of ophthalmic complications (e.g., glaucoma, diabetic retinopathy, macular degeneration, and retinal detachment) was observed among women with a history of RPL (adjusted HR 1.5, 95% CI 1.01–2.2; $p = .04$) [86].

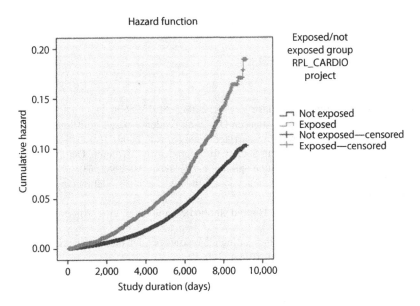

FIGURE 5.2 Kaplan–Meier hazard function analysis curve for cardiovascular hospitalizations of patients with and without RPL. (Adapted from Kessous R, et al., *Am J Obstet Gynecol*, 211, 414.e1–414.e11, 2014.)

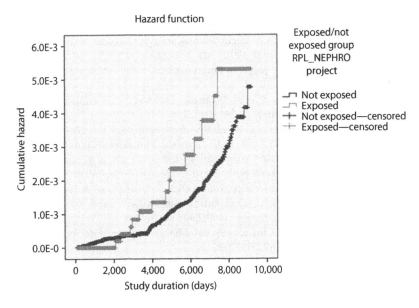

FIGURE 5.3 Kaplan–Meier hazard function analysis curve for renal-related hospitalizations of patients with and without RPL. (Adapted from Kessous R, et al., *Am J Obstet Gynecol*, 211, 414.e1–414.e11, 2014.)

SUMMARY

There are numerous etiologies and underlying maternal conditions that have been associated with RPL. Some of these underlying conditions may have obvious potential future impact on maternal health; however, the association between unexplained RPL and future morbidities is less straightforward. In most cases, patients will experience RPL years earlier than being diagnosed with any chronic illness. Those years could serve as a "window of opportunity" for primary prevention, earlier diagnosis, and intervention, which in turn may prevent or attenuate future potential long-term morbidities. Whether RPL may serve as an important early indicator for future maternal complications, allowing early effective interventions, is yet to be determined.

REFERENCES

1. Rai R, Regan L. Recurrent miscarriage. *Lancet*. 2006;368(9535):601–11.
2. Jauniaux E, Farquharson RG, Christiansen OB, et al. Evidence-based guidelines for the investigation and medical treatment of recurrent miscarriage. *Hum Reprod*. 2006;21(9):2216–22.
3. Practice Committee of the American Society for Reproductive Medicine. Definitions of infertility and recurrent pregnancy loss: A committee opinion. *Fertil Steril*. 2013;99(1):63.
4. Ford HB, Schust DJ. Recurrent pregnancy loss: Etiology, diagnosis, and therapy. *Rev Obstet Gynecol*. 2009;2(2):76–83.
5. Abramson J, Stagnaro-Green A. Thyroid antibodies and fetal loss: An evolving story. *Thyroid*. 2001;11(1):57–63.
6. Brezina PR, Kutteh WH. Classic and cutting-edge strategies for the management of early pregnancy loss. *Obstet Gynecol Clin North Am*. 2014;41(1):1–18.
7. Kutteh WH, Hinote CD. Antiphospholipid antibody syndrome. *Obstet Gynecol Clin North Am*. 2014;41(1):113–32.
8. Allison JL, Schust DJ. Recurrent first trimester pregnancy loss: Revised definitions and novel causes. *Curr Opin Endocrinol Diabetes Obes*. 2009;16(6):446–50.
9. Practice Committee of the American Society for Reproductive Medicine. Evaluation and treatment of recurrent pregnancy loss: A committee opinion. *Fertil Steril*. 2012;98(5):1103–11.
10. Stray-Pedersen B, Stray-Pedersen S. Etiologic factors and subsequent reproductive performance in 195 couples with a prior history of habitual abortion. *Am J Obstet Gynecol*. 1984;148(2):140–46.
11. Liddell HS, Pattison NS, Zanderigo A. Recurrent miscarriage: Outcome after supportive care in early pregnancy. *Aust NZ J Obstet Gynaecol*. 1991;31(4): 320–22.
12. Clifford K, Rai R, Regan L. Future pregnancy outcome in unexplained recurrent first trimester miscarriage. *Hum Reprod*. 1997;12(2):387–9.
13. Kharazmi E, Dossus L, Rohrmann S, et al. Pregnancy loss and risk of cardiovascular disease: A prospective population-based cohort study (EPIC-Heidelberg). *Heart*. 2011;97(1):49–54.
14. Kessous R, Shoham-Vardi I, Pariente G, et al. Recurrent pregnancy loss: A risk factor for long-term maternal atherosclerotic morbidity? *Am J Obstet Gynecol*. 2014;211(4):414.e1–11.
15. Pell JP, Smith GC, Walsh D. Pregnancy complications and subsequent maternal cerebrovascular events: A retrospective cohort study of 119,668 births. *Am J Epidemiol*. 2004; 159(4):336–42.
16. Germain AM, Romanik MC, Guerra I, et al. Endothelial dysfunction: A link among preeclampsia, recurrent pregnancy loss, and future cardiovascular events? *Hypertension*. 2007;49(1):90–95.
17. Stirrat GM. Recurrent miscarriage. *Lancet*. 1990;336(8716):673–5.
18. Nybo Andersen AM, Wohlfahrt J, Christens P, et al. Maternal age and fetal loss: Population based register linkage study. *BMJ*. 2000;320(7251):1708–12.
19. Brigham SA, Conlon C, Farquharson RG. A longitudinal study of pregnancy outcome following idiopathic recurrent miscarriage. *Hum Reprod*. 1999;14(11):2868–71.
20. de la Rochebrochard E, Thonneau P. Paternal age and maternal age are risk factors for miscarriage: Results of a multicentre European study. *Hum Reprod*. 2002;17(6):1649–56.
21. Clifford K, Rai R, Watson H, et al. An informative protocol for the investigation of recurrent miscarriage: Preliminary experience of 500 consecutive cases. *Hum Reprod*. 1994;9(7):1328–32.
22. De Braekeleer M, Dao TN. Cytogenetic studies in couples experiencing repeated pregnancy losses. *Hum Reprod*. 1990;5(5):519–28.
23. American College of Obstetricians and Gynecologists. Management of recurrent pregnancy loss. ACOG Practice Bulletin no. 24, February 2001. (Replaces Technical Bulletin no. 212, September 1995.) *Int J Gynaecol Obstet*. 2002;78(2):179–90.
24. Barber JC, Cockwell AE, Grant E, et al. Is karyotyping couples experiencing recurrent miscarriage worth the cost? *BJOG*. 2010;117(7):885–8.
25. Carp H, Feldman B, Oelsner G, et al. Parental karyotype and subsequent live births in recurrent miscarriage. *Fertil Steril*. 2004;81(5):1296–301.

26. Carp H, Guetta E, Dorf H, et al. Embryonic karyotype in recurrent miscarriage with parental karyotypic aberrations. *Fertil Steril*. 2006;85(2):446–50.
27. Stephenson MD, Awartani KA, Robinson WP. Cytogenetic analysis of miscarriages from couples with recurrent miscarriage: A case-control study. *Hum Reprod*. 2002;17(2):446–51.
28. Ogasawara M, Aoki K, Okada S, et al. Embryonic karyotype of abortuses in relation to the number of previous miscarriages. *Fertil Steril*. 2000;73(2):300–304.
29. Carp H, Toder V, Aviram A, et al. Karyotype of the abortus in recurrent miscarriage. *Fertil Steril*. 2001;75(4):678–82.
30. Royal College of Obstetricians and Gynecologists. The investigation and treatment of couples with recurrent first trimester and second trimester miscarriage. Greentop Guideline no. 17; 2011.
31. Otani T, Roche M, Mizuike M, et al. Preimplantation genetic diagnosis significantly improves the pregnancy outcome of translocation carriers with a history of recurrent miscarriage and unsuccessful pregnancies. *Reprod Biomed Online*. 2006;13(6):869–74.
32. De Wolf F, Carreras LO, Moerman P, et al. Decidual vasculopathy and extensive placental infarction in a patient with repeated thromboembolic accidents, recurrent fetal loss, and a lupus anticoagulant. *Am J Obstet Gynecol*. 1982;142(7):829–34.
33. Rai RS, Regan L, Clifford K, et al. Antiphospholipid antibodies and beta 2-glycoprotein-I in 500 women with recurrent miscarriage: Results of a comprehensive screening approach. *Hum Reprod*. 1995;10(8):2001–5.
34. Kutteh WH, Rote NS, Silver R. Antiphospholipid antibodies and reproduction: The antiphospholipid antibody syndrome. *Am J Reprod Immunol*. 1999;41(2):133–52.
35. Oron G, Ben-Haroush A, Goldfarb R, et al. Contribution of the addition of anti-β2-glycoprotein to the classification of antiphospholipid syndrome in predicting adverse pregnancy outcome. *J Matern Fetal Neonatal Med*. 2011;24(4):606–9.
36. Miyakis S, Lockshin M, Atsumi T, et al. International consensus statement on an update of the classification criteria for definite antiphospholipid syndrome (APS). *J Thromb Haemost*. 2006;4(2):295–306.
37. Empson M, Lassere M, Craig J, et al. Prevention of recurrent miscarriage for women with antiphospholipid antibody or lupus anticoagulant. *Cochrane Database Syst Rev*. 2005;2:CD002859.
38. Stephenson MD, Ballem PJ, Tsang P, et al. Treatment of antiphospholipid antibody syndrome (APS) in pregnancy: A randomized pilot trial comparing low molecular weight heparin to unfractionated heparin. *J Obstet Gynaecol Can*. 2004;26(8):729–34.
39. Ziakas PD, Pavlou M, Voulgarelis M. Heparin treatment in antiphospholipid syndrome with recurrent pregnancy loss: A systematic review and meta-analysis. *Obstet Gynecol*. 2010;115(6):1256–62.
40. Davenport WB, Kutteh WH. Inherited thrombophilias and adverse pregnancy outcomes: A review of screening patterns and recommendations. *Obstet Gynecol Clin North Am*. 2014;41(1):133–44.
41. Shahine L, Lathi R. Recurrent pregnancy loss: Evaluation and treatment. *Obstet Gynecol Clin North Am*. 2015;42(1):117–34.
42. Carp H, Dolitzky M, Tur-Kaspa I, et al. Hereditary thrombophilias are not associated with a decreased live birth rate in women with recurrent miscarriage. *Fertil Steril*. 2002;78(1):58–62.
43. Ke RW. Endocrine basis for recurrent pregnancy loss. *Obstet Gynecol Clin North Am*. 2014;41(1):103–12.
44. Hanson U, Persson B, Thunell S. Relationship between haemoglobin A1C in early type 1 (insulin-dependent) diabetic pregnancy and the occurrence of spontaneous abortion and fetal malformation in Sweden. *Diabetologia*. 1990;33(2):100–104.
45. Mills JL, Simpson JL, Driscoll SG, et al. Incidence of spontaneous abortion among normal women and insulin-dependent diabetic women whose pregnancies were identified within 21 days of conception. *N Engl J Med*. 1988;319(25):1617–23.
46. Greene MF, Hare JW, Cloherty JP, et al. First-trimester hemoglobin A1 and risk for major malformation and spontaneous abortion in diabetic pregnancy. *Teratology*. 1989;39(3):225–31.
47. Jovanovic L, Knopp RH, Kim H, et al. Elevated pregnancy losses at high and low extremes of maternal glucose in early normal and diabetic pregnancy: Evidence for a protective adaptation in diabetes. *Diabetes Care*. 2005;28(5):1113–17.
48. Abalovich M, Gutierrez S, Alcaraz G, et al. Overt and subclinical hypothyroidism complicating pregnancy. *Thyroid*. 2002;12(1):63–8.
49. Cleary-Goldman J, Malone FD, Lambert-Messerlian G, et al. Maternal thyroid hypofunction and pregnancy outcome. *Obstet Gynecol*. 2008;112(1):85–92.

50. Bussen S, Steck T. Thyroid autoantibodies in euthyroid non-pregnant women with recurrent spontaneous abortions. *Hum Reprod.* 1995;10(11):2938–40.

51. Stagnaro-Green A, Glinoer D. Thyroid autoimmunity and the risk of miscarriage. *Best Pract Res Clin Endocrinol Metab.* 2004;18(2):167–81.

52. Rushnorth FH, Backos M, Rai R, et al. Prospective pregnancy outcome in untreated recurrent miscarriers with thyroid autoantibodies. *Hum Reprod.* 2000;15(7):1637–9.

53. Bellver J, Soares SR, Alvarez C, et al. The role of thrombophilia and thyroid autoimmunity in unexplained infertility, implantation failure and recurrent spontaneous abortion. *Hum Reprod.* 2008;23(2):278–84.

54. Esplin MS, Branch DN, Silver R, et al. Thyroid autoantibodies are not associated with recurrent pregnancy loss. *Am J Obstet Gynecol.* 1998; 179 (6 Pt 1): 1583–6.

55. Matalon ST, Blank M, Ornoy A, et al. The association between anti-thyroid antibodies and pregnancy loss. *Am J Reprod Immunol.* 2001;45(2):72–7.

56. Rai R, Backos M, Rushworth F, et al. Polycystic ovaries and recurrent miscarriage: A reappraisal. *Hum Reprod.* 2000;15(3):612–15.

57. Craig LB, Ke RW, Kutteh WH. Increased prevalence of insulin resistance in women with a history of recurrent pregnancy loss. *Fertil Steril.* 2002;78(3):487–90.

58. Glueck CJ, Phillips M, Cameron D, et al. Continuing metformin throughout pregnancy in women with polycystic ovary syndrome appears to safely reduce first-trimester spontaneous abortion: A pilot study. *Fertil Steril.* 2001;75(1):46–52.

59. Jakobowicz DJ, Ivorno MJ, Jakobowicz S, et al. Effects of metformin on early pregnancy loss in the polycystic ovary syndrome. *J Clin Endocrinol Metab.* 2002;87(2):524–9.

60. Glueck CJ, Wang P, Goldenberg N, et al. Pregnancy outcomes among women with polycystic ovary syndrome treated with metformin. *Hum Reprod.* 2002;17(11):2858–64.

61. Palomba S, Orio F, Falbo A, et al. Clomiphene citrate versus metformin as first-line approach for the treatment of anovulation in infertile patients with polycystic ovary syndrome. *J Clin Endocrinol Metab.* 2007;92(9):3498–503.

62. Practice Committee of the American Society for Reproductive Medicine. Current clinical irrelevance of luteal phase deficiency: A committee opinion. *Fertil Steril.* 2015;103(4):e27–32.

63. Salim R, Regan L, Woelfer B, et al. A comparative study of the morphology of congenital uterine anomalies in women with and without a history of recurrent first trimester miscarriage. *Hum Reprod.* 2003;18(1):162–6.

64. Grimbizis GF, Camus M, Tarlatzis BC, et al. Clinical implications of uterine malformations and hysteroscopic treatment results. *Hum Reprod Update.* 2001;7(2):161–74.

65. Lin PC. Reproductive outcomes in women with uterine anomalies. *J Womens Health (Larchmt).* 2004;13(1):33–9.

66. Tomazevic T, Ban-Frangez H, Virant-Klun I, et al. Septate, subseptate and arcuate uterus decrease pregnancy and live birth rates in IVF/ICSI. *Reprod Biomed Online.* 2010;21(5):700–705.

67. Nouri K, Ott J, Huber JC, et al. Reproductive outcome after hysteroscopic septoplasty in patients with septate uterus: A retrospective cohort study and systematic review of the literature. *Reprod Biol Endocrinol.* 2010;8:52.

68. Mollo A, De Franciscis P, Colacurci N, et al. Hysteroscopic resection of the septum improves the pregnancy rate of women with unexplained infertility: A prospective controlled trial. *Fertil Steril.* 2009;91(6):2628–31.

69. Homer HA, Li TC, Cooke ID. The septate uterus: A review of management and reproductive outcome. *Fertil Steril.* 2000;73(1):1–14.

70. Or Y, Appelman Z. Is prophylactic hysteroscopic metroplasty for the septate uterus justified? *Journal of Gynecologic Surgery.* 2014;30(6):325–8.

71. Yu D, Wong YM, Cheong Y, et al. Asherman syndrome: One century later. *Fertil Steril.* 2008;89(4):759–79.

72. Simpson JL. Causes of fetal wastage. *Clin Obstet Gynecol.* 2007;50(1):10–30.

73. Bajekal N, Li TC. Fibroids, infertility and pregnancy wastage. *Hum Reprod Update.* 2000;6(6):614–20.

74. Casini ML, Rossi F, Agostini R, et al. Effects of the position of fibroids on fertility. *Gynecol Endocrinol.* 2006;22(2):106–9.

75. Lund M, Kamper-Jorgensen M, Nielsen HS, et al. Prognosis for live birth in women with recurrent miscarriage: What is the best measure of success? *Obstet Gynecol.* 2012;119(1):37–43.

76. Clark P, Walker ID, Langhorne P, et al. SPIN (Scottish Pregnancy Intervention) study: A multicenter, randomized controlled trial of low-molecular-weight heparin and low-dose aspirin in women with recurrent miscarriage. *Blood*. 2010;115(21):4162–7.

77. Kaandorp S, Goddijn M, Van der Post JA, et al. Aspirin plus heparin or aspirin alone in women with recurrent miscarriage. *N Engl J Med*. 2010; 362(17): 1586–96.

78. The Diabetes Control and Complications Trial Research Group. The effect of intensive treatment of diabetes on the development and progression of long-term complications in insulin-dependent diabetes mellitus. *N Engl J Med*. 1993;329(14):977–86.

79. Nathan DM, Cleary PA, Backlund JY, et al. Intensive diabetes treatment and cardiovascular disease in patients with type 1 diabetes. *N Engl J Med*. 2005;353(25):2643–53.

80. Klein R, Klein BE, Moss SE, et al. Relationship of hyperglycemia to the long-term incidence and progression of diabetic retinopathy. *Arch Intern Med*. 1994;154(19):2169–78.

81. Bash LD, Selvin E, Steffes M, et al. Poor glycemic control in diabetes and the risk of incident chronic kidney disease even in the absence of albuminuria and retinopathy: Atherosclerosis Risk in Communities (ARIC) study. *Arch Intern Med*. 2008;168(22):2440–47.

82. O'Brien T, Dinneen SF, O'Brien PC, et al. Hyperlipidemia in patients with primary and secondary hypothyroidism. *Mayo Clin Proc*. 1993;68(9):860–6.

83. Osterweil D, Syndulko K, Cohen SN, et al. Cognitive function in non-demented older adults with hypothyroidism. *J Am Geriatr Soc*. 1992;40(4):325–35.

84. Rosenow F, McCarthy V, Caruso AC. Sleep apnoea in endocrine diseases. *J Sleep Res*. 1998;7(1):3–11.

85. Charach R, Kessous R, Beharier O, Sheiner E, Davidson E. Is there an association between recurrent pregnancy loss and future risk for female malignancies? *Am J Obstet Gynecol*. 2016;214(1 Suppl):S101.

86. Charach R, Kessous R, Beharier O, Davidson E, Sheiner E. Is there an association between recurrent pregnancy loss and future risk for ophthalmic complications? *Am J Obstet Gynecol*. 2016;241(1 Suppl):S248.

6

Preterm Parturition and Long-Term Maternal Morbidity

**Salvatore Andrea Mastrolia, Shirley Greenbaum, Vered Klaitman,
Ruthy Beer-Weisel, Shiran Zer, Gal Rodavsky, Idit Erez-Weiss, and Offer Erez**

Introduction

Preterm birth accounts for about 7%–12% of all deliveries worldwide; it is the most common cause for neonatal morbidity and mortality, as well as maternal morbidity. In the past, most research interest resulted in the prevention of preterm birth in order to alleviate the complications of prematurity. However, recent evidence suggests that the effects of preterm birth on the future health of both the mother and her offspring go far beyond the preterm delivery itself. The current chapter will describe the epidemiology and underlying mechanisms leading to preterm delivery, its short- and long-term effects on the mother and her neonate, and the methods to prevent preterm parturition.

Epidemiology of Preterm Birth

Definition

Preterm birth is a delivery between fetal viability and 37 completed weeks of gestation [1]. While the upper cutoff of 37 weeks according to menstrual age is well accepted, there is a debate regarding the lower cutoff, which is currently defined as the limit of viability, a point where the risk of neonatal death does not exceed 50% [2,3]. For improved specificity, it can be subdivided into *moderately* or *late preterm* (32–36 completed weeks of gestation), *very preterm* (28–32 weeks), and *extremely preterm* (<28 weeks) [4]. Separate distinctions between spontaneous and medically indicated preterm birth are also used. This level of specificity is important for understanding the prevalence and etiologies of preterm birth and to guide intervention strategies [5].

Prevalence

The prevalence of preterm birth varies from 5% to 18% of all deliveries depending on the geographical and demographical characteristics of the population tested [6,7]. Based on data from 184 countries, the global average preterm birth rate in 2010 was 11.1%, giving a worldwide total of 14.9 million. Prematurity rates varied widely between countries; at a national level, it ranged from about 5% in several Northern European countries to 18% in Malawi. In 88 countries, this rate was lower than 10%. Of the 11 countries with estimated rates of 15% or more in 2010, all but two were in sub-Saharan Africa. The high absolute number of preterm births in Africa and Asia are related, in part, to high fertility and the large number of births in those two regions in comparison with other parts of the world [8]. The prevalence of preterm delivery is highest for low-income countries (11.8%), followed by lower-middle-income countries (11.3%), and lowest for upper-middle-income (9.4%) and high-income (9.3%) countries. Nevertheless, some high-income countries have an increased prevalence of preterm deliveries (e.g., United States, 12.0%; Austria, 10.9%) [9] (Figure 6.1).

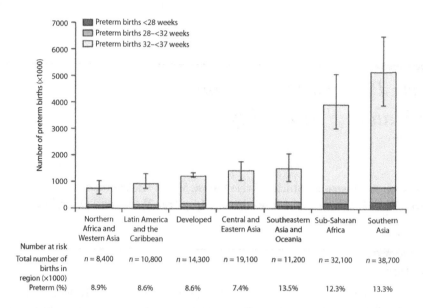

FIGURE 6.1 Estimated preterm births by region and by gestational-age grouping for the year 2010. (Adapted from Blencowe H, et al., *Lancet*, 379(9832), 2162–72, 2012. With permission.)

In the National Vital Statistics Reports for births in 2014, the preterm birth rate (less than 37 weeks) was 9.57% in 2014, which represents a decrease by 8% from 2007. The preterm rate among singleton births has declined 10% since 2007 [10]. Reductions in late-preterm and early-term deliveries from 2007 to 2014 may be related to a heightened understanding of the increased neonatal risk at these gestational ages compared with full-term deliveries, and to subsequent recommendations and efforts to reduce non-medically indicated deliveries before 39 weeks [11,12].

Subtypes of Preterm Births

Preterm delivery is classified by gestational age at delivery and the type of preterm birth.

Classification by Gestational Age at Delivery

Preterm delivery can be defined by the severity of prematurity (also referred to as the *time definition*) [13,14]: (1) extreme prematurity, which occurs before 28 weeks of gestation and accounts for 5% of preterm deliveries; (2) severe prematurity, which occurs from 28 to 31 6/7 weeks and accounts for 15% of all preterm deliveries; (3) moderate prematurity, which relates to deliveries between 32 and 33 6/7 weeks of gestation and occurs in about 20% of preterm births; and (4) near-term birth, which occurs from 34 to 36 6/7 weeks of gestation and is the largest group, including 60%–70% of all preterm deliveries.

The gestational age at which preterm delivery occurs has a direct effect on neonatal morbidity and mortality [15]. Several cutoffs have been proposed to differentiate early- from late-preterm birth. The most commonly used cutoffs are 32 or 34 weeks of gestation. The Centers for Disease Control and Prevention (CDC) has defined 34 weeks of gestation to distinguish between early- and late-preterm delivery [10]. However, the survival rate of neonates born after 32 weeks of gestation is near 100% (Figure 6.2a), and neonatal morbidity substantially declines at this gestational age (Figure 6.2b) [16]. Thus, the use of 32 weeks of gestation as the cutoff for early-preterm birth has been proposed [17]. Although this cutoff may seem appealing, not all countries have well-developed neonatal intensivecare units, and their survival rate at 32 weeks of gestation is lower. Hence, the CDC approach to the definition of early-preterm birth as a delivery before 34 weeks may serve as a better cutoff for clinical and comparative epidemiological studies. Recent data from several sources indicate improvements in survival for extremely premature infants in the United States [18–20] and other international developed nations

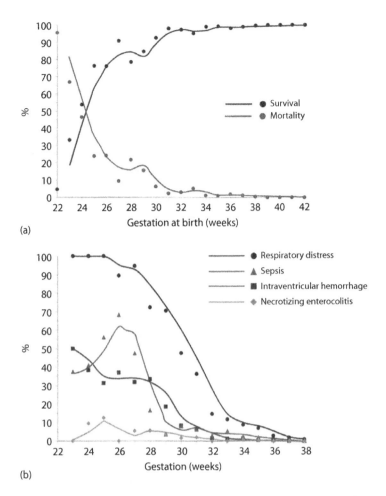

FIGURE 6.2 (a) The association between perinatal mortality and gestational age at delivery. (b) The changes in prematurity complications according to gestational age at delivery among surviving infants. (Adapted from Mercer BM, *Obstet Gynecol*, 101(1), 178–93, 2003. With permission.)

[21–23]. Based on estimates from the neonatal research network [24], 74% of extremely preterm infants survive the initial birth hospitalization [18,19], although each decreasing gestational week has substantial effects on mortality, particularly for infants born at 22 to 25 weeks of gestation [15].

Classification by Type: Spontaneous versus Indicated Preterm Birth

Preterm delivery can be either spontaneous or *indicated* (medically induced) regardless of the gestational age. Spontaneous preterm birth accounts for 75% of all preterm deliveries [25–27] and can be the end result of three main clinical presentations: (1) preterm labor with intact membranes; (2) preterm prelabor rupture of membranes (PROM); and (3) cervical insufficiency [28]. Indicated preterm birth results from maternal or fetal complications that necessitate medical intervention [2,25,29–31]. Although many studies have focused on the rate of preterm birth [32–34], an important consideration is whether these deliveries are the result of spontaneous labor or indicated preterm deliveries. The need for this distinction is based on the premise that the risk factors for recurrent preterm PROM, preterm labor with intact membranes, preeclampsia, and/or SGA are different. However, recent observations suggest that there may be overlaps between these conditions [29,31] so that a patient with an indicated preterm birth may also be at risk of spontaneous preterm birth [29,31]. The converse may also be true (i.e., that a patient with a spontaneous preterm birth is at risk of an indicated preterm birth in a subsequent pregnancy).

Spontaneous Preterm Birth

Spontaneous preterm birth is defined as a labor that begins without prior medical intervention and can present either as a preterm contraction with intact membranes or related diagnoses such as incompetent cervix that leads to preterm delivery. Preterm labor, preterm PROM, and cervical insufficiency are all obstetrical syndromes [35–38]. Each of these pathologies can be derived from several underlying mechanisms including infection, thrombosis, hormonal, autoimmunity, allergy, and others [35–38]. The risk factors for spontaneous preterm birth change according to gestational age at delivery and parity. Previous preterm delivery, vaginal bleeding during the first or second trimester, a positive fetal fibronectin test, and cervical length <25 mm are risk factors for preterm birth before 37, 35, and 32 weeks of gestation [39–41]. Bacterial vaginosis and maternal body mass index (BMI) <19.8 kg/m^2 are associated with an increased risk of preterm birth <32 weeks of gestation, while African American ethnicity is a risk factor for preterm delivery before 37 weeks of gestation. When the risk is stratified according to parity, a low BMI (<19.8) and an increased Bishop score were significantly associated with spontaneous preterm delivery in nulliparous and multiparous women. Black race, poor social environment, and working during pregnancy were associated with increased risk of nulliparous women. However, among multiparous patients, a prior preterm birth overshadows the socioeconomic risk factors and is associated with a twofold increase in the odds of spontaneous preterm delivery for each prior spontaneous preterm birth. Finally, multiple gestations are an independent risk factor for preterm birth regardless of gestational age at delivery or parity [39–41].

Preterm Labor with Intact Membranes   Preterm labor with intact membranes is defined as uterine contraction before 37 completed weeks of gestation that leads to cervical effacement and/or dilatation without rupture of the chorioamniotic membranes [36]. Preterm labor with intact membranes accounts for 40%–45% of all preterm deliveries [13]. Among singleton gestation in the United States, the rate of spontaneous preterm labor declined between the years 1989 and 2000 by 6.5%, from 6.1% in 1989 to 5.7% in 2000. However, when these changes were studied according to ethnic origin, the rate of spontaneous preterm labor leading to preterm birth increased by 2% in Caucasians (from 4.9% in 1989 to 5.0% in 2000) and decreased by 24.8% in African Americans (from 12.1% in 1989 to 9.1% in 2000) [42].

Preterm PROM   Preterm PROM is defined as spontaneous rupture of the chorioamniotic membranes before 37 completed weeks of gestation without labor and accounts for 25% of all preterm deliveries. Among singleton gestation in the United States, the rate of preterm PROM declined between the years 1989 and 2000 by 30.8%, from 1.3% in 1989 to 0.9% in 2000. The rate of preterm PROM has declined in both Caucasians (a 27.2% decrease from 1.1% in 1989 to 0.8% in 2000) and African Americans (a 34.8% decrease from 2.3% in 1989 to 1.5% in 2000) [42]. The three factors that were prominently associated with preterm PROM include the following: (1) a previous preterm delivery [43,44]; (2) a history of vaginal bleeding during the index pregnancy [43–45]; and (3) cigarette smoking [44,45]. Mercer et al. [46] differentiated the risk factors for preterm PROM before 35 weeks of gestation according to parity. Cervical length ≤25 mm was an independent risk factor in nulliparous (OR 9.9, 95% CI 3.8–25.9) as well as in multiparous (OR 4.2, 95% CI 2.0–8.9) women [46]. Independent risk factors for preterm PROM among nulliparous patients included working during pregnancy and medical complications. The independent risk factors for this syndrome among multiparous patients were previous preterm PROM or spontaneous preterm delivery with intact membranes, positive fetal fibronectin in the absence of bacterial vaginosis, and the presence of bacterial vaginosis with a negative fetal fibronectin test [46].

Indicated Preterm Deliveries

Indicated preterm births are preterm deliveries in which the medical team has decided to deliver the patient before term as a result of maternal or fetal indications. They account for about 30%–35% of all preterm births [13]. In the United States, from 1989 to 2000 there was a 46% increase in the rate of indicated preterm births (from 2.6% in 1989 to 3.8% in 2000). During this period the rate of indicated preterm deliveries increased by 56.5% in Caucasians and by 36.6% in African Americans [31,42] (Figure 6.3). The most common diagnoses that precede an indicated preterm birth are preeclampsia

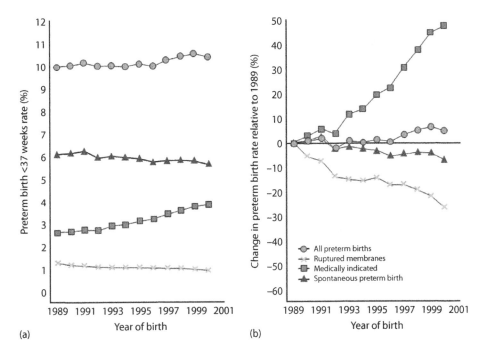

FIGURE 6.3   Rates (a) and relative temporal changes (b) of preterm birth <37 weeks (all races), as well as those resulting from ruptured membrane, medically indicated, and spontaneous preterm birth in the United States from 1989 through 2000. (Adapted from Ananth CV, et al., *Obstet Gynecol*, 105(5), 1084–91, 2005. With permission.)

(40%), fetal distress (25%), intrauterine growth restriction (10%), placental abruption (7%), and fetal demise (7%) (Table 6.1) [27]. Illicit drug use in pregnancy, especially cocaine ingestion, has been associated with indicated preterm birth [47]. Ananth et al. [42] calculated that, from 1989 to 2000, the perinatal mortality rate among preterm birth <37 weeks of gestation in Caucasians decreased by 29%. However, the authors reported that after stratification according to the type of preterm delivery, if indicated preterm births were not included, the decrease in the perinatal mortality rate was only 21%. Thus, the authors concluded that the increase in the rate of indicated preterm deliveries was associated with a reduction in the rate of perinatal death. Of note, among African Americans the major contributors to the reduction in perinatal mortality rate were the reduction in the rate of spontaneous preterm labor and preterm PROM and not the increase in the rate of indicated preterm deliveries [42].

Preterm Parturition Syndrome

Preterm parturition is a syndrome [13,48] resulting from premature activation of the common pathway of parturition, including (1) increased myometrial contractility, (2) cervical ripening/dilatation and effacement, and (3) membrane/decidual activation [13,49]. The activation of human parturition is a result of anatomical, physiological, biochemical, endocrinological, immunological, and clinical events that occur in the mother and/or fetus in both term and preterm labor. In most cases of spontaneous labor at term, there is synchronous activation of the common pathway [49,50]. However, preterm parturition is the clinical presentation of different underlying mechanisms [13], including intrauterine infection [2,17,51,52], uteroplacental ischemia [53,54], uterine overdistension [16,25,26], cervical disease [27–29], allergic phenomena [31–33], and endocrine disorders [34,55] (Figure 6.4).

Since the current taxonomy of disease in obstetrics is based on the clinical presentation of the mother and not on the mechanism of disease responsible for the clinical manifestations, the term *preterm labor* does not relate to the underlying mechanism of disease. This understanding of the biology of preterm

TABLE 6.1

Distribution of Preeclampsia, SGA, Fetal Distress, and Abruption among
Medically Indicated Preterm Birth at <35 Weeks and among Term/Near-Term
Birth

Maternal–Fetal Conditions	Rate among Term/Near-Term Birth at ≥35 weeks (%)	Medically Indicated Preterm Birth at <35 weeks	
		Rate (%)	Adjusted RR (95% CI)
Preeclampsia only	2.9	10.4	6.4 (5.9–7.0)
Preeclampsia + SGA	0.6	5.6	16.8 (15.1–18.7)
Preeclampsia + fetal distress	0.3	3.1	20.6 (17.8–23.8)
Preeclampsia + SGA + fetal distress	0.1	2.6	44.5 (37.7–52.6)
Preeclampsia + abruption	0.02	0.8	63.1 (45.8–86.8)
Preeclampsia + SGA + abruption	0.02	0.5	38.2 (23.2–62.9)
Preeclampsia + fetal distress + abruption	0.01	0.3	83.9 (49.9–141.0)
Preeclampsia + SGA + fetal distress + abruption	0.01	0.2	58.6 (30.2–113.8)
Fetal distress only	4.6	11.4	4.2 (3.8–4.5)
Fetal distress + SGA	0.9	3.3	5.5 (4.8–6.3)
Fetal distress + abruption	0.1	1.6	32.0 (26.1–39.3)
Fetal distress + SGA + abruption	0.02	0.5	29.0 (20.1–42.0)
SGA only	7.9	5.0	0.9 (0.8–1.0)
SGA + abruption	0.1	1.4	21.5 (17.3–26.8)
Placental abruption only	0.3	6.8	37.6 (33.8–41.8)

Source: Ananth CV and Vintzileos AM, *Am J Obstet Gynecol*, 195(6), 1557–63, 2006. With
                permission.

Note: RR is adjusted for the confounding effect of period of birth, maternal age, parity, mater-
                nal race/ethnicity, marital status, maternal education, smoking and alcohol use during
                pregnancy, and prepregnancy BMI.

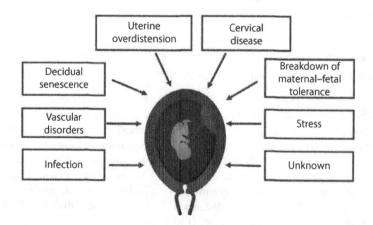

FIGURE 6.4   Proposed mechanisms of disease implicated in spontaneous preterm parturition syndrome. (Adapted from
Romero R, et al., *Science*, 345(6198), 760–765, 2014. With permission.)

parturition is crucial in order to develop clinical strategies to diagnose, treat, and prevent spontaneous preterm parturition [13,49].

Intrauterine Infection and/or Inflammation

Infection and inflammation are the leading mechanisms in the activation of preterm parturition and relate to the activation of the innate immune system [36–41]. Indeed, pyelonephritis and pneumonia are frequently associated with the onset of premature labor and delivery [36–40]. In addition, placenta, fetal membranes, and myometrium might be involved in the inflammatory pathway through the upregulation of several proinflammatory molecules, such as the chemokines IL-1β, TNF-α, and IL-8. These cytokines are elevated in the amniotic fluid and fetal membranes of patients with preterm parturition [42], where they induce prostaglandin production in the fetal membranes and deciduas, leading to the premature initiation of fetal membrane remodeling manifested in the form of preterm PROM [43,44]. In vitro evidence supports this view, showing that the exposure of amniochorion to TNF-α increases the activity of matrix metalloproteinases (MMPs), drives IL-1β and TNF-α production, and induces labor [45]. Similarly, subclinical intrauterine infection is a frequent and important mechanism of disease leading to premature contraction, preterm labor, and preterm birth [2,17,46,47,51,52]. Microbiological and histopathological studies suggest that infection-related inflammation may account for 25%–40% of cases of preterm deliveries. Goncalves et al. [17] studied the rate of positive amniotic fluid cultures for microorganisms in women with preterm labor and intact membranes in 33 studies. The prevalence of microbial invasion of amniotic fluid among patients with preterm labor was 12.8% [17,41] and about 50% of them were polymicrobial. The rate of microbial invasion of the amniotic cavity in patients with preterm labor and intact membrane is gestational-age dependent. It is as high as 45% at 23–26 weeks and decreases to 11.5% at 31–34 weeks of gestation [56]. Thus, the earlier the gestational age at preterm birth, the more likely that microbial invasion of the amniotic cavity is present [56]. In preterm PROM, the prevalence of a positive amniotic fluid culture for microorganisms is approximately 32.4% [17,41]. However, when amniocenteses were performed at the time of the onset of labor, 75% of patients had microbial invasion of the amniotic cavity [57], suggesting that some patients are already infected prior to the clinical rupture of membranes, while others are infected after the membrane has ruptured. The rate of microbial invasion of the amniotic cavity among women presenting with cervical insufficiency in the mid-trimester is around 33% (range 13%–52%) [58,59] and 45%–51% in the early third trimester [59]. In addition, a recent study has demonstrated that while only 8% of patients with cervical insufficiency had a positive amniotic fluid culture, 80% have intra-amniotic inflammation determined by a positive rapid MMP-8 kit [60]. Patients with intra-amniotic inflammation and negative amniotic fluid culture had a shorter amniocentesis-to-delivery interval and a lower gestational age at delivery than patients without intra-amniotic infection/inflammation. In twin gestations, microbial invasion of the amniotic cavity occurs in 11.9% of patients presenting with preterm labor and deliver preterm [51,61].

In addition to the changes observed in the amniotic fluid in cases of infection or inflammation, several studies show the involvement of the cervix and myometrium in these pathologic conditions, in terms of the expression of the mediators of inflammation. Of interest, both IL-6 and IL-8 concentrations are significantly higher in the cervical secretions of women destined to deliver preterm [62]. It is suggested that IL-8 specifically plays a role in cervical ripening by chemoattracting leukocytes such as neutrophils, which produce MMPs and PGE2 [63]. The myometrium also responds to and propagates inflammatory signaling during parturition. During preterm labor, myometrium experiences marked leukocyte invasion [64] along with the increased expression of proinflammatory cytokines such as CXCL8 and IL1b [65].

Uteroplacental Ischemia

Abnormal placentation and vascular lesions in the fetal and maternal sides of the placenta are the second-most prevalent lesions observed in patients who deliver preterm [66,67]. Several possible mechanisms can lead to such findings as vaginal and decidual bleeding, the spontaneous or iatrogenic death of an intrauterine sibling, and uterine vascular changes that are more prevalent in older parturients, such as atherosclerosis. Vascular pathology is one of the mechanisms leading to decidual hemorrhage and subsequent preterm birth. During normal pregnancy, cytotrophoblast invasion physiologically transforms uterine spiral arteries from small-diameter, high-resistance vessels into large-diameter, low-resistance conduits that perfuse the chorionic villi of the placenta [68]. Approximately 30% of patients with preterm labor have placental lesions consistent with maternal vascular underperfusion, and a similar number have failure of physiologic transformation of the myometrial segment of the spiral arteries [68–71]. Arias et al. [72] reported that the rate of vascular lesions in the placentae of patients with preterm labor was 34% and was 35% in those with preterm PROM, in comparison with only in 12% in those of women who delivered at term. The rate of failure of transformation of spiral arteries is higher among patients with preterm labor with intact membranes as well as those with preterm PROM than in patients who delivered at term [70,73–75].

Decidual bleeding is thought to play a role in the pathogenesis of preterm labor and preterm PROM leading to preterm birth. Indeed, hemosiderin deposition, which is regarded as a marker for bleeding, is found in the decidua, and retrochorionic hematoma is present in 37.5% of patients who deliver preterm after PROM between 22 and 32 weeks of gestation, and 36% of patients with preterm delivery and intact membranes [76]. In contrast, these lesions are found only in 0.8% of the placentas of those who deliver at term.

The effect of decidual bleeding on the activation of premature uterine contractions and/or rupture of membranes is thought to be mediated by thrombin [75,77]. The decidua is rich with tissue factor, the most potent activator of the coagulation cascade. Thus, any minor decidual bleeding activates the coagulation cascade, leading to the generation of thrombin [75,78–80]. Indeed, patients with preterm labor as well as those with preterm PROM have a higher median maternal plasma thrombin–antithrombin III concentration than that of women with a normal pregnancy [73,81,82]; and maternal plasma thrombin–antithrombin III complex concentrations in the mid-trimester were lower in patients about to deliver preterm than in those who subsequently delivered at term [83]. Moreover, increased thrombin generation was detected not only in the maternal circulation but also in the amniotic fluid [84]. Women with preterm labor who delivered preterm had a higher median thrombin–antithrombin III concentration than those who delivered at term [84]. This was particularly evident among those without intra-amniotic infection/inflammation, in which elevated amniotic fluid of thrombin antithrombin complex concentrations were associated with a shorter amniocentesis to delivery interval and a lower gestational age at delivery than those with normal or low concentrations of this complex [84]. Thrombin can activate preterm parturition through several mechanisms: (1) it has uterotonic activity (indeed, the administration of whole blood into a nonpregnant uterus generated uterine contractions that were not evident when saline or heparinized blood were introduced into the uterine cavity) [81,85]; (2) thrombin and activated coagulation factor X can induce proinflammatory cytokine production (IL-6 and IL-1), which may lead to prostaglandin generation and premature myometrial activation and contractions [79]; and (3) thrombin activates matrix-degrading enzymes such as MMP-1, MMP-3, and MMP-9 that can degrade the chorioamniotic membranes, leading to the rupture of membranes [78,86].

Uterine Overdistension

Intra-amniotic pressure remains relatively constant throughout gestation despite the growth of the fetus and placenta. As a consequence, women carrying a multiple gestation or with polyhydramnios are at increased risk of spontaneous preterm labor and delivery [87,88]. This has been attributed to progressive myometrial relaxation due to the effects of progesterone and endogenous myometrial relaxants such as nitric oxide [89]. Uterine overdistension can, however, induce increased myometrial contractility [90], prostaglandin release [91], and expression of gap junction protein or connexin-43 [92] as well as oxytocin receptor in the myometrium [93]. The effect of stretch increases in late gestation and is maximal during labor as a consequence of the relative reduction in uterine growth compared with fetal growth and of the declining circulating and/or local concentrations of progesterone [92,94,95]. Stretch may not only induce increased myometrial contractility but may also modify the contractile response through *mechanoelectrical feedback* similar to that reported in the heart. The chorioamniotic membranes are distended by 40% at 25–29 weeks of gestation, 60% at 30–34 weeks of gestation, and 70% at term [96]. Stretching of the membranes in vitro induces histological changes characterized by the elongation of the amnion cells, increased collagenase activity, and the increased production of IL-8 and prostaglandin E_2 [97–99]. Collectively, these observations suggest that mechanical forces associated with uterine overdistension may result in the activation of mechanisms leading to membrane rupture.

Insulin Resistance

There are reports hypothesizing that an alteration in adipocytokines may be involved in the process of preterm labor [100–103]. Moreover, the exact mechanisms leading to preterm birth due to maternal insulin resistance are not clear. It is suggested that insulin resistance may contribute to preterm birth in twin gestations, especially among patients with polycystic ovary syndrome (PCOS). Indeed, the rate of pregnancy complications among patients with PCOS is increased and women with PCOS demonstrated a significantly higher risk of developing gestational diabetes (odds ratio [OR] 2.94, 95% CI 1.70–5.08), gestational hypertension (OR 3.67, 95% CI 1.98–6.81), preeclampsia (OR 3.47, 95% CI 1.95–6.17), and preterm birth (OR 1.75, 95% CI 1.16–2.62) [104]. Their neonates had a significantly higher risk of admission to a neonatal intensivecare unit (OR 2.31, 95% CI 1.25–4.26) and a higher perinatal mortality (OR 3.07, 95% CI 1.03–9.21), unrelated to multiple births [104].

Long-Term Effects of Preterm Parturition on the Mother

The understanding that pregnancy is a stress test to the mother and the development of one of the great obstetrical syndromes can implicate an underlying maternal disease or pathologic process that may resurface later on in life in the form of chronic morbidity was presented about two decades ago and is rapidly evolving. Indeed, the primary evidence originated from the data regarding women who developed preeclampsia and had a higher risk of subsequently developing chronic hypertension [105–107], and those who had gestational diabetes and developed type 2 diabetes later in life [108,109]. Moreover, in a systematic review and meta-analysis of 15 studies, women who had preeclampsia/eclampsia had a significantly higher risk of subsequently developing cardiac disease (relative risk [RR] 2.33, 95% CI 1.95–2.78), cerebrovascular disease (RR 2.03, 95% CI 1.54–2.67), and cardiac mortality (RR 2.29, 95% CI 1.73–3.04). Additionally, there was a gradient relationship between the severity of the hypertensive maternal disease during pregnancy and the risk of subsequent cardiac disease for those with mild preeclampsia (RR 2.00, 95% CI 1.83–2.19) as well as severe preeclampsia (RR 5.36, 95% CI 3.96–7.27). Altogether these findings suggest that the effect of a specific pregnancy complication on subsequent maternal morbidity depends also on its severity [110].

When studying the long-term effects of preterm delivery on maternal health, the phenotype of the preterm delivery must be taken into account—meaning whether it was a spontaneous or indicated preterm birth and whether it was early or late preterm. Nevertheless, the picture is often more complicated as women who delivered an indicated early-preterm birth also have an increased risk of subsequent spontaneous early-preterm delivery and vice versa [31].

Preliminary evidence that mothers who delivered preterm have changes in their cardiovascular parameters in comparison with those who delivered at term is brought by Perng Wei and his associates [111]. This group studied the cardiovascular risk factors in a longitudinal cohort, including systolic and diastolic blood pressure, HDL cholesterol concentrations, and others. The authors [111] report that 3 years following an event of preterm delivery, these patients had higher systolic blood pressure and lower HDL cholesterol concentrations than those who delivered at term, even after adjustment for sociodemographic, perinatal, and lifestyle characteristics as well as blood pressure during the first trimester of the affected pregnancy.

The association between preterm birth and subsequent maternal cardiovascular disease is well documented [48,49,112–119], with an OR that varies between 1.3 and 2.6. This effect was demonstrated in all the parameters that were tested, including: cardiovascular disease (CVD) morbidity, ischemic heart disease (IHD), CVD/IHD mortality, IHD hospitalization and mortality, and CVD/cerebrovascular disease hospitalization or death. Robbins et al. [120] summarized the evidence regarding these parameters in a systematic review, which included 10 studies that were selected for analysis. Women with a history of preterm birth were found to have an increased risk of all the aforementioned outcome measures.

Nevertheless, the simple association between preterm delivery and subsequent maternal CVD and mortality is not sufficient. Given the diversity of the underlying mechanisms of this syndrome and the differences in its precursors, a more systematic approach is needed to address the phenotypic (gestational age at delivery, single episode vs. recurrent disease, spontaneous vs. indicated) and mechanistic (infection, uteroplacental ischemia, neurohormonal problems, insulin resistance) variations and the subsequent development of future maternal CVD or death.

The association between the phenotypic diversity of preterm delivery and subsequent maternal disease is under extensive study. The effect of gestational age at delivery on the risk of subsequent maternal CVD and death was reported in two large cohort studies. The first, by Rich-Edwards et al. [121], a population-based study of Norwegian birth records, studied the effect of gestational age at delivery on the risk of maternal CVD and demonstrated that the hazard ratio (HR) for this long-term sequel declines with advancing gestation, reaching the nadir at 39–41 weeks of gestation. Of interest was the fact that even the deliveries at early term (37–38 weeks of gestation) were associated with an increased risk of subsequent maternal CVD (Figure 6.5). The authors [121] also differentiated between indicated and spontaneous preterm deliveries and reported that at an earlier gestational age, the maternal risk of CVD was higher in women who had an indicated rather than spontaneous preterm birth. The second study, by Bonamy et al. [113], was a population-based cohort of Swedish women. They stratified the patients according to gestational age at delivery and reported that the adjusted HR for the future maternal risk of women who delivered <28 weeks was 2.58 (95% CI 1.7–3.93), 2.62 (95% CI 2.04–3.36) for 28–31 weeks, and 1.45 (95% CI 1.26–1.64) for 32–36 weeks, in comparison with delivery at term. The authors [113] also reported that they found an interaction term between birth weight and gestational age at delivery. Hence the delivery of a fetus that is two standard deviations below the mean birth rate for gestational age before 28 weeks was associated with an adjusted HR of 3.59 (95% CI 2.44–5.27) for future maternal CVD in comparison with an appropriate-for-gestational-age fetus born at term (Figure 6.6).

The comparison between the effect of a single or recurrent event of premature delivery is not extensively studied. Catov et al. [114] demonstrated that women with recurrent preterm deliveries had a substantially higher HR for atherosclerosis and cardiovascular disease/death than those with a single episode of preterm birth. Lykke et al. [117] reported a minor difference between the two groups, but women with recurrent preterm birth were still at higher risk of IHD than those with a single episode [114,116]. Kessous et al. [119] reported a linear association between recurrent preterm birth and future simple cardiovascular events as well as total cardiovascular hospitalizations (Table 6.2).

The third epidemiologic characteristic of preterm birth is the difference between spontaneous or indicated preterm births and their association with the future maternal risk of CVD. Most studies

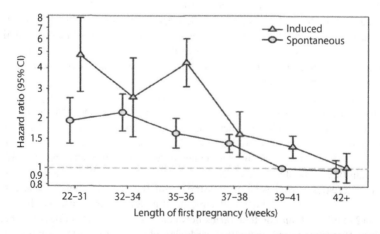

FIGURE 6.5   Hazard ratios (95% CIs) for cardiovascular disease mortality by gestational length and precursor of preterm delivery (spontaneous vs. indicated) of first pregnancy (Norwegian Medical Birth Registry). (Adapted from Rich-Edwards JW, et al., *Am J Obstet Gynecol*, 213(4), 518.e1–518.e8, 2015. With permission.)

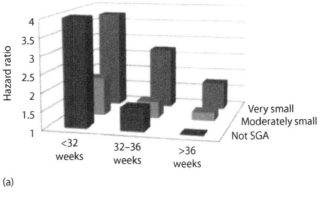

(a)

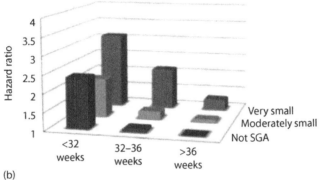

(b)

FIGURE 6.6 Hazard ratios for maternal coronary heart disease (a) and cerebrovascular events (b) in Swedish women stratified according to presence of small-for-gestational-age (SGA) and preterm birth in their first delivery, 1983 to 2005 ($n = 923,686$), and adjusted for confounding factors (maternal age, birth year, highest income, and highest education level before first delivery, country of birth, pregestational hypertension, pregestational diabetes mellitus, gestational diabetes mellitus, gestational hypertension, and preeclampsia/eclampsia). (Adapted from Bonamy AKE, et al., *Circulation*, 124, 2839–2846, 2011. With permission.)

are adjusted for the presence of preeclampsia and other factors for indicated preterm birth in their risk calculations. Kessous et al. [119] demonstrated that in comparison with patients who delivered at term, women with indicated preterm deliveries had a higher OR for simple cardiovascular events and total cardiovascular hospitalizations, and those who had a spontaneous preterm delivery had a higher OR for simple, complex, and total cardiovascular events. Moreover, the authors performed a Mantel–Haenszel test, and reported that after correction for preeclampsia, IUGR, induction of labor, and preterm PROM, there is still a higher risk of CVD in women who deliver preterm. Actual comparison between indicated and spontaneous preterm deliveries and the maternal risk of future CVD morbidity was performed by Rich-Edwards et al., who demonstrated a substantially increased risk of this future complication among patients who had an indicated preterm delivery (Figure 6.7). Indeed, in comparison with spontaneous delivery at term, the HR for CV mortality was higher in women with indicated preterm delivery (HR 3.7, 95% CI 2.9–4.8) and those with spontaneous preterm birth (HR 1.7, 95% CI 1.5–2.0). Altogether, these findings suggest that indicated preterm delivery may carry a higher risk of future maternal CVD.

The contribution of the specific underlying mechanisms leading to premature birth to the maternal risk of subsequent CVD was not studied. One could infer that placental lesions leading to maternal underperfusion (e.g., atherosis, which is regarded as the atherosclerotic disease of the maternal side of the placenta) may be associated with such elevation in the risk of future disease, but there is no current information in the literature to support this postulation.

TABLE 6.2

A Comparison of the Incidence of Cardiovascular-Related Hospitalizations and Morbidity between Patients with a History of More than Two, Just One, and No PTDs (with Use of the χ^2 Test for Trends)

	PTD (%)			
Variable	0 (*n* = 41,916)	1 (*n* = 5,217)	≥2 (*n* = 775)	*p* Value
Cardiac noninvasive diagnostic procedures	1.1	1.4	1.2	.150
Cardiac invasive diagnostic procedures	0.4	0.4	0.6	.582
Simple cardiovascular events	2.5	3.6	4.1	.001
Complex cardiovascular events	0.1	0.4	0.3	.001
Total cardiovascular hospitalizations	3.5	5.0	5.5	.001

Source: Kessous R, et al., PTD and future risk of cardiovascular disease, *Am J Obstet Gynecol*, 209(4), 368.e1–368.e8, 2013. With permission.
Abbreviation: PTD: preterm delivery.

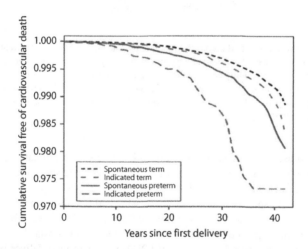

FIGURE 6.7   Cumulative survival free from CVD mortality in the 40 years after the first delivery, stratified by gestational length and precursor of birth (spontaneous vs. medically indicated delivery) in a cohort of Norwegian women. (Data from the Norwegian Medical Birth Registry). (Adapted from Rich-Edwards JW, et al., *Am J Obstet Gynecol*, 213(4), 518. e1–518.e8, 2015. With permission.)

CONCLUSIONS

Preterm birth is associated with an increased risk of subsequent maternal cardiovascular disease and mortality. This risk is related to the phenotype of the preterm birth whether it spontaneous or indicated, a single episode or recurrent, and early or late. There is evidence that the severity of the phenotype, meaning very early disease with concomitantly affected fetal growth, increases the risk of subsequent maternal CVD.

There is a gap in the literature regarding the effect of the underlying mechanisms leading to premature delivery and the subsequent maternal risk of CVD.

The clinical implication of the information presented herein is that women who had a preterm birth should be consulted regarding their future risk and be followed accordingly. This information may give the opportunity to initiate prevention programs that will affect the overall occurrence of CVD in this group.

REFERENCES

1. Duryea EL, McIntire DD, Leveno KJ. The rate of preterm birth in the United States is affected by the method of gestational age assignment. *Am J Obstet Gynecol.* 2015;213(2):231.e1–5.
2. Mazaki-Tovi S, Romero R, Kusanovic JP, et al. Recurrent preterm birth. *Semin Perinatol.* 2007;31(3):142–58.
3. Tucker J, McGuire W. ABC of preterm birth Epidemiology of preterm birth. *BMJ.* 2004;329:675–8.
4. World Health Organization. *Preterm Birth.* 2015. WHO Press, Geneva. Switzerland 2015.
5. Simmons LE, Rubens CE, Darmstadt GL, Gravett MG. Preventing preterm birth and neonatal mortality: Exploring the epidemiology, causes, and interventions. *Semin Perinatol.* 2010;34(6):408–15.
6. Hamilton BE, Martin JA, Osterman MJK, Curtin SC, Mathews TJ. Births: Final data for 2014. *Natl Vital Stat Rep.* 2015;64(12):2007–14.
7. Romero R, Dey SK, Fisher SJ. Preterm labor: One syndrome, many causes. *Science.* 2014;345(6198):760–65.
8. Blencowe H, Cousens S, Chou D, et al. Born too soon: The global epidemiology of 15 million preterm births. *Reprod Health.* 2013;10(Suppl 1):S2.
9. Blencowe H, Cousens S, Oestergaard MZ, et al. National, regional, and worldwide estimates of preterm birth rates in the year 2010 with time trends since 1990 for selected countries: A systematic analysis and implications. *Lancet.* 2012;379(9832):2162–72.
10. Hamilton BE, Martin JA, Osterman MJK, Curtin SC, Matthews TJ. Births: Final data for 2014. *Natl Vital Stat Rep.* 2015;64(12):1–64.
11. Oshiro BT, Kowalewski L, Sappenfield W, et al. A multistate quality improvement program to decrease elective deliveries before 39 weeks of gestation. *Obstet Gynecol.* 2013;121(5):1025–31.
12. American College of Obstetricians and Gynecologists. Nonmedically indicated early-term deliveries. Committee Opinion no. 561. *Obs Gynecol.* 2013;121:911–15.
13. Goldenberg RL, Culhane JF, Iams JD, Romero R. Epidemiology and causes of preterm birth. *Lancet.* 2008;371(9606):75–84.
14. Goldenberg RL, Gravett MG, Iams J, et al. The preterm birth syndrome: Issues to consider in creating a classification system. *Am J Obstet Gynecol.* 2012;206(2):113–18.
15. Patel RM. Short- and long-term outcomes for extremely preterm infants. *Am J Perinatol.* 2016; 33(3):318–28.
16. Mercer BM. Preterm premature rupture of the membranes. *Obstet Gynecol.* 2003;101(1):178–93.
17. Slattery MM, Morrison JJ. Preterm delivery. *Lancet.* 2002;360(9344):1489–97.
18. Stoll BJ, Hansen NI, Bell EF, et al. Trends in care practices, morbidity, and mortality of extremely preterm neonates, 1993–2012. *JAMA.* 2015;314(10):1039–51.
19. Patel RM, Kandefer S, Walsh MC, et al. Causes and timing of death in extremely premature infants from 2000 through 2011. *N Engl J Med.* 2015;372(4):331–40.
20. Horbar JD, Carpenter JH, Badger GJ, et al. Mortality and neonatal morbidity among infants 501 to 1500 grams from 2000 to 2009. *Pediatrics.* 2012;129(6):1019–26.
21. Ancel PY, Goffinet F, Kuhn P, et al. Survival and morbidity of preterm children born at 22 through 34 weeks' gestation in France in 2011. *JAMA Pediatr.* 2015;169(3):230.
22. Shah PS, Sankaran K, Aziz K, et al. Outcomes of preterm infants <29 weeks gestation over 10-year period in Canada: A cause for concern? *J Perinatol.* 2012;32(2):132–8.
23. Ishii N, Kono Y, Yonemoto N, Kusuda S, Fujimura M. Outcomes of infants born at 22 and 23 weeks' gestation. *Pediatrics.* 2013;132(1):62–71.
24. Su BH, Hsieh WS, Hsu CH, Chang JH, Lien R, Lin CH. Neonatal outcomes of extremely preterm infants from Taiwan: Comparison with Canada, Japan, and the USA. *Pediatr Neonatol.* 2015;56(1):46–52.

25. Meis PJ, Michielutte R, Peters TJ, et al. Factors associated with preterm birth in Cardiff, Wales. *Am J Obstet Gynecol*. 1995;173(2):597–602.
26. Meis PJ, Ernest JM, Moore M Lou, Michielutte R, Sharp PC, Buescher PA. Regional program for prevention of premature birth in northwestern North Carolina. *Am J Obstet Gynecol*. 1987;157(3):550–56.
27. Meis PJ, Goldenberg RL, Mercer BM, et al. The preterm prediction study: Risk factors for indicated preterm births. *Am J Obstet Gynecol*. 1998;178(3):562–7.
28. McElrath TF, Hecht JL, Dammann O, et al. Pregnancy disorders that lead to delivery before the 28th week of gestation: An epidemiologic approach to classification. *Am J Epidemiol*. 2008;168(9):980–89.
29. Ananth CV, Getahun D, Peltier MR, Salihu HM, Vintzileos AM. Recurrence of spontaneous versus medically indicated preterm birth. *Am J Obstet Gynecol*. 2006;195(3):643–50.
30. Ananth CV, Vintzileos AM. Maternal-fetal conditions necessitating a medical intervention resulting in preterm birth. *Am J Obstet Gynecol*. 2006;195(6):1557–63.
31. Ananth CV, Vintzileos AM. Epidemiology of preterm birth and its clinical subtypes. *J Matern Fetal Neonatal Med*. 2006;19(12):773–82.
32. Centers for Disease Control and Prevention. Preterm singleton births: United States, 1989–1996. *MMWR Morb Mortal Wkly Rep*. 1999;48(9):185–9.
33. Joseph KS, Kramer MS, Marcoux S, et al. Determinants of preterm birth rates in Canada from 1981 through 1983 and from 1992 through 1994. *N Engl J Med*. 1998;339(20):1434–9.
34. Vintzileos AM, Ananth C V, Smulian JC, Scorza WE, Knuppel RA. The impact of prenatal care in the United States on preterm births in the presence and absence of antenatal high-risk conditions. *Am J Obstet Gynecol*. 2002;187(5):1254–7.
35. Romero R, Espinoza J, Kusanovic JP, et al. The preterm parturition syndrome. *BJOG*. 2006;113(Suppl):17–42.
36. Romero R, Sepulveda W, Baumann P, et al. The preterm labor syndrome: Biochemical, cytologic, immunologic, pathologic, microbiologic, and clinical evidence that preterm labor is a heterogeneous disease. *Am J Obstet Gynecol*. 1993;168(1):288.
37. Romero R. Prenatal medicine: The child is the father of the man. *J Matern Fetal Neonatal Med*. 2009;22(8):636–9.
38. Romero R, Athayde N, Maymon E, Pacora P, Bahado-Singh R. Premature rupture of the membranes. In: Reece A, Hobbins J, eds, *Medicine of the Fetus and Mother*. Philadelphia, PA: JB Lippincott; 1998: 1581–625.
39. Mercer B, Goldenberg R, Das A. The preterm prediction study: A clinical risk assessment system . *Am J Obstet Gynecol*. 1996;1885–95.
40. Goldenberg RL, Iams JD, Mercer BM, et al. The preterm prediction study: The value of new vs standard risk factors in predicting early and all spontaneous preterm births. NICHD MFMU Network. *Am J Public Health*. 1998;88(2):233–8.
41. Mercer BM, Goldenberg RL, Moawad AH, et al., and National Institute of Child Health and Human Development Maternal–Fetal Medicine Units Network. The preterm prediction study: Effect of gestational age and cause of preterm birth on subsequent obstetric outcome. *Am J Obstet Gynecol*. 1999; 181 (5 Pt 1): 1216–21.
42. Ananth CV, Joseph KS, Oyelese Y, Demissie K, Vintzileos AM. Trends in preterm birth and perinatal mortality among singletons: United States, 1989 through 2000. *Obstet Gynecol*. 2005;105(5):1084–91.
43. Ladfors L, Mattsson LA, Eriksson M, Milsom I. Prevalence and risk factors for prelabor rupture of the membranes (PROM) at or near-term in an urban Swedish population. *J Perinat Med*. 2000;28(6):491–6.
44. Harger JH, Hsing AW, Tuomala RE, et al. Risk factors for preterm premature rupture of fetal membranes: A multicenter case-control study. *Am J Obstet Gynecol*. 1990;163(1):130–37.
45. Spinillo A, Nicola S, Piazzi G, Ghazal K, Colonna L, Baltaro F. Epidemiological correlates of preterm premature rupture of membranes. *Int J Gynecol Obstet*. 1994;47(1):7–15.
46. Mercer BM, Goldenberg RL, Meis PJ, et al. The Preterm Prediction Study: Prediction of preterm premature rupture of membranes through clinical findings and ancillary testing. *Am J Obstet Gynecol*. 2000;183(3):738–45.
47. Shiono PH, Klebanoff MA, Nugent RP, et al. The impact of cocaine and marijuana use on low birth weight and preterm birth: A multicenter study. *Am J Obstet Gynecol*. 1995;172:19–27.
48. Nardi O, Zureik M, Courbon D, Ducimetiere P, Clavel-Chapelon F. Preterm delivery of a first child and subsequent mothers: Risk of ischaemic heart disease; A nested case-control study. *Eur J Cardiovasc Prev Rehabil*. 2006;13(2):281–3.

49. Smith GC, Pell JP, Walsh D. Pregnancy complications and maternal risk of ischaemic heart disease: A retrospective cohort study of 129,290 births. *Lancet*. 2001;357:2002–6.
50. Moster D, Lie RT, Markestad T. Long-term medical and social consequences of preterm birth. *N Engl J Med*. 2008;359(3):262–73.
51. Romero R, Mazor M, Munoz H, Gomez R, Galasso M, Sherer DM. The preterm labor syndrome. *Ann NY Acad Sci*. 1994;734:414–29.
52. Martin JA, Hamilton BE, Sutton PD, et al. Births: Final data for 2006. *Natl Vital Stat Rep*. 2009;57(7):1–104.
53. Martin JA, Hamilton BE, Sutton PD, et al. Births: Final data for 2005. *Natl Vital Stat Rep*. 2007;56(6):1–103.
54. Martin JA, Hamilton BE, Sutton PD, Ventura SJ, Menacker F, Munson ML. Births: Final data for 2003. *Natl Vital Stat Rep*. 2005;54(2):1–116.
55. Romero R, Espinoza J, Mazor M, Chaiworapongsa T. The preterm parturition syndrome. In: Critchely H, Bennett P, Thornton S, eds. *Preterm Birth*. London: RCOG Press; 2004: 28–60.
56. Menard MK, Newman RB, Keenan A, Ebelingc M. Prognostic significance of prior preterm twin delivery on subsequent singleton pregnancy. *Am J Obstet Gynecol*. 1996;174(5):1429–32.
57. Bloom SL, Yost NP, McIntire DD, Leveno KJ. Recurrence of preterm birth in singleton and twin pregnancies. *Obstet Gynecol*. 2001;98(3):379–85.
58. Rydhstroem H. Gestational duration in the pregnancy after a preterm twin delivery. *Am J Obstet Gynecol*. 1998;178(1):136–9.
59. Lee SE, Romero R, Park CW, Jun JK, Yoon BH. The frequency and significance of intraamniotic inflammation in patients with cervical insufficiency. *Am J Obs Gynecol*. 2008;198(6):633.e1–8.
60. Kiwi R, Neuman M, Merkatz I, Selim M, Lysikiewicz A. Determination of the elastic properties of the cervix. *Obstet Gynecol*. 1998;71(4):568–74.
61. Page E. Incompetent internal Os of the cervix causing late abortion and premature labor: Technic for surgical repair. *Obstet Gynecol*. 1958;12(5):509–15.
62. Romero R, Espinoza J, Erez O, Hassan S. The role of cervical cerclage in obstetric practice: Can the patient who could benefit from this procedure be identified? *Am J Obs Gynecol*. 2006;194(1):1–9.
63. Craig CJ. Congenital abnormalities of the uterus and foetal wastage. *S Afr Med J*. 1973;47(42):2000–2005.
64. Levine RU, Berkowitz KM. Conservative management and pregnancy outcome in diethylstilbestrol-exposed women with and without gross genital tract abnormalities. *Am J Obstet Gynecol*. 1993;169(5):1125–9.
65. Ludmir J, Landon MB, Gabbe SG, Samuels P, Mennuti MT. Management of the diethylstilbestrol-exposed pregnant patient: A prospective study. *Am J Obstet Gynecol*. 1987;157(3):665–9.
66. Salafia CM, Vogel CA, Vintzileos AM, Bantham KF, Pezzullo J, Silberman L. Placental pathologic findings in preterm birth. *Am J Obstet Gynecol*. 1991;165(4):934–8.
67. Kim YM, Bujold E, Chaiworapongsa T, et al. Failure of physiologic transformation of the spiral arteries in patients with preterm labor and intact membranes. *Am J Obs Gynecol*. 2003;189(4):1063–9.
68. Finland M, Dublin TD. Pneumococcic pneumonias complicating pregnancy and the puerperium. *J Am Med Assoc*. 1939;112(11):1027.
69. Gilles HM, Lawson JB, Sibolas M, Voller A, Allan N. Malaria, anaemia and pregnancy. *Ann Trop Med Parasit*. 1969;63(2):245–63.
70. Herd N, Jordan T. An investigation of malaria during pregnancy in Zimbabwe. *Cent Afr J Med*. 1981;27(4):62–8.
71. Hibbard L, Thrupp L, Summeril S, Smale M, Adams R. Treatment of pyelonephritis in pregnancy. *Am J Obstet Gynecol*. 1967;98(5):609–15.
72. Arias F, Rodriquez L, Rayne SC, Kraus FT. Maternal placental vasculopathy and infection: Two distinct subgroups among patients with preterm labor and preterm ruptured membranes. *Am J Obs Gynecol*. 1993;168(2):585–91.
73. Kass E. Maternal urinary tract infection. *NY State J Med*. 1962;1:2822–6.
74. Madinger NE, Greenspoon JS, Ellrodt AG. Pneumonia during pregnancy: Has modern technology improved maternal and fetal outcome? *Am J Obs Gynecol*. 1989;161(3):657–62.
75. McLane CM. Pyelitis of pregnancy. *Am J Obstet Gynecol*. 1939;38(1):117–23.
76. Oxorn H. The changing aspects of pneumonia complicating pregnancy. *Am J Obstet Gynecol*. 1955;70(5):1057–63.

77. Stevenson CS. Treatment of thyphoid in pregnancy with choeamphenicol (Chloromycetin®). *J Am Med Assoc*. 1951;146(13):1190.
78. Wing ES. The intra-uterine transmission of thyphoid. *JAMA*. 1930;95(6):405.
79. Gonçalves LF, Chaiworapongsa T, Romero R. Intrauterine infection and prematurity. *Ment Retard Dev Disabil Res Rev*. 2002;8(1):3–13.
80. Minkoff H. Prematurity: Infection as an etiologic factor. *Obs Gynecol*. 1983;62(2):137–44.
81. Bang B. The etiology of epizootic abortion. *J Comp Pathol Ther*. 1897;10:125–149.
82. Fidel PL, Romero R, Wolf N, et al. Systemic and local cytokine profiles in endotoxin-induced preterm parturition in mice. *Am J Obstet Gynecol*. 1994;170(5):1467–75.
83. Kullander S. Fever and parturition an experimental study in rabbits. *Acta Obstet Gynecol Scand*. 1977;56(s66):77–85.
84. McDuffie RS, Sherman MP, Gibbs RS. Amniotic fluid tumor necrosis factor-alpha and interleukin-1 in a rabbit model of bacterially induced preterm pregnancy loss. *Am J Obs Gynecol*. 1992;167(6):1583–8.
85. McKay DG, Wong TC. The effect of bacterial endotoxin on the placenta of the rat. *Am J Pathol*. 1963;42(3):357–77.
86. Reider RF, Thomas L. Studies on the mechanisms involved in the production of abortion by endotoxin. *J Immunol*. 1960;84(2):189–93.
87. Romero R, Munoz H, Gomez R, et al. Antibiotic therapy reduces the rate of infection-induced preterm delivery and perinatal mortality. *Am J Obstet Gynecol*. 1994;170(1):390.
88. Skarnes RC, Harper MJK. Relationship between endotoxin-induced abortion and the synthesis of prostaglandin F. *Prostaglandins*. 1972;1(3):191–203.
89. Takeda Y, Tsuchiya I. Studies on the pathological changes caused by the injection of the Shwartzman filtrate and the endotoxin into pregnant rabbits. *Jap J Exper Med*. 1953;21:9–16.
90. Zahl PA, Bjerknes C. Induction of decidua-placental hemorrhage in mice by the endotoxins of certain gram-negative bacteria. *Exp Biol Med*. 1943;54(3):329–32.
91. Gomez R, Ghezzi F, Romero R, Muñoz H, Tolosa JE, Rojas I. Premature labor and intra-amniotic infection: Clinical aspects and role of the cytokines in diagnosis and pathophysiology. *Clin Perinatol*. 1995;22(2):281–342.
92. Romero R, Salafia CM, Athanassiadis AP, et al. The relationship between acute inflammatory lesions of the preterm placenta and amniotic fluid microbiology. *Am J Obstet Gynecol*. 1992;166(5):1382–8.
93. Romero R, Espinoza J, Chaiworapongsa T, Kalache K. Infection and prematurity and the role of preventive strategies. *Semin Neonatol*. 2002;7(4):259–74.
94. Romero R, Mazor M. Infection and preterm labor. *Clin Obs Gynecol*. 1988;31(3):553–84.
95. Alanen A. Polymerase chain reaction in the detection of microbes in amniotic fluid. *Ann Med*. 1998;30(3):288–95.
96. Leitich H, Bodner-Adler B, Brunbauer M, Kaider A, Egarter C, Husslein P. Bacterial vaginosis as a risk factor for preterm delivery: A meta-analysis. *Am J Obs Gynecol*. 2003;189(1):139–47.
97. Vidaeff AC, Ramin SM. From concept to practice: The recent history of preterm delivery prevention; Part II. Subclinical infection and hormonal effects. *Am J Perinatol*. 2006;23(2):75–84.
98. Newton ER, Piper J, Peairs W. Bacterial vaginosis and intraamniotic infection. *Am J Obs Gynecol*. 1997;176(3):672–7.
99. Ralph SG, Rutherford AJ, Wilson JD. Influence of bacterial vaginosis on conception and miscarriage in the first trimester: Cohort study. *BMJ*. 1999;319(7204):220–3.
100. Watts DH, Krohn MA, Hillier SL, Eschenbach DA. Bacterial vaginosis as a risk factor for post-cesarean endometritis. *Obs Gynecol*. 1990;75(1):52–8.
101. Chaim W, Mazor M, Leiberman JR. The relationship between bacterial vaginosis and preterm birth: A review. *Arch Gynecol Obs*. 1997;259(2):51–8.
102. Watts DH, Eschenbach DA, Kenny GE. Early postpartum endometritis: The role of bacteria, genital mycoplasmas, and *Chlamydia trachomatis*. *Obs Gynecol*. 1989;73(1):52–60.
103. McDonald HM, O'Loughlin JA, Vigneswaran R, et al. Impact of metronidazole therapy on preterm birth in women with bacterial vaginosis flora (*Gardnerella vaginalis*): A randomised, placebo controlled trial. *Br J Obstet Gynaecol*. 1997;104(12):1391–7.
104. Carey JC, Klebanoff MA, Hauth JC, et al., and National Institute of Child Health and Human Development Network of Maternal-Fetal Medicine Units. Metronidazole to prevent preterm delivery in pregnant women with asymptomatic bacterial vaginosis. *N Engl J Med*. 2000;342(8):534–40.

105. Chesley LC, Annitto JE, Cosgrove RA. The remote prognosis of eclamptic women. *Am J Obstet Gynecol.* 1976;124(5):446–59.
106. Diehl CL, Brost BC, Hogan MC, et al. Preeclampsia as a risk factor for cardiovascular disease later in life: Validation of a preeclampsia questionnaire. *Am J Obstet Gynecol.* 2008;198(5):e11–13.
107. Bellamy L, Casas J-P, Hingorani AD, Williams DJ. Pre-eclampsia and risk of cardiovascular disease and cancer in later life: Systematic review and meta-analysis. *BMJ.* 2007;335(7627):974.
108. Lee AJ, Hiscock RJ, Wein P, Walker SP, Permezel M. Gestational diabetes mellitus: Clinical predictors and long-term risk of developing type 2 diabetes; A retrospective cohort study using survival analysis. *Diabetes Care.* 2007;30:878–83.
109. Metzger BE. Long-term outcomes in mothers diagnosed with gestational diabetes mellitus and their offspring. *Clin Obstet Gynecol.* 2007;50(4):972–9.
110. McDonald SD, Malinowski A, Zhou Q, Yusuf S, Devereaux PJ. Cardiovascular sequelae of preeclampsia/eclampsia: A systematic review and meta-analyses. *Am Heart J.* 2008;156:918–30.
111. Perng W, Stuart J, Rifas-Shiman SL, Rich-Edwards JW, Stuebe A, Oken E. Preterm birth and long-term maternal cardiovascular health. *Ann Epidemiol.* 2015;25(1):40–45.
112. Smith GD, Whitley E, Gissler M, Hemminki E. Birth dimensions of offspring, premature birth, and the mortality of mothers. *Lancet.* 2000;356(9247):2066–7.
113. Bonamy AKE, Parikh NI, Cnattingius S, Ludvigsson JF, Ingelsson E. Birth characteristics and subsequent risks of maternal cardiovascular disease: Effects of gestational age and fetal growth. *Circulation.* 2011;124:2839–46.
114. Catov JM, Wu CS, Olsen J, Sutton-Tyrrell K, Li J, Nohr EA. Early or recurrent preterm birth and maternal cardiovascular disease risk. *Ann Epidemiol.* 2010;20(8):604–9.
115. Hastie CE, Smith GCS, Mackay DF, Pell JP. Maternal risk of ischaemic heart disease following elective and spontaneous pre-term delivery: Retrospective cohort study of 750,350 singleton pregnancies. *Int J Epidemiol.* 2011;40(4):914–9.
116. Lykke JA, Langhoff-Roos J, Lockwood CJ, Triche EW, Paidas MJ. Mortality of mothers from cardiovascular and non-cardiovascular causes following pregnancy complications in first delivery. *Paediatr Perinat Epidemiol.* 2010;24(4):323–30.
117. Lykke JA, Paidas MJ, Damm P, Triche EW, Kuczynski E, Langhoff-Roos J. Preterm delivery and risk of subsequent cardiovascular morbidity and type-II diabetes in the mother. *BJOG.* 2010;117(3):274–81.
118. Catov JM, Newman AB, Roberts JM, et al. Preterm delivery and later maternal cardiovascular disease risk. *Epidemiology.* 2007;18(6):733–9.
119. Kessous R, Shoham-Vardi I, Pariente G, Holcberg G, Sheiner E. An association between preterm delivery and long-term maternal cardiovascular morbidity. *Am J Obstet Gynecol.* 2013;209(4):368.e1–8.
120. Robbins CL, Hutchings Y, Dietz PM, Kuklina EV, Callaghan WM. History of preterm birth and subsequent cardiovascular disease: A systematic review. *Am J Obstet Gynecol.* 2014;210(4):285–97.
121. Rich-Edwards JW, Klungsoyr K, Wilcox AJ, Skjaerven R. Duration of pregnancy, even at term, predicts long-term risk of coronary heart disease and stroke mortality in women: A population-based study. *Am J Obstet Gynecol.* 2015;213(4):518.e1–8.

7

Renal Function Tests during Pregnancy and Long-Term Risk of Atherosclerotic Morbidity

Leah Shalev and Talya Wolak

Introduction

Pregnancy is a physiological challenge of the human organism because it requires significant adaptation in order to enable the normal growth of the fetus. Metabolic, cardiovascular, and renal alterations are profound. Maladaptation may jeopardize both the mother and the fetus. Lately, there has been growing evidence that maladaptation not only has hazardous effects during the pregnancy period but is associated with increased cardiovascular morbidity later during nonpregnant life.

Normal Kidney Function during Pregnancy

Normal pregnancy is characterized by profound alterations in almost every maternal organ system in order to accommodate the demands of the fetoplacental unit. Like other organs, the kidneys and lower urinary tract are affected both in anatomy and function.

Physiological Changes in Renal Structure and Function

Both kidneys increase in size by 1.0–1.5 cm during pregnancy [1]. Kidney volume increases by up to 30%, primarily due to an increase in renal vascular and interstitial volume (Table 7.1). The renal pelvises, caliceal systems, and ureters may be dilated as early as the first trimester, suggesting that the dilation is due not only to mechanical pressure but also to hormonal changes [2].

Normal pregnancy is characterized by widespread vasodilation, with increased arterial compliance and decreased systemic vascular resistance. These global hemodynamic changes are accompanied by increases in renal perfusion and the glomerular filtration rate (GFR), changing the reference range for many indices of renal function (such as creatinine, urea, and uric acid [UA]) at very early stages of the pregnancy.

GFR rises markedly during pregnancy, primarily due to elevations in cardiac output and renal blood flow, which increases by 80% above nonpregnant levels. Studies in both rodents and humans suggest that the increase in GFR results from enhanced glomerular plasma flow, rather than increased intraglomerular capillary pressure. Furthermore, there are no histological changes or changes in the number of nephrons.

The increase in GFR is observed within 1 month of conception and peaks at approximately 40%–50% above baseline levels by the early second trimester, then declines slightly toward term [3]. Failure to achieve the appropriate decrease in creatinine will result in both pregnancy-induced hypertension [4] as well as long-term atherosclerotic complications [5].

TABLE 7.1

Renal Changes during Pregnancy: Structural and Functional

Renal size	Increase
Renal pelvises, caliceal systems, and ureters	Dilatation
Glomerular filtration rate	Increase
Renal perfusion	Increase
Nephron number	No chance
Plasma: Creatinine, urea, uric acid, and potassium	Decrease

Decrease of Vascular Resistance

Angiotensin II, Norepinephrine

The mechanisms for decreased vascular resistance and increased renal plasma flow during pregnancy are not fully understood. Reduced vascular responsiveness to vasopressors such as angiotensin II, nor-epinephrine, and vasopressin is well documented [6]. Nitric oxide synthesis increases during normal pregnancy and may contribute to the systemic and renal vasodilation and the fall in blood pressure [7,8].

Relaxin

The ovarian hormone and vasodilator relaxin appears to be a key upstream mediator of enhanced nitric oxide signaling in pregnancy. Relaxin is a peptide hormone in the insulin family; it is normally produced in the corpus luteum, and in pregnancy it is secreted in large amounts by the placenta and decidua in response to human chorionic gonadotropin (hCG) [9]. Relaxin increases endothelin and nitric oxide production in the renal circulation, leading to generalized renal vasodilation, decreased renal afferent and efferent arteriolar resistance, and a subsequent increase in renal blood flow and GFR. This action of endothelin is mediated via the ETB receptor subtype that results in dilatation (in contrast to endothelin action as a vasoconstrictor, which is mediated via the ETA receptor subtype) [9]. In rats, the chronic administration of relaxin mimics the renal hemodynamic changes of pregnancy (20%–40% increase in GFR and renal plasma flow); these changes can be abolished by the administration of a nitric oxide synthase inhibitor [10], the administration of antirelaxin antibodies, or even oophorectomy [11].

Renal Function and Serum Biochemical Profile in Pregnant Woman

How to Monitor GFR

Management of pregnant women with preeclampsia or preexisting kidney disease requires an understanding of whether the GFR (and therefore, disease severity) is changing or stable; knowledge of the absolute value of the GFR is not usually needed.

Serum Creatinine

Changes in GFR are best identified by monitoring changes in the serum creatinine concentration. A rising serum creatinine concentration implies a reduction in GFR, a falling level indicates improvement, and a stable value usually reflects stable function. Among women with normal or near-normal serum creatinine at baseline, a small rise in serum creatinine reflects a marked reduction in GFR.

Urine Creatinine

The assessment of renal function with a 24-hour urine collection for creatinine clearance is cumbersome for the patient and is of limited accuracy in pregnancy [12]. Overcollection and undercollection of 24-hour urine samples appear to be more common in pregnancy than in nonpregnant women. This may be due, in part, to urinary stasis from dilatation of the lower urinary tract in pregnancy; several hundred milliliters of urine can be trapped in the dilated ureters, resulting in a significant lapse between urine formation and urine collection.

Modification of diet in renal disease (MDRD) equation: Estimates of GFR based on the MDRD equation are also inaccurate during pregnancy; studies of GFR with measured values obtained by inulin clearance (the gold standard for GFR) in early and late normal pregnancy and in pregnancies complicated by renal disease or preeclampsia show that MDRD substantially underestimates GFR during pregnancy and cannot be recommended for use in clinical practice [13,14].

In conclusion, the best way to monitor renal function during pregnancy is by serum creatinine.

Biochemical Profile

Creatinine and Urea

The physiologic increase in GFR during pregnancy results in a decrease in serum creatinine concentration, which falls by an average of 0.4 mg/dL (35 μmol/L) to a normal range of 0.4–0.8 mg/dL (35–70 μmol/L). Thus, a serum creatinine of 1.0 mg/dL (88 μmol/L), while normal in a nonpregnant individual, reflects renal impairment in a pregnant woman. Blood urea nitrogen (BUN) levels fall to approximately 8–10 mg/dL (2.9–3.9 mmol/L) for the same reason.

Osmolality and Sodium

The plasma osmolality in normal pregnancy falls to a new set point of about 270 mOsmol/kg, with a proportional decrease in plasma sodium concentration that is 4–5 mEq/L below nonpregnancy levels. The physiological responses to changes in osmolality above or below the new set point (i.e., thirst and the release of antidiuretic hormone [ADH] from the pituitary) are intact [15]. The reduced set point for plasma osmolality has been attributed to pregnancy-related vasodilation and resultant arterial underfilling, which stimulates ADH release and thirst. However, there is evidence that hyponatremia in pregnancy is mediated by hormonal factors. The fall in plasma sodium concentration during pregnancy correlates closely with increased production of hCG [16,17]. Furthermore, the administration of hCG to normal women during the luteal phase of the menstrual cycle can induce a similar resetting of the thresholds for ADH release and thirst [17,18]. Rather than acting directly, hCG appears to produce these changes via the release of relaxin [10]. As an example, hyponatremia in pregnant rats can be corrected by the administration of antirelaxin antibodies or by oophorectomy [11]. As noted previously, relaxin also plays an important role in the increased GFR in pregnancy. Attempts to correct the physiologic hyponatremia of pregnancy are both unnecessary (the change is mild and asymptomatic) and ineffective. This physiological hyponatremia is a marker for appropriate relaxin-induced vasodilatation. Resetting of the osmostat means that the plasma sodium concentration will be maintained at the new level despite variations in water or sodium intake. The plasma sodium concentration spontaneously rises to prepregnancy levels within 1–2 months after delivery [15,16].

Uric Acid

Serum UA declines in early pregnancy because of the rise in GFR, volume expansion, and the uricosuric effects of estrogen, reaching a nadir of 2.0–3.0 mg/dL (119–178 μmol/L) by 22–24 weeks [19]. Thereafter, the UA level begins to rise, reaching nonpregnant levels by term. The late-gestational rise in UA is attributed to the increased renal tubular absorption of urate.

Potassium

The plasma potassium levels during pregnancy are influenced by opposite forces. High levels of circulating aldosterone favor potassium excretion. On the other hand, high levels of progesterone serve as an antagonist to the mineralocorticoid receptor [20]. Pregnant women retain about 350 mmol of potassium. However, most of it is stored as an intracellular cation in the fetal space as well as in the placenta and uterus [21]. The net result of all described mechanisms on plasma potassium level is not fully understood, albeit the normal range for potassium during pregnancy is lower than nonpregnancy.

Glucose and Organic Substance

Pregnancy is associated with reductions in the fractional reabsorption of glucose, amino acids, and beta microglobulin, which results in higher rates of urinary excretion. Thus, pregnant patients may exhibit glucosuria and aminoaciduria in the absence of hyperglycemia or renal disease.

The different reference ranges for the mentioned indices reflect the normal kidney and vasculature adaptation to pregnancy. Failure of these indices to decrease may indicate the presence of occult vascular and renal abnormalities. These abnormalities might be a risk of pregnancy-induced complications such as gestational hypertension and gestational diabetes mellitus (GDM), and may even predict atherosclerotic-related morbidity in future nonpregnant life [5].

Biochemical Profile and Pregnancy Complications

Potassium: GDM and Gestational Hypertension

A cohort analysis ($n = 8114$ deliveries) performed at the largest medical center in the south of Israel linked appropriately high levels of potassium during the beginning of pregnancy to a higher prevalence of GDM and preeclampsia in later stages [22]. A significant linear association was documented between potassium levels in the first half of the pregnancy and the prevalence of GDM ($n = 604$) in the second half of the pregnancy: 6.3% in the $K \leq 3.5$ mEq/L group, 6.6% in the $K = 3.50–3.99$ mEq/L group, and 8.2% in the $K > 4$ mEq/L group ($p = .008$). A statistically significant difference for the rate of severe preeclampsia ($n = 103$) was noted between the groups: 0.4% in the $K \leq 3.5$ mEq/L group, 0.9% in the $K = 3.5–3.99$ mEq/L group, 1.3% in the $K = 4.0–4.99$ mEq/L group, and 1.5% in the $K \geq 5$ mEq/L group ($p = .027$). Specifically, $K > 5$ mEq/L was noted as a significant risk factor for both severe preeclampsia and GDM (Figure 7.1).

Gestational Diabetes Mellitus

The link between potassium, GDM, and hypertensive disorders during pregnancy was described two decades ago. As an intracellular cation, potassium is considered to play a role in pregnancy adaptation and in the pathogenesis of GDM and preeclampsia [23,24]. During normal pregnancy, a progressive insulin resistance develops, reaching levels nearly as high as those measured in type 2 diabetes mellitus. Insulin resistance in normal pregnancy is secondary to the insulin-desensitizing effects of the hormonal products of the placenta and to maternal adiposity. In order to overcome the enhanced insulin resistance there is proliferation of pancreatic beta cells and increased insulin secretion [25]. Insulin resistance begins near mid-pregnancy (although both human and animal models demonstrated that islet cell proliferation and insulin resistance are already present in the first trimester). The main function of insulin

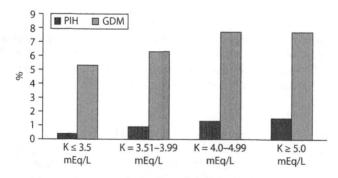

FIGURE 7.1   Prevalence of severe preeclampsia and GDM against various potassium groups. There is significant linear-by-linear association between potassium level during the first half of the pregnancy and the prevalence of severe preeclampsia and GDM ($p = .008$) in the second half of the pregnancy ($p = .027$). PIH: pregnancy-induced hypertension. (Adapted from Wolak T, et al., *J Matern Fetal Neonatal Med*, 23(9), 994–8, 2010).

is to increase the entrance of glucose into the cells, thus preventing hyperglycemia. However, insulin also increases the entrance of potassium into the cells. Accordingly, low potassium levels might be a surrogate marker for the appropriate increase in insulin levels during pregnancy due to augmentation in pancreatic beta islet cell function and number.

Gestational Hypertension and Preeclampsia

Potassium metabolism might shed light on normal versus abnormal vascular and renal function during pregnancy. Normal plasma potassium levels are mainly regulated by renal potassium excretion. Most of the secretion of potassium by the kidney is achieved by the principle cells of the collecting duct. The factors that increase potassium excretion include high aldosterone level, high distal delivery of sodium to the collecting duct, and high negativity of the lumen in the collecting duct [26]. As mentioned previously, potassium metabolism during pregnancy is influenced by additional factors. During normal pregnancy the secretion of aldosterone is enhanced [27]; one of the causes for this increase is splanchnic and systemic vasodilatation. In addition, the rise in GFR increases the distal delivery of sodium, thereby increasing the excretion of potassium. These effects are only partially negated by the high levels of progesterone, which acts as a mineralocorticoid receptor blocker [28] and by that decreases the full effect of aldosterone on the kidney, avoiding severe potassium wastage.

In conclusion, relatively low plasma potassium levels may indicate that appropriate vascular, renal, and pancreatic adaptation occurred. Failure to decrease potassium during the early stage of pregnancy was found to be an independent risk factor for both preeclampsia and GDM in the second half of pregnancy.

Uric Acid

Because of its role in metabolic syndrome in the nonpregnant population, UA has also been evaluated as an early marker for GDM and gestational hypertension in the pregnant patient.

Gestational diabetes mellitus: Two studies [29,30] to date have suggested that elevated UA in the first trimester was associated with a higher rate of GDM. A significant linear association was documented between UA level in the first 20 weeks and the prevalence of GDM and mild preeclampsia. From a total of 5077 births, 7.6% ($n = 417$) suffered from GDM. The lowest and highest prevalence of GDM were found in the UA ≤ 2.4 mEq/L group (6.3%) and the UA > 5.5 mEq/L group (10.5%) ($p < .001$), respectively. Mild preeclampsia was diagnosed in 3.4% ($n = 185$) of the pregnancies from the UA ≤ 2.4 mEq/L group, 3.3% from the UA $= 2.5–4.0$ mEq/L group, 5.3% from the UA $= 4.1–5.5$ mEq/L group, and 4.5% from the UA > 5.5 mEq/L group ($p < .001$) [27] (Figure 7.2). However, both studies were not able to demonstrate that UA was a risk factor independent of obesity.

Gestational hypertension: Elevated UA has been shown not only to be a marker of essential hypertension but also to play a causal role in its pathogenesis by mediating oxidative stress, activating the

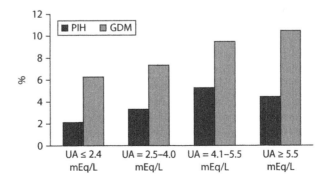

FIGURE 7.2 Uric acid levels and the prevalence of GDM and the prevalence of mild preeclampsia. There is significant linear-by-linear association between UA value in the first half of the pregnancy and the prevalence of GDM ($p < .001$) and mild preeclampsia ($p < .001$). (Adapted from Wolak T, et al., *Hypertens Pregnancy*, 31(3), 307–15, 2012).

renin–angiotensin system, and causing endothelial dysfunction. In pregnancy, hyperuricemia has been strongly associated with preeclampsia, often predating the clinical signs to as early as 10 weeks of gestation. Hyperuricemia accompanying hypertensive disorders (with or without proteinuria) may be linked to adverse fetal outcomes such as preterm birth and growth restriction. To date, UA is strongly associated with preeclampsia.

GDM and hypertensive disorders during pregnancy are more common in women with metabolic syndrome and are accordingly associated with a higher incidence of future chronic hypertension, type 2 diabetes mellitus, and cardiovascular disease [31]. In the nonpregnant population, UA is receiving growing attention as a surrogate marker of cardiovascular morbidity and as a cardiovascular atherosclerotic risk factor [32]. It might be suggested that UA is a link between GDM and hypertension and future cardiovascular morbidity.

Biochemical Profile during Pregnancy and Late Atherosclerotic Morbidity

It is well known that metabolic abnormalities during pregnancy are harbingers of future morbidity. For example, GDM and hypertensive disorders of pregnancy are predictors of cardiovascular disease and metabolic syndrome in future nonpregnant life [33–35].

For example, a large-scale retrospective study found that women with hypertensive disorders during pregnancy were at high risk of end-stage renal disease. The risk was much greater for women who had preeclampsia or eclampsia than for those who had gestational hypertension alone [36]. An opposite association has been found as well.

Likewise, Kessous et al., in a population-based study, compared the incidence of long-term atherosclerotic morbidity in a cohort of women who delivered in the years 1988–2012 [33]. A significant linear association was noted between the severity of preeclampsia (no preeclampsia, mild preeclampsia, severe preeclampsia, and eclampsia) and renal disease (0.1% vs. 0.2% vs. 0.5% vs. 1.1%, respectively; $p = .001$; Figure 7.3a), as well as cardiovascular disease (2.7% vs. 4.5% vs. 5.2% vs. 5.7%, respectively; $p = .001$) (Figure 7.3b).

However, milder, subclinical changes during pregnancy may also predict such morbidity. In a retrospective study of 27,000 women, failure to lower creatinine and urea during pregnancy was associated with hospitalizations for cardiovascular reasons years after the pregnancy [5]. A recent case-control study including women who gave birth during 2000–2012 investigated whether renal function during pregnancy can serve as a surrogate marker for the risk of developing atherosclerotic-related morbidity [32]. This population was divided into cases of women who were subsequently hospitalized for atherosclerotic morbidity during the study period and age-matched controls. The mean follow-up period was about 60 months. Multivariate analyses showed that creatinine of ≥ 1.01 mg/dL was associated with a significantly increased risk of hospitalization due to cardiovascular events (adjusted HR 2.91, CI 1.37–6.19; $p = .005$) and a urea level of ≤ 20 mg/dL was independently associated with a reduced prevalence of cardiovascular hospitalization (adjusted HR 0.62, CI 0.57–0.86; $p = .001$). The opposite correlation exists as well (Figure 7.4). Women who suffered a hypertensive pregnancy disorder were found to have higher UA levels decades after the index pregnancy. This association was independent of family predisposition, as normotensive sisters of these women were examined as well and were found to have a normal UA level [37]. Two other studies confirmed the importance of UA as well as potassium during pregnancy. It was demonstrated that high potassium and UA levels during pregnancy are both independent predictors of long-term atherosclerotic morbidity [38,39].

Endothelial dysfunction may be a mechanism that unifies pregnancy-related disorders and future cardiovascular morbidity. Endothelial dysfunction refers to the disturbed endothelial control of vascular tone, increased permeability, and the abnormal expression of procoagulants. These abnormalities are effected by many mechanisms, of which the decreased production of endothelial-derived vasodilators such as nitric oxide and prostacyclin, the increased production of vasoconstrictors such as endothelins and thromboxanes, and the increased vascular reactivity of angiotensin II are the most important. Oxidative stress, meaning an imbalance between the presence of reactive oxygen species and antioxidants, is a

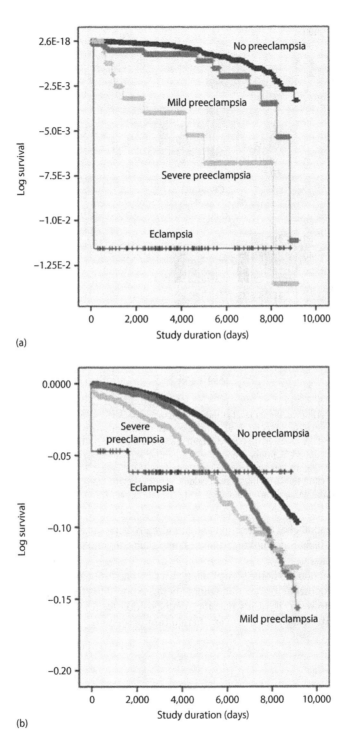

FIGURE 7.3 Long-term renal and cardiovascular morbidity according to the severity of preeclampsia. Kaplan–Meier survival curves for the cumulative incidence of (a) renal and (b) cardiovascular hospitalizations following the index birth in the following groups: no preeclampsia, mild preeclampsia, severe preeclampsia, and eclampsia. Patients with a history of any form of preeclampsia had a significantly higher risk of cumulative cardiovascular and renal events during the whole follow-up period. (Adapted from Kessous R, et al., *Heart*, 101(6), 442–6, 2015.)

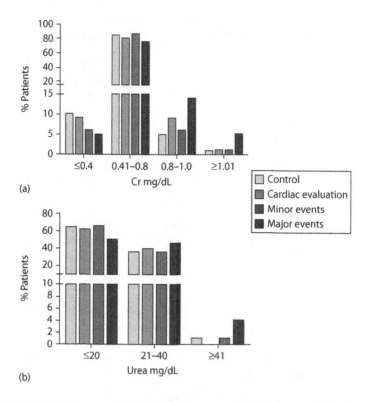

(a)

(b)

FIGURE 7.4   High creatinine and urea level at index pregnancy associated with increased risk of long-term atherosclerotic morbidity. (a) The prevalence of controls vs. cardiac evaluation, minor events, and major events was the highest in the Cr ≤ 0.4 mg/dL group and the lowest in the 0.8–1.0 mg/dL group and the Cr ≥ 1.01 mg/dL group ($p < .001$ linear-by-linear association). Major events: $n = 367$; minor events: $n = 205$; cardiac evaluations: $n = 90$. (b) The prevalence of controls vs. cardiac evaluation, minor events, and major events was the highest in the urea ≤ 20 mg/dL group and the lowest when urea exceeded 20 mg/dL ($p = .017$ linear-by-linear association). Major events: $n = 367$; minor events: $n = 204$; cardiac evaluations: $n = 90$. Cr: creatinine. (Adapted from Wolak T, et al., *Nephrology (Carlton)*, 21(2), 116–21, 2016.)

strong promoter of endothelial dysfunction and has already been proved to be caused by known cardiovascular risk factors including smoking, diabetes, hypertension, and hyperlipidemia. UA is also emerging as an oxidative factor.

Endothelial dysfunction lies at the base of many diseases and is not always initiated by the same events (men can develop endothelial dysfunction without being exposed to pregnancy) and does not target only one vascular bed. However, it seems that the predisposition to develop endothelial dysfunction may become evident at different stages in life and herald future, seemingly unrelated morbidity.

SUMMARY

In conclusion, renal and cardiovascular systems go through major changes during pregnancy in order to adjust to the special needs of the mother and the fetus. These normal physiologic changes in kidney and vascular structure are essential. In order to protect the mother from gestational hypertension there is vasodilatation, increased renal blood flow, and a significant increase in GFR. In order to prevent the development of diabetes, there is an increase in the ability of the pancreas to secrete insulin. Failure to go through these adequate changes may result in occult subclinical abnormalities that will be expressed only by abnormal serum markers (elevated creatinine, urea, UA, and potassium), and in more severe cases, the development of gestational hypertension, preeclampsia, and GDM. Usually after delivery there is a resolution of pregnancy-induced complications. However, failure to achieve this vascular renal adjustment during pregnancy is a recognized risk factor for future atherosclerotic morbidity (Figure 7.5).

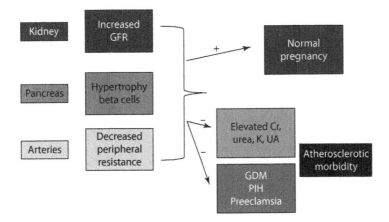

FIGURE 7.5   Physiological adjustment of the kidneys, pancreas, and vascular system during normal pregnancy. Normal adjustment will result in normal pregnancy, while failure to go through appropriate renal, pancreatic, and vascular changes will be reflected in abnormal biochemical markers and even in pregnancy-induced complications. These pregnancy abnormalities are risk factors for atherosclerotic morbidity later during nonpregnant life. K: potassium.

The connection between pregnancy-related morbidity and future atherosclerotic diseases is so strong that the American Cardiology Society guidelines include this information in the assessment of the patients' cardiovascular risk [40].

REFERENCES

1. Bailey RR, Rolleston GL. Kidney length and ureteric dilatation in the puerperium. *J Obstet Gynaecol Br Commonw*. 1971;78(1):55–61.
2. Beydoun SN. Morphologic changes in the renal tract in pregnancy. *Clin Obstet Gynecol*. 1985;28(2):249–56.
3. Davison JM, Dunlop W. Renal hemodynamics and tubular function normal human pregnancy. *Kidney Int*. 1980;18(2):152–61.
4. Wolak T, Sergienko R, Wiznitzer A, Paran E, Sheiner E. Creatinine level as a predictor of hypertensive disorders during pregnancy. *Br J Biomed Sci*. 2011;68(3):112–15.
5. Wolak T, Shoham-Vardi I, Sergienko R, Sheiner E. Renal function during pregnancy may predict risk of future hospitalization due to atherosclerotic-related morbidity. *Nephrology (Carlton)*. 2016 Feb;21(2):116–21.
6. Gant NF, Chand S, Whalley PJ, MacDonald PC. The nature of pressor responsiveness to angiotensin II in human pregnancy. *Obstet Gynecol*. 1974;43(6):854.
7. Danielson LA, Conrad KP. Acute blockade of nitric oxide synthase inhibits renal vasodilation and hyperfiltration during pregnancy in chronically instrumented conscious rats. *J Clin Invest*. 1995;96(1):482–90.
8. Deng A, Engels K, Baylis C. Impact of nitric oxide deficiency on blood pressure and glomerular hemodynamic adaptations to pregnancy in the rat. *Kidney Int*. 1996;50(4):1132–8.
9. Conrad KP, Jeyabalan A, Danielson LA, Kerchner LJ, Novak J. Role of relaxin in maternal renal vasodilation of pregnancy. *Ann NY Acad Sci*. 2005;1041:147–54.
10. Danielson LA, Sherwood OD, Conrad KP. Relaxin is a potent renal vasodilator in conscious rats. *J Clin Invest*. 1999;103(4):525–33.
11. Novak J, Danielson LA, Kerchner LJ, et al. Relaxin is essential for renal vasodilation during pregnancy in conscious rats. *J Clin Invest*. 2001;107(11):1469–75.
12. Côté A-M, Firoz T, Mattman A, Lam EM, von Dadelszen P, Magee LA. The 24-hour urine collection: Gold standard or historical practice? *Am J Obstet Gynecol*. 2008;199(6):625.e1–6.
13. Smith MC, Moran P, Ward MK, Davison JM. Assessment of glomerular filtration rate during pregnancy using the MDRD formula. *BJOG*. 2008;115(1):109–12.

14. Alper AB, Yi Y, Webber LS, et al. Estimation of glomerular filtration rate in preeclamptic patients. *Am J Perinatol*. 2007;24(10):569–74.
15. Lindheimer MD, Barron WM, Davison JM. Osmoregulation of thirst and vasopressin release in pregnancy. *Am J Physiol*. 1989; 257 (2 Pt 2): F159–69.
16. Lindheimer MD, Barron WM, Davison JM. Osmotic and volume control of vasopressin release in pregnancy. *Am J Kidney Dis*. 1991;17(2):105–11.
17. Davison JM, Shiells EA, Philips PR, Lindheimer MD. Serial evaluation of vasopressin release and thirst in human pregnancy: Role of human chorionic gonadotrophin in the osmoregulatory changes of gestation. *J Clin Invest*. 1988;81(3):798–806.
18. Davison JM, Shiells EA, Philips PR, Lindheimer MD. Influence of humoral and volume factors on altered osmoregulation of normal human pregnancy. *Am J Physiol*. 1990; 258 (4 Pt 2): F900–907.
19. Lind T, Godfrey KA, Otun H, Philips PR. Changes in serum uric acid concentrations during normal pregnancy. *Br J Obstet Gynaecol*. 1984;91(2):128–32.
20. Couette B, Lombes M, Baulieu EE, Rafestin-Oblin ME. Aldosterone antagonists destabilize the mineralocorticosteroid receptor. *Biochem J*. 1992;282(Pt 3):697–702.
21. Lindheimer MD, Richardson DA, Ehrlich EN, Katz AI. Potassium homeostasis in pregnancy. *J Reprod Med*. 1987;32(7):517–22.
22. Wolak T, Sergienko R, Wiznitzer A, Ben Shlush L, Paran E, Sheiner E. Low potassium level during the first half of pregnancy is associated with lower risk for the development of gestational diabetes mellitus and severe pre-eclampsia. *J Matern Fetal Neonatal Med*. 2010;23(9):994–8.
23. Tranquilli AL, Bilancia F, Valensise H, Garzetti GG, Romanini C. Intracellular potassium in normal and pathological pregnancy: I. Regulation of transport and concentration. *Ann Ostet Ginecol Med Perinat*. 1989;110(5):226–8.
24. Tranquilli AL, La Palombara C, Rabini RA, Leocani B, Testa I, Romanini C. Intracellular potassium in normal and pathological pregnancy: II. Experimental results. *Ann Ostet Ginecol Med Perinat*. 1989;110(5):229–35.
25. Buchanan TA, Xiang AH. Gestational diabetes mellitus. *J Clin Invest*. 2005;115(3):485–91.
26. Greenlee M, Wingo CS, McDonough AA, Youn JH, Kone BC. Narrative review: Evolving concepts in potassium homeostasis and hypokalemia. *Ann Intern Med*. 2009;150(9):619–25.
27. Godard C, Gaillard R, Vallotton MB. The renin–angiotensinal–dosterone system in mother and fetus at term. *Nephron*. 1976;17(5):353–60.
28. Quinkler M, Meyer B, Bumke-Vogt C, et al. Agonistic and antagonistic properties of progesterone metabolites at the human mineralocorticoid receptor. *Eur J Endocrinol*. 2002;146(6):789–99.
29. Wolak T, Sergienko R, Wiznitzer A, Paran E, Sheiner E. High uric acid level during the first 20 weeks of pregnancy is associated with higher risk for gestational diabetes mellitus and mild preeclampsia. *Hypertens Pregnancy*. 2012;31(3):307–15.
30. Laughon SK, Catov J, Provins T, Roberts JM, Gandley RE. Elevated first-trimester uric acid concentrations are associated with the development of gestational diabetes. *Am J Obstet Gynecol*. 2009;201(4):402.e1–5.
31. Pouta A, Hartikainen AL, Sovio U, et al. Manifestations of metabolic syndrome after hypertensive pregnancy. *Hypertension*. 2004;43(4):825–31.
32. Brodov Y, Behar S, Goldenberg I, Boyko V, Chouraqui P. Usefulness of combining serum uric acid and C-reactive protein for risk stratification of patients with coronary artery disease (Bezafibrate Infarction Prevention [BIP] study). *Am J Cardiol*. 2009;104(2):194–8.
33. Kessous R, Shoham-Vardi I, Pariente G, Sergienko R, Sheiner E. Long-term maternal atherosclerotic morbidity in women with pre-eclampsia. *Heart*. 2015;101(6):442–6.
34. Beharier O, Shoham-Vardi I, Pariente G, et al. Gestational diabetes mellitus is a significant risk factor for long-term maternal renal disease. *J Clin Endocrinol Metab*. 2015;100(4):1412–16.
35. Kessous R, Shoham-Vardi I, Pariente G, Sherf M, Sheiner E. An association between gestational diabetes mellitus and long-term maternal cardiovascular morbidity. *Heart*. 2013;99(15):1118–21.
36. Wang IK, Muo CH, Chang YC, et al. Association between hypertensive disorders during pregnancy and end-stage renal disease: A population-based study. *CMAJ*. 2013;185(3):207–13.
37. Weissgerber TL, Milic NM, Turner ST, et al. Uric acid: A missing link between hypertensive pregnancy disorders and future cardiovascular disease? *Mayo Clin Proc*. 2015;90(9):1207–16.

38. Wolak T, Shoham-Vardi I, Sergienko R, Sheiner E. High potassium level during pregnancy is associated with future cardiovascular morbidity. *J Matern Fetal Neonatal Med*. 2016;29(6):1021–4.
39. Wolak T, Shoham-Vardi I, Sergienko R, Sheiner E. High Uric acid levels during pregnancy linked to increased risk for future atherosclerotic-related hospitalization. *J Clin Hypertens (Greenwich)*. 2015;17(6):481–5.
40. Mosca L, Benjamin EJ, Berra K, et al. Effectiveness-based guidelines for the prevention of cardiovascular disease in women: 2011 update; A guideline from the American Heart Association. *Circulation*. 2011;123(11):1243–62.

8

Pregnancy and Depression: The Tip of the Iceberg?

Samantha Meltzer-Brody

Introduction

For many women, the perinatal period (pregnancy and postpartum) is the trigger for the first onset of a mood disorder. Depression during pregnancy, or *antenatal depression*, is an important public health concern with serious consequences for mother and fetus [1]. The prevalence of antenatal depression ranges between 14% and 23% [2]. Importantly, depression during pregnancy has been documented to be one of the greatest risk factors for development of *postpartum depression* (PPD) [3] and PPD is one of the primary causes of maternal death from suicide and is also associated with infanticide [4].

There has been recent international recognition that screening for antenatal and postpartum depression is important. For example, in January 2016, the U.S. Preventive Services Task Force (USPSTF) recommended, for the first time, that women be screened for depression during pregnancy and after giving birth [5]. This echoes the 2007 guidelines for Antenatal and Postnatal Mental Health by the U.K. National Institute for Health and Care Excellence (NICE) [6]. However, with screening comes an imperative to deliver effective health care in a wide range of systems. Therefore, it is critical to examine the consequences of perinatal psychiatric illness. This chapter will focus specifically on maternal mood and anxiety symptoms during pregnancy and the consequent medical and psychiatric complications on both mother and fetus. It will also discuss current theories on screening, the underlying pathophysiology of antenatal depression, and potential treatments.

Screening

The clinical presentation of perinatal depression has unique characteristics compared with depression that occur outside of the perinatal period. Symptoms of severe anxiety and rumination can manifest as the primary clinical concern and significantly impact functioning [7,8]. The recognition of anxiety as a hallmark feature of perinatal depression led to the development of the Edinburgh Postnatal Depression Scale (EPDS) by Cox et al. [9]. The EPDS is the most widely used and validated screening tool for depressive symptoms in pregnant and postpartum women [9]. It has demonstrated good reliability and validity: the reported split-half reliability of the EPDS is 0.88 and the standardized Cronbach's alpha coefficient is 0.87 [9]. Each item is scored on a four-point Likert scale ranging from 0 to 3. Therefore, the total scores range from 0 to 30, with greater scores reflecting worse symptom severity. Extensive validation studies have shown that a cutoff score ≥ 12 indicates symptom severity consistent with major depression, while a cutoff ≥ 10 has been used to include probable cases of minor depression that require additional clinical monitoring [10].

Recent work examining the use of the EPDS during pregnancy demonstrates that a positive score on the EPDS may identify women with potentially serious mental disorders other than depression, including bipolar disorder and anxiety disorders such as obsessive compulsive disorder (OCD) [11]. Further, other work using large-scale consortium data and the EPDS further indicates that the onset of depression or anxiety symptoms during pregnancy in expectant mothers may be a key predictor of risk of more severe postpartum depression [12].

Pathophysiology: Hormone Sensitivity and Genetic Contributions

The literature documents that sensitivity to the hormonal fluctuations that normally occur during pregnancy are a major part of the pathophysiology of perinatal mood disorders [13,14] (Box 8.1). Genetic vulnerability also strongly contributes to risk, and there is very promising new work that supports increased heritability for perinatal depression. Recent work by Viktorin et al. demonstrated in two samples that the heritability of perinatal depression is far greater than that of major depression outside of the perinatal period [15]. This is the largest heritability study of perinatal depression to date and extends the previous literature on the heritability of perinatal depression. Other genetic studies of perinatal depression are as follows: there are two family studies that showed clustering in families for PPD [16,17], an Australian twin study [18], and one PPD genome-wide linkage study [19]. There has also been interest in working to identify noninvasive biomarkers during pregnancy that predict for PPD and would allow for the development of new preventive strategies and treatments that could dramatically decrease suffering for women and their families. While these studies have not been replicated to date in large samples, they remain a highly promising area of investigation [20–22].

Psychiatric and Medical Complications during Pregnancy and Risk of Postpartum Depression

Untreated antenatal depression is a major risk factor for postpartum depression [23] and increases the risk of recurrent psychiatric illness [24,25]. Women with antenatal depression in pregnancy are less likely to participate in recommended prenatal care practices and more likely to engage in risky health behaviors (e.g., substance abuse) [26], thereby increasing the risk of adverse obstetrical outcomes [27]. Fetal exposure to maternal suicide attempts is associated with mental retardation and serious congenital abnormalities [28].

A careful review of the literature indicates that medical complications occurring during pregnancy and/or childbirth have been *inconsistently* linked to postpartum psychiatric disorders [29]. These include complications of pregnancy such as preeclampsia [30], hyperemesis gravidarum (severe nausea and vomiting) [31,32], gestational diabetes [33], and gestational hypertension [34,35], as well as obstetrical complications including postpartum hemorrhage [36,37], cesarean section (CS) [38–40], and preterm birth [41] (Box 8.2). These pregnancy and obstetrical complications occur relatively commonly: the prevalence

---

BOX 8.1   PATHOPHYSIOLOGY OF PERINATAL MOOD DISORDERS

- Sensitivity to the hormonal fluctuations during pregnancy
- Genetic vulnerability: increased heritability for perinatal depression

---

BOX 8.2   OBSTETRICAL COMPLICATIONS THAT MIGHT INCREASE THE RISK OF POSTPARTUM DEPRESSION

- Preeclampsia
- Hyperemesis gravidarum
- Gestational diabetes
- Gestational hypertension
- Postpartum hemorrhage
- Cesarean section
- Preterm birth

of preeclampsia is 5%–8% of all pregnancies [42], preterm birth is ~10% [43,44], and gestational diabetes is up to 9% [45]. Medical complications during pregnancy and/or at delivery may be distinguishing features for the onset and degree of severity of postpartum psychiatric disorders [12].

Maternal Obesity

Obesity as a risk factor for poor maternal and child outcomes has attracted recent attention due to the rising prevalence and the clear association in the literature between inflammation and depression. There are two lines of inquiry: the first examines whether weight gain during pregnancy is associated with longer-term obesity and depression [46]. The second line of inquiry has documented an association between anxiety and mood symptoms during pregnancy and the development of postpartum obesity [47,48]. These studies suggest that antenatal anxiety and depression may be important risk factors for retained weight gain postpartum. Postpartum weight retention is associated with long-term metabolic disease risk [49,50], thereby making antenatal anxiety and depression important targets for intervention.

Pathophysiology of Obstetrical Complications of Antenatal Depression

Maternal depression during pregnancy can also have significant negative consequences on the fetus [51]. There is an emerging literature on the peptides and proteins that are produced by both the brain and placenta. These peptides and proteins may have important roles in the development of the fetal central nervous system and placental functioning [52] and may explain the increased risk in adverse obstetrical events observed in women with antenatal depression. For example, there are decreased levels of neurotrophic growth factor (NGF) in the placental tissue of women with untreated depression during pregnancy [53]. NGF plays an important role in neuronal cell survival and differentiation [54], and women with altered placenta levels have been found to have an increased risk of pregnancy complications compared with control women. Interestingly, altered placental levels of NGF were also found in antidepressant-exposed women [53]. Thus, NGF may play an important role in the risk of miscarriage or preterm birth [55].

Further, two mechanisms required to sustain fetal growth—placental angiogenesis and vascular remodeling—depend on matrix metalloproteinases (MMPs) [56]. MMPs have major roles in both adult neurogenesis and neuroprotection as well as placental angiogenesis and vascular remodeling [57]. MMPs are secreted as latent enzymes and are either activated or inhibited by other proteins. In particular, plasminogen activator inhibitor (PAI)-1 plays an important role in the inhibition of critical proteins involved in angiogenesis (i.e., plasmin and plasminogen) and has been reported to be elevated in mothers with depression [52].

Antenatal Depression and Fetal Stress

Maternal antenatal depression has been associated with physiological effects on the fetus. When pregnant women experience significant anxiety stress, anxiety, or depression, their children are at increased risk of development of psychopathology, leading to the *transmission of risk* paradigm that is felt to play a prominent role above and beyond that of the inheritance of specific gene variants [58–61]. The mechanism by which maternal stress is communicated to the fetus is an area of intense research and no definitive answers have been identified to date.

The literature shows that children exposed to perinatal (either during pregnancy or postpartum) maternal depression have higher cortisol levels than infants of mothers who were not depressed [62–64], and this finding continues through adolescence [64]. Importantly, the treatment of maternal depression during pregnancy appears to help normalize infant cortisol levels [65]. These findings may partially explain the mechanism for an increased vulnerability to psychopathology in children of mothers with perinatal depression [66].

Treatment of Antenatal Depression

Pregnant women with antenatal depression must be treated in order to prevent adverse outcomes [67]. For expectant mothers with mild-to-moderate depressive illness, psychotherapy is indicated as a first-line treatment option [68,69]. There is a strong evidence base for the efficacy of psychotherapeutic interventions, including interpersonal psychotherapy (IPT) [70–73], partner-assisted IPT [73], cognitive behavioral therapy [74,75], and group psychoeducation [76,77].

For expectant mothers with severe depressive and anxiety symptoms that cause impairment in functioning, pharmacotherapy is often used [68,78]. Antidepressant medication (ADM) is considered an effective strategy for perinatal depression and, while the risk of fetal exposure remains controversial, for some women ADM is much more accessible than psychotherapy [79]. A new epidemiological report of ADM use in US Medicaid-eligible women (2000–2007) documented that nearly 1 in 12 women used ADM during pregnancy [80–82]. Consequently, this is an area with ongoing debate about the potential associations between ADM use in pregnancy, maternal depression and anxiety, and adverse fetal outcomes (i.e., preterm birth, primary persistent pulmonary hypertension of the newborn, risk of autism, ADHD, and cardiac effects) [83–86].

There is an ever-growing number of large systematic reviews and meta-analyses demonstrating that the absolute risks associated with antidepressant exposure during pregnancy to be small, but still present [84,87,88]. There is also evidence for the efficacy of both newer antidepressants (selective serotonin reuptake inhibitors [SSRIs]) and older tricyclic antidepressants in the treatment of antenatal depression and anxiety [89,90]. Benzodiazepines are also commonly used for the treatment of anxiety during pregnancy and are considered relatively safe [91–93]. As this is an area of significant controversy, treatment decisions about antenatal depression must be made on an individual case-by-case basis, with careful consideration of decision risks to mother and fetus [94].

Due to the controversy, expectant mothers may be faced with unpleasant stigma and experience shame if they decide to continue taking their antidepressant or other psychotropic medication during pregnancy in order to maintain their own mental health. This is a stressful and difficult situation that would be much less likely to occur if the pregnant woman was seeking treatment for a different medical illness such as diabetes or hypertension [95]. Good communication between patient and provider is critical to ensure that the most effective and individually tailored treatment plan is developed.

Lastly, because of the controversy surrounding antidepressant use during pregnancy, there is a great need for other evidence-based treatments for antenatal for depression and anxiety. There is current research focused on bright-light therapy in antenatal depression [96] and the administration of repetitive transcranial magnetic stimulation (rTMS) during pregnancy [97,98].

CONCLUSIONS

The perinatal period is a profound time in a woman's life that poses multiple risks, including the onset of mood and anxiety disorders. Perinatal mood and anxiety disorders are first-rank public health problems. We currently have a poor understanding of who will develop perinatal anxiety and depression. Thus, it is very difficult to effectively counsel women about perinatal psychiatric illness and provide prospective intervention to at-risk women. Moreover, the clinical presentation of perinatal mood disorders during pregnancy is heterogeneous, and treatment cannot be delivered on a one-size-fits-all basis. Careful consideration of medical comorbidities must be part of assessment and treatment. Therefore, a well-defined classification of phenomena in perinatal psychiatric illness based on symptom profiles is crucial to advance our understanding of underlying causes and specialized treatment approaches. Future research is needed to improve our understanding of the pathophysiology of perinatal mood disorders, including genetic and other biological mechanisms implicated in the etiology of maternal perinatal depression and subsequent fetal stress during pregnancy. It is vital that our field pursues this type of investigation so that new preventive strategies and treatments are developed that could dramatically decrease suffering for women and their families.

REFERENCES

1. Grote NK, Bridge JA, Gavin AR, Melville JL, Iyengar S, Katon WJ. A meta-analysis of depression during pregnancy and the risk of preterm birth, low birth weight, and intrauterine growth restriction. *Arch Gen Psychiatry*. 2010;67(10):1012–24.
2. Gaynes B, Gavin N, Meltzer-Brody S. Perinatal depression: Prevalence, screening accuracy and screening outcomes. *Evid Rep Technol Assess*. 2005;119:1–8.
3. Gavin NI, Gaynes BN, Lohr KN, Meltzer-Brody S, Gartlehner G, Swinson T. Perinatal depression: A systematic review of prevalence and incidence. *Obstet Gynecol*. 2005; 106 (5 Pt 1): 1071–83.
4. Lindahl V, Pearson J, Colpe L. Prevalence of suicidality during pregnancy and the postpartum. *Arch Womens Ment Health*. 2005;8(2):77–87.
5. Siu AL, Force USPST, Bibbins-Domingo K, et al. Screening for depression in adults: US Preventive Services Task Force recommendation statement. *JAMA*. 2016;315(4):380–7.
6. National Collaborating Center for Mental Health. *Antenatal and Postnatal Mental Health: The NICE Guideline on Clinical Management and Service Guidance*. Leicester, UK: British Psychological Society and the Royal College of Psychiatrists; 2007.
7. Abramowitz JS, Meltzer-Brody S, Leserman J, et al. Obsessional thoughts and compulsive behaviors in a sample of women with postpartum mood symptoms. *Arch Womens Ment Health*. 2010;13(6):523–30.
8. Bernstein IH, Rush AJ, Yonkers K, et al. Symptom features of postpartum depression: Are they distinct? *Depress Anxiety*. 2008;25(1):20–26.
9. Cox JL, Holden JM, Sagovsky R. Detection of postnatal depression. Development of the 10-item Edinburgh Postnatal Depression Scale. *Br J Psychiatry*. 1987;150:782–6.
10. Meltzer-Brody S, Boschloo L, Jones I, Sullivan PF, Penninx BW. The EPDS-lifetime: Assessment of lifetime prevalence and risk factors for perinatal depression in a large cohort of depressed women. *Arch Womens Ment Health*. 2013;16(6):465–73.
11. Lydsdottir LB, Howard LM, Olafsdottir H, Thome M, Tyrfingsson P, Sigurdsson JF. The mental health characteristics of pregnant women with depressive symptoms identified by the Edinburgh Postnatal Depression Scale. *J Clin Psychiatry*. 2014;75(4):393–8.
12. Postpartum Depression: Action Towards Causes and Treatment (PACT) Consortium. Heterogeneity of postpartum depression: A latent class analysis. *Lancet Psychiatry*. 2015;2(1):59–67.
13. Bloch M, Schmidt PJ, Danaceau M, Murphy J, Nieman L, Rubinow DR. Effects of gonadal steroids in women with a history of postpartum depression. *Am J Psychiat*. 2000;157(6):924–30.
14. Schiller CE, Meltzer-Brody S, Rubinow DR. The role of reproductive hormones in postpartum depression. *CNS Spectr*. 2015;20(1):48–59.
15. Viktorin A, Meltzer-Brody S, Kuja-Halkola R, et al. Heritability of perinatal depression and genetic overlap with nonperinatal depression. *Am J Psychiatry*. 2016;173(2):158–65.
16. Murphy-Eberenz K, Zandi PP, March D, et al. Is perinatal depression familial? *J Affect Disord*. 2006;90(1):49–55.
17. Forty L, Jones L, Macgregor S, et al. Familiality of postpartum depression in unipolar disorder: Results of a family study. *Am J Psychiatry*. 2006;163(9):1549–53.
18. Treloar SA, Martin NG, Bucholz KK, Madden PA, Heath AC. Genetic influences on post-natal depressive symptoms: Findings from an Australian twin sample. *Psychol Med*. 1999;29(3):645–54.
19. Mahon PB, Payne JL, MacKinnon DF, et al. Genome-wide linkage and follow-up association study of postpartum mood symptoms. *Am J Psychiatry*. 2009;166(11):1229–37.
20. Mehta D, Quast C, Fasching PA, et al. The 5-HTTLPR polymorphism modulates the influence on environmental stressors on peripartum depression symptoms. *J Affect Disord*. 2012;136(3):1192–7.
21. Guintivano J, Arad M, Gould TD, Payne JL, Kaminsky ZA. Antenatal prediction of postpartum depression with blood DNA methylation biomarkers. *Mol Psychiatry*. 2013; May;19(5):560–7.
22. Osborne L, Clive M, Kimmel M, et al. Replication of epigenetic postpartum depression biomarkers and variation with hormone levels. *Neuropsychopharmacology*. 2016;41(6):1648–58.
23. Viguera AC, Tondo L, Koukopoulos AE, Reginaldi D, Lepri B, Baldessarini RJ. Episodes of mood disorders in 2,252 pregnancies and postpartum periods. *Am J Psychiatry*. 2011;168(11):1179–85.
24. McMahon C, Barnett B, Kowalenko N, Tennant C. Psychological factors associated with persistent postnatal depression: Past and current relationships, defence styles and the mediating role of insecure attachment style. *J Affect Disord*. 2005;84(1):15–24.

25. Dipietro JA, Costigan KA, Sipsma HL. Continuity in self-report measures of maternal anxiety, stress, and depressive symptoms from pregnancy through two years postpartum. *J Psychosom Obstet Gynaecol*. 2008;29(2):115–24.

26. Flynn HA, Davis M, Marcus SM, Cunningham R, Blow FC. Rates of maternal depression in pediatric emergency department and relationship to child service utilization. *Gen Hosp Psychiatry*. 2004;26(4):316–22.

27. Ibanez G, Charles MA, Forhan A, et al. Depression and anxiety in women during pregnancy and neonatal outcome: Data from the EDEN mother–child cohort. *Early Hum Dev*. 2012;88(8):643–9.

28. Petik D, Czeizel B, Banhidy F, Czeizel AE. A study of the risk of mental retardation among children of pregnant women who have attempted suicide by means of a drug overdose. *J Inj Violence Res*. 2012;4(1):10–19.

29. Blom EA, Jansen PW, Verhulst FC, et al. Perinatal complications increase the risk of postpartum depression. The Generation R Study. *BJOG*. 2010;117(11):1390–98.

30. Bergink V, Laursen TM, Johannsen BM, Kushner SA, Meltzer-Brody S, Munk-Olsen T. Pre-eclampsia and first-onset postpartum psychiatric episodes: A Danish population-based cohort study. *Psychol Med*. 2015;45(16):3481–9.

31. Poursharif B, Korst LM, Fejzo MS, MacGibbon KW, Romero R, Goodwin TM. The psychosocial burden of hyperemesis gravidarum. *J Perinatol*. 2008;28(3):176–81.

32. Buyukkayaci Duman N, Ozcan O, Bostanci MO. Hyperemesis gravidarum affects maternal sanity, thyroid hormones and fetal health: A prospective case control study. *Arch Gynecol Obstet*. 2015;292(2):307–312.

33. Barakat S, Martinez D, Thomas M, Handley M. What do we know about gestational diabetes mellitus and risk for postpartum depression among ethnically diverse low-income women in the USA? *Arch Womens Ment Health*. 2014;17(6):587–92.

34. Rigo J, Jr., Kecskemeti A, Molvarec A, Lefkovics E, Szita B, Baji I. [233-POS]: Postpartum depression and anxiety in hypertensive disorders of pregnancy. *Pregnancy Hypertension*. 2015;5(1):117–18.

35. Bijlenga D, Koopmans CM, Birnie E, et al. Health-related quality of life after induction of labor versus expectant monitoring in gestational hypertension or preeclampsia at term. *Hypertens Pregnancy*. 2011;30(3):260–74.

36. Thompson JF, Roberts CL, Ellwood DA. Emotional and physical health outcomes after significant primary post-partum haemorrhage (PPH): A multicentre cohort study. *Aust NZ J Obstet Gynaecol*. 2011;51(4):365–71.

37. Sentilhes L, Gromez A, Clavier E, Resch B, Descamps P, Marpeau L. Long-term psychological impact of severe postpartum hemorrhage. *Acta Obstet Gynecol Scand*. 2011;90(6):615–20.

38. Houston KA, Kaimal AJ, Nakagawa S, Gregorich SE, Yee LM, Kuppermann M. Mode of delivery and postpartum depression: The role of patient preferences. *Am J Obstet Gynecol*. 2015;212(2):229.e1–7.

39. Sword W, Landy CK, Thabane L, et al. Is mode of delivery associated with postpartum depression at 6 weeks: A prospective cohort study. *BJOG*. 2011;118(8):966–77.

40. Hannah ME, Whyte H, Hannah WJ, et al. Maternal outcomes at 2 years after planned cesarean section versus planned vaginal birth for breech presentation at term: The international randomized Term Breech Trial. *Am J Obstet Gynecol*. 2004;191(3):917–27.

41. Helle N, Barkmann C, Bartz-Seel J, et al. Very low birth-weight as a risk factor for postpartum depression four to six weeks postbirth in mothers and fathers: Cross-sectional results from a controlled multicentre cohort study. *J Affect Disord*. 2015;180:154–61.

42. Leffert LR. What's new in obstetric anesthesia? Focus on preeclampsia. *Int J Obstet Anesth*. 2015;24(3):264–71.

43. Horgan MJ. Management of the late preterm infant: Not quite ready for prime time. *Pediatr Clin North Am*. 2015;62(2):439–51.

44. Delnord M, Blondel B, Zeitlin J. What contributes to disparities in the preterm birth rate in European countries? *Curr Opin Obstet Gynecol*. 2015;27(2):133–42.

45. DeSisto CL, Kim SY, Sharma AJ. Prevalence estimates of gestational diabetes mellitus in the United States, Pregnancy Risk Assessment Monitoring System (PRAMS), 2007–2010. *Prev Chronic Dis*. 2014;11:130415.

46. Phelan S. Pregnancy: A "teachable moment" for weight control and obesity prevention. *Am J Obstet Gynecol*. 2009;202:135.e1–8.

47. Bogaerts AF, Van den Bergh BR, Witters I, Devlieger R. Anxiety during early pregnancy predicts post-partum weight retention in obese mothers. *Obesity (Silver Spring)*. 2010;21(9):1942–9.
48. Pedersen P, Baker JL, Henriksen TB, et al. Influence of psychosocial factors on postpartum weight retention. *Obesity (Silver Spring)*. 2011;19(3):639–46.
49. Rooney B, Schauberger C. Excess pregnancy weight gain and long-term obesity: One decade later. *Obstet Gynecol*. 2002;100(2):245–52.
50. Rooney BL, Schauberger CW, Mathiason MA. Impact of perinatal weight change on long-term obesity and obesity-related illnesses. *Obstet Gynecol*. 2005;106(6):1349–56.
51. Gentile S. Untreated depression during pregnancy: Short- and long-term effects in offspring: A systematic review. *Neuroscience*. 2015;305:15–25.
52. Hoirisch-Clapauch S, Brenner B, Nardi AE. Adverse obstetric and neonatal outcomes in women with mental disorders. *Thromb Res*. 2015;135(Suppl 1):S60–63.
53. Kaihola H, Olivier J, Poromaa IS, Akerud H. The effect of antenatal depression and selective serotonin reuptake inhibitor treatment on nerve growth factor signaling in human placenta. *PLoS One*. 2015;10(1):e0116459.
54. Kawamura K, Kawamura N, Sato W, Fukuda J, Kumagai J, Tanaka T. Brain-derived neurotrophic factor promotes implantation and subsequent placental development by stimulating trophoblast cell growth and survival. *Endocrinology*. 2009;150(8):3774–82.
55. Dhobale MV, Pisal HR, Mehendale SS, Joshi SR. Differential expression of human placental neurotrophic factors in preterm and term deliveries. *Int J Dev Neurosci*. 2013;31(8):719–23.
56. Cohen M, Meisser A, Bischof P. Metalloproteinases and human placental invasiveness. *Placenta*. 2006;27(8):783–93.
57. Verslegers M, Lemmens K, Van Hove I, Moons L. Matrix metalloproteinase-2 and -9 as promising benefactors in development, plasticity and repair of the nervous system. *Prog Neurobiol*. 2013;105:60–78.
58. Bale TL, Baram TZ, Brown AS, et al. Early life programming and neurodevelopmental disorders. *Biol Psychiatry*. 2010;68(4):314–9.
59. Van den Bergh BR, Marcoen A. High antenatal maternal anxiety is related to ADHD symptoms, externalizing problems, and anxiety in 8- and 9-year-olds. *Child Dev*. 2004;75(4):1085–97.
60. O'Donnell KJ, Glover V, Barker ED, O'Connor TG. The persisting effect of maternal mood in pregnancy on childhood psychopathology. *Dev Psychopathol*. 2014;26(2):393–403.
61. O'Connor TG, Monk C, Burke AS. Maternal affective illness in the perinatal period and child development: Findings on developmental timing, mechanisms, and intervention. *Curr Psychiatry Rep*. 2016;18(3):24.
62. Diego MA, Field T, Hernandez-Reif M, Cullen C, Schanberg S, Kuhn C. Prepartum, postpartum, and chronic depression effects on newborns. *Psychiatry*. 2004;67(1):63–80.
63. Essex MJ, Klein MH, Cho E, Kalin NH. Maternal stress beginning in infancy may sensitize children to later stress exposure: Effects on cortisol and behavior. *Biol Psychiatry*. 2002;52(8):776–84.
64. Halligan SL, Herbert J, Goodyer IM, Murray L. Exposure to postnatal depression predicts elevated cortisol in adolescent offspring. *Biol Psychiatry*. 2004;55(4):376–81.
65. Brennan PA, Pargas R, Walker EF, Green P, Newport DJ, Stowe Z. Maternal depression and infant cortisol: Influences of timing, comorbidity and treatment. *J Child Psychol Psychiatry*. 2008;49(10):1099–107.
66. O'Connor TG, Ben-Shlomo Y, Heron J, Golding J, Adams D, Glover V. Prenatal anxiety predicts individual differences in cortisol in pre-adolescent children. *Biol Psychiatry*. 2005;58(3):211–17.
67. Meltzer-Brody S, Jones I. Optimizing the treatment of mood disorders in the perinatal period. *Dialogues Clin Neurosci*. 2015;17(2):207–18.
68. Yonkers KA, Wisner KL, Stewart DE, et al. The management of depression during pregnancy: A report from the American Psychiatric Association and the American College of Obstetricians and Gynecologists. *Obstet Gynecol*. 2009;114(3):703–13.
69. Yonkers KA, Vigod S, Ross LE. Diagnosis, pathophysiology, and management of mood disorders in pregnant and postpartum women. *Obstet Gynecol*. 2011;117(4):961–77.
70. Stuart S, O'Hara MW. Treatment of postpartum depression with interpersonal psychotherapy. *Arch Gen Psychiatry*. 1995;52(1):75–6.
71. Grote NK, Swartz HA, Geibel SL, Zuckoff A, Houck PR, Frank E. A randomized controlled trial of culturally relevant, brief interpersonal psychotherapy for perinatal depression. *Psychiatr Serv*. 2009;60(3):313–21.

72. Zlotnick C, Miller IW, Pearlstein T, Howard M, Sweeney P. A preventive intervention for pregnant women on public assistance at risk for postpartum depression. *Am J Psychiatry*. 2006;163(8):1443–5.

73. Brandon AR, Ceccotti N, Hynan LS, Shivakumar G, Johnson N, Jarrett RB. Proof of concept: Partner-assisted interpersonal psychotherapy for perinatal depression. *Arch Womens Ment Health*. 2012;15(6):469–80.

74. Cooper PJ, Murray L, Wilson A, Romaniuk H. Controlled trial of the short- and long-term effect of psychological treatment of post-partum depression: I. Impact on maternal mood. *Br J Psychiatry*. 2003;182:412–9.

75. Chabrol H, Teissedre F, Saint-Jean M, Teisseyre N, Roge B, Mullet E. Prevention and treatment of post-partum depression: A controlled randomized study on women at risk. *Psychol Med*. 2002;32(6):1039–47.

76. Honey KL, Bennett P, Morgan M. A brief psycho-educational group intervention for postnatal depression. *Br J Clin Psychol*. 2002;41(Pt 4):405–9.

77. Morgan M, Matthey S, Barnett B, Richardson C. A group programme for postnatally distressed women and their partners. *J Adv Nurs*. 1997;26(5):913–20.

78. Einarson A. Antidepressants and pregnancy: Complexities of producing evidence-based information. *CMAJ*. 2010;182(10):1017–18.

79. O'Mahen HA, Flynn HA. Preferences and perceived barriers to treatment for depression during the perinatal period. *J Womens Health (Larchmt)*. 2008;17(8):1301–9.

80. Wisner KL, Appelbaum PS, Uhl K, Goldkind SF. Pharmacotherapy for depressed pregnant women: Overcoming obstacles to gathering essential data. *Clin Pharmacol Ther*. 2009;86(4):362–5.

81. Oberlander TF, Gingrich JA, Ansorge MS. Sustained neurobehavioral effects of exposure to SSRI antidepressants during development: Molecular to clinical evidence. *Clin Pharmacol Ther*. 2009;86(6):672–7.

82. Warburton W, Hertzman C, Oberlander TF. A register study of the impact of stopping third trimester selective serotonin reuptake inhibitor exposure on neonatal health. *Acta Psychiatr Scand*. 2010;121(6):471–9.

83. Huybrechts KF, Palmsten K, Avorn J, et al. Antidepressant use in pregnancy and the risk of cardiac defects. *N Engl J Med*. 2014;370(25):2397–407.

84. Ross LE, Grigoriadis S. Selected pregnancy and delivery outcomes after exposure to antidepressant medication. *JAMA Psychiatry*. 2014;71(6):716–17.

85. Clements CC, Castro VM, Blumenthal SR, et al. Prenatal antidepressant exposure is associated with risk for attention-deficit hyperactivity disorder but not autism spectrum disorder in a large health system. *Mol Psychiatry*. 2014;20(6):727–34.

86. Croen LA, Grether JK, Yoshida CK, Odouli R, Hendrick V. Antidepressant use during pregnancy and childhood autism spectrum disorders. *Arch Gen Psychiatry*. 2011;68(11):1104–12.

87. Suri R, Lin AS, Cohen LS, Altshuler LL. Acute and long-term behavioral outcome of infants and children exposed in utero to either maternal depression or antidepressants: A review of the literature. *J Clin Psychiatry*. 2014;75(10):e1142–52.

88. O'Connor E, Rossom RC, Henninger M, Groom HC, Burda BU. Primary care screening for and treatment of depression in pregnant and postpartum women: Evidence report and systematic review for the US Preventive Services Task Force. *JAMA*. 2016;315(4):388–406.

89. Wisner KL, Hanusa BH, Perel JM, et al. Postpartum depression: A randomized trial of sertraline versus nortriptyline. *J Clin Psychopharmacol*. 2006;26(4):353–60.

90. Newport DJ, Hostetter A, Arnold A, Stowe ZN. The treatment of postpartum depression: Minimizing infant exposures. *J Clin Psychiatry*. 2002;63(Suppl 7):31–44.

91. Burt VK, Suri R, Altshuler L, Stowe Z, Hendrick VC, Muntean E. The use of psychotropic medications during breast-feeding. *Am J Psychiatry*. 2001;158(7):1001–9.

92. Buist A, Norman TR, Dennerstein L. Breastfeeding and the use of psychotropic medication: A review. *J Affect Disord*. 1990;19(3):197–206.

93. Kelly LE, Poon S, Madadi P, Koren G. Neonatal benzodiazepines exposure during breastfeeding. *J Pediatr*. 2012;161(3):448–51.

94. Jones I, McDonald L. Living with uncertainty: Antidepressants and pregnancy. *Br J Psychiatry*. 2014;205(2):103–4.

95. Meltzer-Brody S. Treating perinatal depression: Risks and stigma. *Obstet Gynecol*. 2014;124(4):653–4.

96. Wirz-Justice A, Bader A, Frisch U, et al. A randomized, double-blind, placebo-controlled study of light therapy for antepartum depression. *J Clin Psychiatry*. 2011;72(7):986–93.

97. Kim DR, Sockol L, Barber JP, et al. A survey of patient acceptability of repetitive transcranial magnetic stimulation (TMS) during pregnancy. *J Affect Disord*. 2011;129(1–3):385–90.

98. Zhang X, Liu K, Sun J, Zheng Z. Safety and feasibility of repetitive transcranial magnetic stimulation (rTMS) as a treatment for major depression during pregnancy. *Arch Womens Ment Health*. 2010;13(4):369–70.

9

Pregnancy and Thromboembolic Morbidity

Zeva Daniela Herzog, Aaron Herzog, and Eyal Sheiner

Introduction

Venous thromboembolism (VTE), which encompasses both deep vein thrombosis (DVT) and pulmonary embolism (PE), is an important cause of maternal morbidity and mortality. VTE is a significant cause of maternal death in resource-rich countries, with a case fatality rate for PE in pregnancy at 2.4% [1]. Alongside the short-term morbidity and mortality associated with VTE, long-term consequences such as post-thrombotic syndrome (PTS), which can vary from edema and skin changes to recurrent thrombosis and ulceration, should not be disregarded [2].

Normal pregnancy is accompanied by a physiologic change in hemostasis, leading to a state of hypercoagulability. This change may have evolved as a protective measure against the dangers of maternal hemorrhage [3,4]. This chapter will review the overall epidemiologic significance of VTE and pregnancy, risk factors for women with VTE both antepartum and postpartum, with a special focus on long-term outcomes.

Public awareness of VTE is exceedingly low in comparison with other diseases (such as diabetes and stroke). One recent study found that only 25% of respondents knew what DVT is, and far fewer understood its symptoms or risk factors [5]. Rates of VTE are relatively low in the overall population and are concentrated largely in the elderly, with the mean age of incidence estimated at 59–76 years [6,7]. For comparison, in 2008, over half of all births in the United States were to women their 20s [8].

Conclusions from two recent large prospective cohort studies in the United States found that a minimum of 1 in 12 middle-aged adults will experience VTE during their remaining lifetime [5]. In fact, rates of VTE have been declining in the last 50 years, from 28 per 10,000 women of reproductive age (20–49 years) in 1959–1960 to 2 per 10,000 in 2012 [6,9,10]. Only 2.0%–2.4% of all VTE cases in women are related to pregnancy or the postpartum period [6].

Pregnancy-Related Incidence of VTE

The risk of thromboembolic events is significantly increased in pregnant women compared with non-pregnant women, averaging to be about 4.0–4.6 times higher in age-matched pregnant women [11,12]. The absolute risk of DVT and/or PE in pregnant women was assessed in a recent review [6] of 15 studies in developed countries to be between 2.7 and 12.2 per 10,000 deliveries, with a median of 5.7 per 10,000 across all studies (Figure 9.1). Similarly, a number of studies from various developed countries from 1998 to 2008 found the incidence of thromboembolic events to range from 4.9 to 17.2 per 10,000 deliveries [13–19]. Another 2015 meta-analysis [20] applied a random-effects model to estimate the pooled incidence of VTE in pregnancy, which returned a rate of 1.2 per 1000 deliveries.

Of note, these values were calculated from studies conducted overwhelmingly in developed countries/regions (United States, Europe, Hong Kong, and Korea), limiting the worldwide generalizability. A 2009 study was done among Sudanese women [21]; however, according to the meta-analysis from Kourlaba et al. [20], results from this study were not "well described." Superficial vein thrombosis occurs more often than DVT or PE in pregnancy [22] but is less investigated due its mainly self-limiting course.

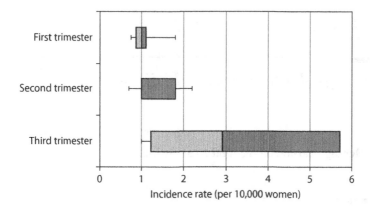

FIGURE 9.1   Incidence of VTE stratified by pregnancy trimester. (Adapted from Parunov LA, et al., *Birth Defects Res C Embryo Today*, 105(3), 167–184, 2015.)

VTE Distribution across Pregnancy and Postpartum

Out of all VTEs, there is a even 50:50 split between occurrences during the antepartum period and postpartum period, of which 58%–75% present as DVT and 20%–25% present as PE [15,18,23–25]. General consensus agrees that the average number of VTEs is the same in the first and second trimester, and increases dramatically in the third trimester [20] (Figure 9.2). Several studies show that the risk of VTE compared with nonpregnant women is six to nine times higher during the third trimester [6,9,11,12,19,26]. Furthermore, VTE risk increases dramatically after delivery [9,11,18,26–28], likely due to vascular damage [29]. Specifically, VTE during puerperium (defined as six weeks postdelivery) occurs 60 times more often than in nonpregnant women [30].

Incidence of Pulmonary Embolism versus Deep Vein Thrombosis

In terms of distribution between DVT and PE, a retrospective study [11] assessing pregnancies from 1966 to 1995 found the incidence of postpartum DVT to be even higher than antepartum (351.4 vs. 85.2 per 100,000). PE occurred 15 times more often in the first 3 months postpartum than during pregnancy (159.7 vs. 10.6 per 100,000). More recent studies support these findings, including a retrospective cohort study [31] that found that 26% of all VTE events occurred during puerperium, of which the majority of

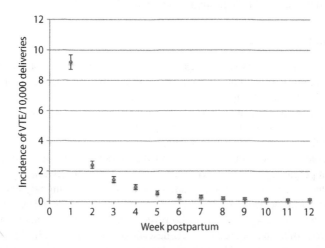

FIGURE 9.2   Incidence of VTE stratified by week postpartum. (Adapted from Tepper NK, et al. *Obstet Gynecol*, 23(5), 987–996, 2014.)

cases presented as DVT. In that study, PE was reported to occur three times more often during puerperium than later postpartum.

Generally, PEs commonly present with symptoms of DVT. However, while the frequency of PE found in patients with symptomatic DVT was found to be from 40% to 50%, PE associated with silent DVT occurs in about 30% of patients [32,33]. Identification of at-risk women with PE is incredibly important, especially because of the greatly decreased survival rate in PE compared with isolated DVT.

Case Mortality Rates

According to the 2014 WHO review of maternal mortality [34], the percentage of maternal deaths due to embolism (arterial and venous) is 3.2% worldwide, whereas it comprises about 14% in developed countries. The majority of these events are due to VTE (80%) and the rest are arterial (20%) [15]. Based on the ratio of 80:20 venous to arterial events, VTE is therefore the cause of 10%–12% of maternal deaths [6,35]. This value is supported by data from a study [15] that found VTE accounting for 1.1 maternal deaths per 100,000 deliveries.

Maternal death caused by PE can be prevented best by early detection of DVT; however, symptoms (tachypnea, dyspnea, tachycardia, and leg swelling) can be found physiologically in pregnancy, and thus may hinder diagnosis. Therefore, early clinical suspicion of DVT in pregnant women and an understanding of risk factors for DVT are both critical to preventing maternal morbidity and mortality.

Pathophysiology

Virchow's triad for the risk of thrombosis (hypercoagulable state, venous stasis, endothelial injury) is present throughout pregnancy and the postpartum period. These changes, and therefore the risk of VTE, start at conception and may not normalize until over 6 to 8 weeks postpartum [36,37].

During early pregnancy hormonal changes lead to a hypercoagulable state. Levels of anticoagulants (specifically free protein S) and fibrinolytic activators decrease, whereas concentrations of fibrinogen, von Willebrand factor, plasminogen activator inhibitors (types 1 and 2) and coagulation factors VII, X, and VIII all increase. Factors II, V, and IX do not change concentration significantly [6,23,38] (Table 9.1).

There are two factors contributing to increased venous stasis of the lower extremities during pregnancy: increased venous capacitance and large vein compression [16,39]. First, venous flow velocity is reduced by 50% starting from 25 to 29 weeks of gestation [32]. Second, as pregnancy progresses, the

TABLE 9.1

Physiologic Changes in Coagulation System during Pregnancy

Procoagulants	Change
Fibrinogen	↑
Factors X, VII, VIII	↑
von Willebrand factor	↑
Plasminogen activator inhibitor 1 and 2	↑
Factors II, V, IX	⟷
Anticoagulants	
Free protein S	↓
Protein C	↓
Antithrombin III	⟷

Sources: James AH, *Birth Defects Res C Embryo Today*, 105(3), 159–166, 2015; Parunov LA, et al., *Birth Defects Res C Embryo Today*, 105(3), 167–184, 2015; American College of Obstetricians and Gynecologists, *Obstet Gynecol*, 118(3), 718–729, 2011.

uterus puts increased pressure on the pelvic veins, causing decreased blood circulation and leading to venous stasis [40,41].

The most common location for DVT during pregnancy is in the proximal left lower extremity (70%–90% occur in the iliofemoral veins), and it is most likely to be massive [19]. In comparison, distal thromboses do occur, but are equally likely on the right side as the left. The actual mechanism for proximal left-sided predominance is unknown, and cannot be explained by uterine enlargement in early pregnancy. A possible mechanism is relative stenosis of the left common iliac vein between the lumbar vertebral body and the right common iliac artery [32,35,42].

This phenomenon of pelvic vein thrombosis is very specific to DVT during pregnancy, accounting for approximately 10%–12% of pregnancy-associated DVT, while occurring in less than 1% of DVT in general. Of note, DVT rarely occurs in the upper extremity; during pregnancy, upper-extremity DVT is likely associated with ovarian hyperstimulation syndrome secondary to the use of assisted reproductive technologies [25,43].

Risk Factors

Past History of Thrombosis

The strongest risk factor for pregnancy-related VTE is a previous thromboembolic event (Tables 9.2 and 9.3). This correlates with between 15% and 25% of all pregnancy-related thromboembolic events [1,6]. The greatest risk occurs when women with a history of VTE do not receive thromboprophylaxis during and after pregnancy.

Unsurprisingly, multiple studies [44–46] support this, showing an increased risk of recurrent VTE over those who did receive anticoagulants. However, according to a recent meta-analysis [6] only 5%–15% of pregnancy-related VTE was linked with a past history of thrombosis (as opposed to 40%–50% attributable to thrombophilia). This is likely due to the low incidence in pregnant women and appropriate prophylactic treatment [6].

TABLE 9.2

Risk Factors for Pregnancy-Related VTE

Thrombophilias	Obstetric Complications	Patient Characteristics or Conditions
Antithrombin deficiency	Preeclampsia	Advanced maternal age >35
Protein C	Gestational diabetes	Smoking
Protein S	Cesarean delivery	African American race
Factor V Leiden	Stillbirth	Heart conditions
Sickle cell trait/disease	Postpartum infection	Systemic lupus erythematosus
Prothrombin gene (20210) mutation	Antepartum hemorrhage	Diabetes mellitus
Fibrinogen gamma (FGG) 10034T variant	Postpartum hemorrhage	Hypertension
Non-O blood group	Transfusion	Inflammatory bowel disease
	Preterm birth	History of superficial thrombophlebitis
		Varicose veins
		Immobility
		Multiple gestation
		Obesity
		Hyperemesis

Source: James AH, *Birth Defects Res C Embryo Today*, 105(3), 159–166, 2015.

TABLE 9.3

Risk Factors for Postpartum VTE Stratified by Time of Occurrence

Variable	VTE	Timing
Maternal age	+++	P,AP
Birth weight (mean, kg)	+++	P,AP
Previous cesarean delivery	+	P,AP
Recurrent abortions	+++	P,AP
Grand multiparity (5+)	+++	P,AP
Obesity	+++	P,AP
Smoking	+++	P,AP
Gestational diabetes mellitus	+++	P,AP
Pregnancy-related hypertension	+++	P,AP
Cesarean delivery	+++	P > AP*
Peripartum hysterectomy	++	P > AP**
Blood products transfusion	+	P > AP***
Placental abruption	+	P,AP
Low birth weight (2.5 kg)	+++	P,AP
Gestational age <36 weeks	+++	P,AP
Stillbirth (%)	+++	P,AP

Source: Waldman M, et al., *J Matern Fetal Neonatal Med*, 28(1), 1–5, 2014.
Notes: P: puerperium; AP: after puerperium (<10 years); +/*: data is suggestive $(p > .05)$; ++/**: significant to $p < .05$; +++/***: significant to $p < .01$.

Thrombophilia

The second-most prominent risk factors for VTE are acquired or inherited hemostatic predispositions to thrombosis—in short, thrombophilia. The association between thrombophilia and adverse pregnancy outcomes in general is widely variable. Although Parunov et al. found that approximately 40%–50% of all postpartum VTE cases are associated with thrombophilia [6], the risk of VTE is highly variable by type of thrombophilia, ranging from 5% to 33% [12,39]. Predictably, the highest-risk profile is found in antiphospholipid antibody syndrome (APLS), with pregnancy-related VTE reported in 5% of women with clinical APLS and a past history of VTE, despite anticoagulant prophylaxis [41].

Obstetric Complications

Several obstetric complications have been identified over the years to be associated with an increased risk of VTE. However, reservations should be used when consulting older data, as guidelines and practice in the use of thromboprophylaxis have changed over time [6]. In general, the following complications have been associated with increased risk: gestational diabetes mellitus [31], preeclampsia [6,18,19,48], cesarean section [16,24], stillbirth [31], postpartum infections [49], bleeding during and after pregnancy [18,19,39], and peripartum hysterectomy [31,39,50]. Of note, in developed countries the rates of postpartum infection have decreased over time, possibly lessening the significance of this factor in recent years [50].

A possibly confounding association with some of the aforementioned risk factors is the receipt of blood products due to selected conditions such as cesarean delivery and postpartum hemorrhage. Multiple studies [2,15,19,31,51] have identified blood transfusions as an early contributor to VTE in puerperium. It is also possible that this increased impact of transfusions in the development of VTE is due to the red blood cell packing and preservation process, which could increase their aggregation tendency [52].

However, the converse may still be true, in which the risk associated with blood transfusions is in fact solely due to its association with the aforementioned risk factors [50].

A recent epidemiologic review [6] makes some novel observations about the risk factors identified in previous studies. Despite the fact that VTE risk after preeclampsia and cesarean section is not high compared with thrombophilia, due to the high incidence they still contribute to a large percentage of VTE events.

Likewise, although the risk of VTE in eclampsia is high, rates of eclampsia are quite low in developed countries, and thus it is only associated with a very small percentage of VTE overall. Additionally, authors concluded that preeclampsia on its own is not associated with antepartum VTE risk, it is only significant when associated with immobilization due to bed rest. However, they did find that preeclampsia is directly associated with VTE during the postpartum period.

Patient Characteristics

According to a number of population-based retrospective studies, many patient characteristics are associated with an increased risk of VTE, such as advanced maternal age >35 [17,39,53], smoking [18,19,48], autoimmune disease (e.g., SLE, dermatomyositis) [54], grand multiparity [31], pregnancy-related hypertension [31], and obesity [15,31,55–57].

Calculations from one study [58] predict that almost one-third of all VTE events could be prevented by weight loss, and this statistic should not be ignored in the case of pregnant obese women. Obesity has consistently been found to be a significant risk factor for VTE in pregnancy [15,31,55–57], and obese patients are more likely than others to suffer from post-thrombotic syndrome (PTS) after DVT [59].

After adjustment for other risk factors, multiple studies [17,31,39,60,61] have found differences in ethnicity or race to significantly impact pregnancy-related VTE risk. For example, medical comorbidities such as hypertension, sickle cell disease, and protein S and antithrombin deficiency are more common in black women with adverse pregnancy outcomes, whereas other thrombophilias are more common among white women [61].

Risk Factor Distribution in Early- versus Late-Postpartum VTE

The risk of postpartum VTE has been found to last up to 12 weeks postdelivery in women with certain complications but is significantly higher during puerperium [62,63]. Clinical practice can potentially be improved if there is a higher level of understanding of which risk factors are associated with early versus late VTE in the postpartum period.

The recent cohort study by Waldman et al. mentioned earlier [31] stratifies risk factors by the outcome of early- versus late-postpartum VTE. Of note, early and late VTE were found to share similar risk factors, with the exception of cesarean section and blood transfusion, which were more specific for early VTE. This is consistent with the aforementioned suggestion that the storage of RBC may cause increased aggregation and therefore increase propensity for VTE [52].

Long-Term Impact

Implications for Quality of Life

Quality of life (QoL) can be impaired via a multitude of factors, but most commonly, post-VTE patients suffer from impaired daily activities such as walking, reduced or inability to work, and comorbidities such as venous claudication [64]. All of this information, however, is from studies of patients with VTE unrelated to pregnancy. Extrapolating these conclusions to outcomes of pregnancy-related VTE is not ideal due to the vast differences in comorbidities and risk factors for disability between the two populations.

Unfortunately, there is a paucity of data when looking specifically at long-term outcomes from antepartum and postpartum VTE. Three studies by the same group have looked at the continuing impact of VTE related to pregnancy [64–66].

One study [64] was a cross-sectional case-control study using self-reported data from Norwegian women who gave birth between 1990 and 2003. The women were given the Ferrans and Powers QoL Index and the General Health Questionnaire to complete in the presence of a health-care professional, as well as a self-reported Villalta score to assess presence or absence of PTS. The final results of the study showed no significant difference in QoL between the two groups after adjustment for probable confounders (e.g., education, age, smoking, BMI, income). An earlier study by the same group using the Venous Insufficiency Epidemiological and Economic Study (VEINES) QoL/symptoms questionnaire had found a significant effect on QoL [65]. However, there were a few specific findings that were significantly different between the cases and controls even after adjusting for possible confounders. Cases had increased frequency of pain other than in lower limbs and felt more physically worn out after a day's work.

This study also found that cases reporting PTS demonstrated a strongly significant difference in long-term QoL, a finding consistent with a third study from the same group [66]. Even after adjusting for possible confounders, these women reported poorer health overall. They had pain not related to lower limbs more often, had more skin and psychiatric problems, used analgesic drugs and allergy medication more frequently, and spent more time on sick leave in comparison with those without PTS.

Post-Thrombotic Syndrome

VTE unrelated to pregnancy has known negative consequences, and also can cause morbidity, diminished QoL, and loss in functional status. This is particularly apparent if the individual suffers from PTS, which includes findings of leg edema, pain, skin discoloration, and less frequently, ulcers [65]. A few studies of VTE unrelated to pregnancy have identified PTS as the most significant predictor for reduced QoL [67–69]. An additional, harmful consequence of PE is chronic thromboembolic pulmonary hypertension, which occurs in 0.4%–4.0% of patients with PE, and thus likely has some significance for women with pregnancy-related PE [1].

VTE Recurrence

One meta-analysis [70] did assess the risk of recurrence of VTE in cases of provocation by a transient risk factor, of which pregnancy was included, compared with unprovoked cases. Although they did not separate out pregnancy from the rest of the data, their overall assessment was that the risk of recurrence is lowest in cases of VTE provoked by surgery, intermediate in cases provoked by a nonsurgical risk factor (e.g., estrogen therapy, leg injury, a long flight), and highest in unprovoked cases.

The risk of recurrence after unprovoked VTE is seven times higher than after surgically related VTE, and 1.5 times higher after nonsurgically provoked VTE. Pregnancy-related VTE was listed in the unprovoked category, but it actually falls in both the surgical and nonsurgical categories depending on whether a Caesarian was performed [70]. Therefore, it is possible that the risk of recurrence after pregnancy-related VTE is actually lower than in post-unprovoked VTE.

Research exploring the risk of recurrence during subsequent pregnancies has not produced conclusive data [71], particularly after first-time pregnancy-associated VTE events. However, findings include a low risk of recurrent antepartum VTE [44] and up to a threefold increase in the overall risk of recurrent thrombosis after pregnancy [45,72].

Another study [73] found women with unprovoked VTE had a significantly higher long-term risk of recurrent VTE compared with women with pregnancy-associated VTE, but a lower risk of recurrent VTE during a subsequent pregnancy. More specifically, this study found that 35% of recurrent VTE events that occurred between 6 months and 5 years after the first event were during a subsequent pregnancy in the pregnancy-associated VTE group, whereas this occurred in only 8.7% of the unprovoked group.

TABLE 9.4

Long-Term Complications following Pregnancy-Related VTE

Post-thrombotic syndrome
Chronic thromboembolic pulmonary hypertension
VTE recurrence
Increased pain (other than in lower limbs)
Physically worn out after a day's work

In terms of known, nontransient risk factors such as thrombophilia, studies have shown that it is still unclear whether thrombophilia specifically increases the risk of recurrent pregnancy-associated VTE [74]. All together, these studies suggest that women with pregnancy-associated VTE are particularly susceptible to developing VTE during subsequent pregnancies.

CONCLUSIONS

The long-term impact of pregnancy-related VTE can be defined by a combination of factors including the risk or frequency of recurrence, QoL, and the amount of ensuing comorbidities (Table 9.4). The risk of VTE recurrence is clinically important because it determines whether women with previous thrombosis should receive anticoagulation therapy during and after subsequent pregnancies. Patients with pregnancy-related VTE were more likely to have an increased frequency of pain other than in the lower limbs and felt more physically worn out after a day's work. Specifically, PTS is a strong predictor of long-term health consequences for pregnancy-related VTE.

REFERENCES

1. James AH. Thrombosis in pregnancy and maternal outcomes. *Birth Defects Res C Embryo Today*. 2015;105(3):159–66.
2. Liu S, Rouleau J, Joseph KS, et al. Epidemiology of pregnancy-associated venous thromboembolism: A population-based study in Canada. *J Obstet Gynaecol Can*. 2009;31(7):611–20.
3. Buzaglo N, Harlev A, Sergienko R, Sheiner E. Risk factors for early postpartum hemorrhage (PPH) in the first vaginal delivery, and obstetrical outcomes in subsequent pregnancy. *J Matern Neonatal Med*. 2015;28(8):932–7.
4. Sheiner E, Sarid L, Levy A, Seidman DS, Hallak M. Obstetric risk factors and outcome of pregnancies complicated with early postpartum hemorrhage: A population-based study. *J Matern Fetal Neonatal Med*. 2005;18(3):149–54.
5. Bell EJ, Lutsey PL, Basu S, et al. Lifetime risk of venous thromboembolism in two cohort studies. *Am J Med*. 2016;129(3):339.e19–26.
6. Parunov LA, Soshitova NP, Ovanesov MV, Panteleev MA, Serebriyskiy II. Epidemiology of venous thromboembolism (VTE) associated with pregnancy. *Birth Defects Res C Embryo Today*. 2015;105(3):167–84.
7. Samama MM. An epidemiologic study of risk factors for deep vein thrombosis in medical outpatients: The Sirius study. *Arch Intern Med*. 2000;160(22):3415–20.
8. Murphy P, Phillips G, Hall A, Brooks S. *Women's Health Stats and Facts*. 2011 http://www.acog.org/~/media/NewsRoom/MediaKit.pdf.
9. Sultan AA, West J, Tata LJ, Fleming KM, Nelson-Piercy C, Grainge MJ. Risk of first venous thromboembolism in and around pregnancy: A population-based cohort study. *Br J Haematol*. 2012;156(3):366–73.
10. Coon WW, Willis PW, Keller JB. Venous thromboembolism and other venous disease in the Tecumseh Community Health Study. *Circulation*. 1973;48:839–46.
11. Heit JA, Kobbervig CE, James AH, Petterson TM, Bailey KR, Melton LJ. Trends in the incidence of venous thromboembolism during pregnancy or postpartum: A 30-year population-based study. *Ann Intern Med*. 2005;143(10):697–706.
12. Pomp ER, Lenselink AM, Rosendaal FR, Doggen CJM. Pregnancy, the postpartum period and prothrombotic defects: Risk of venous thrombosis in the MEGA study. *J Thromb Haemost*. 2008;6(4):632–7.

13. James AH. Pregnancy-associated thrombosis. *Hematology Am Soc Hematol Educ Program.* 2009;1:277–85.

14. Andersen BS, Steffensen FH, Sørensen HT, Nielsen GL, Olsen J. The cumulative incidence of venous thromboembolism during pregnancy and puerperium: An 11 year Danish population-based study of 63,300 pregnancies. *Acta Obstet Gynecol Scand.* 1998;77(2):170–73.

15. James AH, Jamison MG, Brancazio LR, Myers ER. Venous thromboembolism during pregnancy and the postpartum period: Incidence, risk factors, and mortality. *Am J Obstet Gynecol.* 2006;194(5):1311–15.

16. Gherman RB, Goodwin TM, Leung B, Byrne JD, Hethumumi R, Montoro M. Incidence, clinical characteristics, and timing of objectively diagnosed venous thromboembolism during pregnancy. *Obstet Gynecol.* 1999; 94 (5 Pt 1): 730–34.

17. Lindqvist P, Dahlbäck B, Maršál K. Thrombotic risk during pregnancy: A population study. *Obstet Gynecol.* 1999;94(4):595–9.

18. Simpson EL, Lawrenson RA, Nightingale AL, Farmer RD. Venous thromboembolism in pregnancy and the puerperium: Incidence and additional risk factors from a London perinatal database. *BJOG.* 2001;108(1):56–60.

19. Jacobsen AF, Skjeldestad FE, Sandset PM. Incidence and risk patterns of venous thromboembolism in pregnancy and puerperium: A register-based case-control study. *Am J Obstet Gynecol.* 2008;198(2):233. e1–7.

20. Kourlaba G, Relakis J, Kontodimas S, Holm MV, Maniadakis N. A systematic review and meta-analysis of the epidemiology and burden of venous thromboembolism among pregnant women. *Int J Gynaecol Obstet.* 2015;132(1):4–10.

21. Gader AA, Haggaz AED, Adam I. Epidemiology of deep venous thrombosis during pregnancy and puerperium in Sudanese women. *Vasc Health Risk Manag.* 2009;5(1):85–7.

22. McColl MD, Ramsay JE, Tait RC, et al. Risk factors for pregnancy associated venous thromboembolism. *Thromb Haemost.* 1997;78(4):1183–8.

23. American College of Obstetricians and Gynecologists. Thromboembolism in pregnancy. ACOG Practice Bulletin no. 123. *Obstet Gynecol.* 2011;118(3):718–29.

24. Blanco-Molina A, Rota LL, Di Micco P, et al. Venous thromboembolism during pregnancy, postpartum or during contraceptive use. *Thromb Haemost.* 2010;103(2):306–11.

25. Ray JG, Chan WS. Deep vein thrombosis during pregnancy and the puerperium: A meta-analysis of the period of risk and the leg of presentation. *Obstet Gynecol Surv.* 1999;54(4):265–71.

26. Virkus RA, Løkkegaard ECL, Bergholt T, Mogensen U, Langhoff-Roos J, Lidegaard Ø. Venous thromboembolism in pregnant and puerperal women in Denmark 1995–2005: A national cohort study. *Thromb Haemost.* 2011;106(2):304–9.

27. Soomro RM, Bucur IJ, Noorani S. Cumulative incidence of venous thromboembolism during pregnancy and puerperium: A hospital-based study. *Angiology.* 2002;53(4):429–34.

28. Jang MJ, Bang S, Oh D. Incidence of venous thromboembolism in Korea: From the health insurance review and assessment service database. *J Thromb Haemost.* 2011;9(1):85–91.

29. Brown HL, Hiett AK. Deep vein thrombosis and pulmonary embolism in pregnancy: Diagnosis, complications, and management. *Clin Obstet Gynecol.* 2010;53(2):345–59.

30. Marik PE. Venous thromboembolism in pregnancy. *Clin Chest Med.* 2010;31(4):731–40.

31. Waldman M, Sheiner E, Sergienko R, Shoham-Vardi I. Can we identify risk factors during pregnancy for thrombo-embolic events during the puerperium and later in life? *J Matern Fetal Neonatal Med.* 2015;28(9):1005–9.

32. Marik PE, Plante LA. Venous thromboembolic disease and pregnancy. *N Engl J Med.* 2008;359(19):2025–33.

33. Meignan M, Rosso J, Gauthier H, et al. Systematic lung scans reveal a high frequency of silent pulmonary embolism in patients with proximal deep venous thrombosis. *Arch Intern Med.* 2000;160(2):159–64.

34. Say L, Chou D, Gemmill A, et al. Global causes of maternal death: A WHO systematic analysis. *Lancet Glob Heal.* 2014;2(6):e323–33.

35. James AH. Venous thromboembolism in pregnancy. *Arterioscler Thromb Vasc Biol.* 2009;29(3):326–31.

36. Bremme KA. Haemostatic changes in pregnancy. *Best Pract Res Clin Haematol.* 2003;16(2):153–68.

37. Jackson E, Curtis KM, Gaffield ME. Risk of venous thromboembolism during the postpartum period: A systematic review. *Obstet Gynecol.* 2011;117(3):691–703.

38. Martineau M, Nelson-Piercy C. Venous thromboembolic disease and pregnancy. *Postgrad Med J.* 2009;85(1007):489–94.

39. Ralli E, Zezza L, Caserta D. Pregnancy and venous thromboembolism. *Curr Opin Obstet Gynecol.* 2014;26(6):469–75.

40. Goodrich SM, Wood JE. Peripheral venous distensibility and velocity of venous blood flow during pregnancy or during oral contraceptive therapy. *Am J Obstet Gynecol.* 1964;90:740–44.

41. Wright H, Osborn S, Edmunds D. Changes in the rate of flow of venous blood in the leg during pregnancy, measured with radioactive sodium. *Surg Gynecol Obs.* 1950;90:481–5.

42. Bourjeily G, Paidas M, Khalil H, Rosene-Montella K, Rodger M. Pulmonary embolism in pregnancy. *Lancet (London).* 2010;375(9713):500–512.

43. James AH. Prevention and treatment of venous thromboembolism in pregnancy. *Clin Obstet Gynecol.* 2012;55(3):774–87.

44. Brill-Edwards P, Ginsberg JS, Gent M, et al. Safety of withholding heparin in pregnant women with a history of venous thromboembolism: Recurrence of clot in this pregnancy study group. *N Engl J Med.* 2000;343(20):1439–44.

45. De Stefano V, Martinelli I, Rossi E, et al. The risk of recurrent venous thromboembolism in pregnancy and puerperium without antithrombotic prophylaxis. *Br J Haematol.* 2006;135(3):386–91.

46. Roeters van Lennep JE, Meijer E, Klumper FJCM, Middeldorp JM, Bloemenkamp KWM, Middeldorp S. Prophylaxis with low-dose low-molecular-weight heparin during pregnancy and postpartum: Is it effective? *J Thromb Haemost.* 2011;9(3):473–80.

47. Bramham K, Hunt B, Germain S, et al. Pregnancy outcome in different clinical phenotypes of antiphospholipid syndrome. *Lupus.* 2009;19(1):58–64.

48. Larsen TB, Sørensen HT, Gislum M, Johnsen SP. Maternal smoking, obesity, and risk of venous thromboembolism during pregnancy and the puerperium: A population-based nested case-control study. *Thromb Res.* 2007;120(4):505–9.

49. James AH, Tapson VF, Goldhaber SZ. Thrombosis during pregnancy and the postpartum period. *Am J Obstet Gynecol.* 2005;193(1):216–9.

50. Ghaji N, Boulet SL, Tepper N, Hooper W. Trends in venous thromboembolism among pregnancy-related hospitalizations, United States, 1994–2009. *Am J Obstet Gynecol.* 2013;209(5):433.e1–8.

51. Danilenko-Dixon DR, Heit JA, Silverstein MD, et al. Risk factors for deep vein thrombosis and pulmonary embolism during pregnancy or post partum: A population-based, case-control study. *Am J Obstet Gynecol.* 2001;184(2):104–10.

52. Ho J, Sibbald WJ, Chin-Yee IH. Effects of storage on efficacy of red cell transfusion: When is it not safe? *Crit Care Med.* 2003;31(12 Suppl):S687–97.

53. Bates SM. Pregnancy-associated venous thromboembolism: Prevention and treatment. *Semin Hematol.* 2011;48(4):271–84.

54. Bleau N, Patenaude V, Abenhaim HA. Risk of venous thromboembolic events in pregnant patients with autoimmune diseases: A population-based study. *Clin Appl Thromb.* 2016;22(3):285–91 [E-pub 2014 Oct 7].

55. Drife J. Deep venous thrombosis and pulmonary embolism in obese women. *Best Pract Res Clin Obstet Gynaecol.* 2015;29(3):365–76.

56. Jensen TB, Gerds TA, Grøn R, et al. Risk factors for venous thromboembolism during pregnancy. *Pharmacoepidemiol Drug Saf.* 2013;22(12):1283–91.

57. Virkus RA, Løkkegaard E, Lidegaard Ø, et al. Risk factors for venous thromboembolism in 1.3 million pregnancies: A nationwide prospective cohort. *PLoS One.* 2014;9(5):e96495.

58. Pomp ER, le Cessie S, Rosendaal FR, Doggen CJM. Risk of venous thrombosis: Obesity and its joint effect with oral contraceptive use and prothrombotic mutations. *Br J Haematol.* 2007;139(2):289–96.

59. Tick LW, Kramer MHH, Rosendaal FR, Faber WR, Doggen CJM. Risk factors for post-thrombotic syndrome in patients with a first deep venous thrombosis. *J Thromb Haemost.* 2008;6(12):2075–81.

60. Blondon M, Harrington LB, Righini M, Boehlen F, Bounameaux H, Smith NL. Racial and ethnic differences in the risk of postpartum venous thromboembolism: A population-based, case-control study. *J Thromb Haemost.* 2014;12(12):2002–9.

61. Philipp CS, Faiz AS, Beckman MG, et al. Differences in thrombotic risk factors in black and white women with adverse pregnancy outcome. *Thromb Res.* 2014;133(1):108–11.

62. Tepper NK, Boulet SL, Whiteman MK, et al. Postpartum venous thromboembolism: Incidence and risk factors. *Obstet Gynecol.* 2014;123(5):987–96.

63. Kamel H, Navi BB, Sriram N, Hovsepian DA, Devereux RB, Elkind MSV. Risk of a thrombotic event after the 6-week postpartum period. *N Engl J Med*. 2014;370(14):1307–15.
64. Wik HS, Jacobsen AF, Sandvik L, Sandset PM. Long-term impact of pregnancy-related venous thrombosis on quality-of-life, general health and functioning: Results of a cross-sectional, case-control study. *BMJ Open*. 2012;2(6).
65. Wik HS, Enden TR, Jacobsen AF, Sandset PM. Long-term quality of life after pregnancy-related deep vein thrombosis and the influence of socioeconomic factors and comorbidity. *J Thromb Haemost*. 2011;9(10):1931–6.
66. Wik HS, Jacobsen AF, Sandvik L, Sandset PM. Prevalence and predictors for post-thrombotic syndrome 3 to 16 years after pregnancy-related venous thrombosis: A population-based, cross-sectional, case-control study. *J Thromb Haemost*. 2012;10(5):840–47.
67. Klok FA, van Kralingen KW, van Dijk APJ, et al. Quality of life in long-term survivors of acute pulmonary embolism. *Chest*. 2010;138(6):1432–40.
68. van Korlaar IM, Vossen CY, Rosendaal FR, et al. The impact of venous thrombosis on quality of life. *Thromb Res*. 2004;114(1):11–18.
69. Kahn SR, Shbaklo H, Lamping DL, et al. Determinants of health-related quality of life during the 2 years following deep vein thrombosis. *J Thromb Haemost*. 2008;6(7):1105–12.
70. Iorio A, Kearon C, Filippucci E, et al. Risk of recurrence after a first episode of symptomatic venous thromboembolism provoked by a transient risk factor: A systematic review. *Arch Intern Med*. 2010;170(19):1710–16.
71. Bates SM, Greer IA, Middeldorp S, Veenstra DL, Prabulos AM, Vandvik PO. VTE, thrombophilia, antithrombotic therapy, and pregnancy: Antithrombotic therapy and prevention of thrombosis, 9th ed: American College of Chest Physicians evidence-based clinical practice guidelines. *Chest*. 2012;141(2 Suppl):e691S–e736S.
72. Pabinger I, Grafenhofer H, Kyrle PA, et al. Temporary increase in the risk for recurrence during pregnancy in women with a history of venous thromboembolism. *Blood*. 2002;100(3):1060–62.
73. White RH, Chan WS, Zhou H, Ginsberg JS. Recurrent venous thromboembolism after pregnancy-associated versus unprovoked thromboembolism. *Thromb Haemost*. 2008;100(2):246–52.
74. James AH, Grotegut CA, Brancazio LR, Brown H. Thromboembolism in pregnancy: Recurrence and its prevention. *Semin Perinatol*. 2007;31(3):167–75.

10

Cholestasis and Long-Term Maternal Morbidity

Hanns-Ulrich Marschall

Introduction

Cholestasis is an impairment of bile formation and/or bile flow, which may clinically present with fatigue, pruritus, and jaundice. Biochemical markers include increases in serum alkaline phosphatase (ALP) and gamma-glutamyltranspeptidase (γGT), followed by conjugated hyperbilirubinemia at more advanced stages [1]. Cholestasis may be classified as extrahepatic, caused by mechanical obstruction due to bile duct stones, tumors, cysts, or strictures, or intrahepatic, resulting from hepatocellular functional defects or from obstructive lesions of the intrahepatic biliary tract distal from bile canaliculi [1].

In women of childbearing age, the most prevalent diseases with intrahepatic cholestasis are intrahepatic cholestasis of pregnancy (ICP), primary biliary cholangitis (PBC), and primary sclerosing cholangitis (PSC).

In ICP, the liver does not show any morphological changes; thus, the intrahepatic cholestasis is based on a functional, and after delivery fully reversible, defect. PBC is histologically characterized by immune destruction of the interlobular bile ducts resulting in a gradually progressive ductopenia, whereas in PSC, inflammation, fibrosis, and destruction of the intrahepatic and extrahepatic bile ducts occurs with multiple areas of stricturing in the biliary tree.

Intrahepatic Cholestasis of Pregnancy

ICP is the most common pregnancy-specific liver disease, with reported incidence rates between 0.2% and 2.0% in different countries [2–4]. In some populations and in women with a multiple pregnancy, incidence rates up to 22% have been reported. The characteristics of ICP are presented in Table 10.1 and include otherwise unexplained pruritus in the late-second and third trimesters of pregnancy, elevated bile acids, and spontaneous clinical and biochemical normalization within a few weeks after delivery. Transaminases (ALT/AST) are elevated in about 80% of cases. ALP levels are of limited diagnostic value due to large amounts of the placental isoform in the third trimester. The levels of γGT are commonly normal. An elevation of bilirubin is found in 10%–20% of women with ICP and may indicate a severe form. Overt jaundice is more suggestive of viral hepatitis [5].

The etiology of ICP is multifactorial, with genetic, environmental, and hormonal factors playing important roles. The central role of hormonal factors is supported by the higher incidence of cholestasis in twin pregnancies and the fact that predisposed women often suffered from pruritus when taking oral contraceptives. It has been suggested that the combination of increased synthesis and impaired biliary excretion of sulfated progesterone metabolites is closely associated with the severity of pruritus. Heterozygous mutations and polymorphisms in the bile acid transporters and membrane integrity genes ABCB4, ABCB11, and ATP8B1 and their regulating nuclear receptor FXR may result in ICP in the increased hormonal milieu of pregnancy [2,3,6]. Modern management of ICP consists of symptomatic treatment of pruritus with ursodeoxycholic acid (UDCA) and early elective delivery, although evidence from randomized controlled trials for this common practice is still missing [5].

TABLE 10.1

Diagnostic Criteria of Intrahepatic Cholestasis of Pregnancy

1	Otherwise unexplained pruritus in late-second and third trimester
2	Elevated bile acids (10–14 µmol/L; repeated testing might be necessary) and/or transaminases
3	Spontaneous relief of pruritus and complete normalization of biochemical aberrations within a few weeks after delivery

Fetal and Maternal Risks in Intrahepatic Cholestasis of Pregnancy

ICP is an established risk condition for the unborn child (Table 10.2). Recent data indicate that ICP also puts the mother at risk (Table 10.3).

Fetal Risks

ICP is associated with preterm delivery and poor perinatal outcome [7], including intrauterine fetal death (IUFD) [2]. In the largest prospective observational study from Sweden, which identified 693 cases of ICP among 45,485 pregnancies, a 1%–2% increase in risk of spontaneous preterm labor, asphyxial events (defined as operative delivery due to asphyxia, Apgar score <7 at 5 minutes, or arterial cord pH <7.05), or meconium staining of the amniotic fluid and/or placenta and membranes was observed for every additional µmol/L of maternal serum bile acids [8]. However, this study did not find an increase in adverse outcomes in mild ICP and moderately elevated bile acid levels (10–40 µmol/L) compared with women with pruritus but normal bile acid levels (<10 µmol/L). A recent retrospective study from the Netherlands analyzed the outcome of 215 women with ICP that was classified as mild (bile acids 10–39 µmol/L), moderate (bile acids 40–99 µmol/L), or severe (bile acids >100 µmol/L). Spontaneous preterm birth (19.0%), meconium-stained fluid (47.6%), and perinatal death (9.5%) occurred significantly more often in cases with severe ICP [9] (Table 10.2).

Stillbirth is the most feared complication of ICP. The overall risk of stillbirth in ICP is difficult to estimate as its etiology is unknown and fetal autopsy is usually normal [2]. A recent large prospective population-based case-control study from the United Kingdom confirmed the increased risk of IUFD at least in severe ICP, defined as serum bile acids >40 µmol/L (adjusted OR 2.58, 95% CI 1.03–6.49) [10]. A doubling of serum bile acid levels correlated with a 200% increase in the risk of IUFD, and also other fetal complications increased with increasing serum bile acid levels. Of note, 7 of the reported 10 ICP cases of stillbirth had coexisting pregnancy complications, such as preeclampsia ($n = 2$), gestational diabetes ($n = 3$), and nonspecified complications [10].

Preeclampsia and gestational diabetes both are common complications of pregnancy that increase the risk of ICP about threefold [7,11].

TABLE 10.2

Fetal Risks of Intrahepatic Cholestasis of Pregnancy

	%[a]
Spontaneous preterm labor	30–40
Iatrogenic preterm delivery	30–60
Meconium staining of amniotic fluid and placenta	20–80
Intrauterine fetal death (stillbirth)	<1

[a] Incidence rates from various studies.

TABLE 10.3

Maternal Risks of Intrahepatic
Cholestasis of Pregnancy

	Risk[a]
Later Hepatobiliary Disease	2.62
Hepatitis C/chronic hepatitis	4.16
Fibrosis/cirrhosis	5.11
Gallstone disease/cholangitis	2.72
Cholangitis	4.22
Liver cancer	3.61
Biliary tree cancer	2.62
Later Autoimmune Disease	1.28
Diabetes mellitus	1.47
Thyroid disease	1.30
Psoriasis	1.27
Inflammatory polyarthropathies	1.32
Crohn's disease	1.55
Later Cardiovascular Disease	1.12

[a] Hazard ratios compared with pregnant women without ICP.

Maternal Risks

Long-standing severe cholestasis may be complicated by steatorrhea and vitamin K deficiency, leading to postpartum hemorrhage. Otherwise, for the mother, ICP has for a long time only been considered as an annoying but not serious condition that spontaneously resolves after delivery.

However, ICP obviously is not such a benign condition for the mother: studies from Finland [12] and Sweden [13] showed that women with ICP have a three- to five-times-increased risk of hepatobiliary diseases such as hepatitis C, cirrhosis, and gallstones.

The Swedish study analyzed data of women with births between 1973 and 2009 registered in the Swedish Medical Birth Register. By linkage with the Swedish Patient Register, 11,388 women with ICP were identified who were matched to 113,893 women without this diagnosis. Diagnosis of preexisting or later hepatobiliary disease was obtained from the patient register. Women with ICP were more often diagnosed with later hepatobiliary disease (HR 2.62, 95% CI 2.47–2.77; increment at 1% per year), hepatitis C or chronic hepatitis (HR 4.16, 95% CI 3.14–5.51, and 5.96, 95% CI 3.43–10.33, respectively), fibrosis/cirrhosis (HR 5.11, 3.29–7.96), or gallstone disease or cholangitis (HR 2.72, 95% CI 2.55–2.91, and 4.22, 95% CI 3.13–5.69, respectively), compared with women without ICP ($p < .0001$ for all HRs). Later ICP was more common in women with prepregnancy hepatitis C (OR 5.76, 95% CI 1.30–25.44; $p = .021$), chronic hepatitis (OR 8.66, 95% CI 1.05–71.48; $p = .045$), and gallstone disease (OR 3.29, 95% CI 2.02–5.36; $p < .0001$). Thus, an increased risk of hepatobiliary disease was found both before and after ICP diagnosis and was not related to age at first ICP, number of earlier pregnancies, or smoking status [13] (Table 10.3).

In an extension of the Swedish population-based study, it was found that women once diagnosed with ICP had an increased risk for later liver and biliary tree cancer (HR 3.61, 95% CI 1.68–7.77, and 2.62, 95% CI 1.26–5.46, respectively). Even after adjusting for a diagnosis of hepatitis C, which was very strongly associated with liver cancer (HR 31.23, 95% CI 9.90–99.52; $p < .001$), women with ICP were still at increased risk of later liver malignancy (HR 2.66, 95% CI 1.16–6.12; $p = .021$) [14] (Table 10.3).

From these data it is concluded that although pruritus without skin affection in the late-second and third trimesters of pregnancy together with elevated bile acids and/or transaminases is highly predictive of ICP, other liver diseases need to be excluded, in particular hepatitis C. The high prevalence of hepatitis C infection in women with ICP may be due to an enhanced susceptibility to hepatitis C infection in ICP and vice versa. Prevalent hepatitis C infection may also worsen cholestatic pruritus under high estrogen and progesterone loads of late pregnancy when potentially itch-related enzymes such as autotaxin are also markedly elevated [15]. Mothers should be followed up for the normalization of liver function test 6–12 weeks after delivery, irrespective of persisting pruritus, and referred to a hepatologist for further evaluation if elevated [5].

The Swedish study also found ICP to be associated with later immune-mediated diseases (HR 1.28, 95% CI 1.19–1.38), and specifically, diabetes mellitus (HR 1.47, 95% CI 1.26–1.72), thyroid disease (HR 1.30, 95% CI 1.14–1.47), psoriasis (HR 1.27, 95% CI 1.07–1.51), inflammatory polyarthropathies (HR 1.32, 95% CI 1.11–1.58), and Crohn's disease (HR 1.55, 95% CI 1.14–2.10), but not ulcerative colitis (HR 1.21, 95% CI 0.93–1.58). Women with ICP also had a small increased risk of later cardiovascular disease (HR 1.12, 95% CI 1.06–1.19), in particular if the woman with ICP also suffered from preeclampsia [14]. At this point, no specific conclusion or advice to a pregnant woman diagnosed with ICP can be given based on these data. ICP at least is not associated with genetic markers of autoimmunity [6] (Table 10.3).

Contraception after Delivery

Although estrogen has been linked to ICP, it is possible for women with a prior history of ICP to use combined oral contraceptives, as most progesterone-containing contraception is not associated with hepatic impairment. However, these women should be advised of the risk of pruritus and elevated liver enzymes when using combined pills. They can commence oral contraceptives with low-dose estrogen or progesterone-only products once the liver tests have normalized following delivery.

Primary Biliary Cholangitis

PBC is an autoimmune liver disease that primarily (90%) affects women, most of them older than 40 years, while pregnancies are rare. The course of PBC is good for those (about two out of three) who respond to treatment with ursodeoxycholic acid (UDCA) with the normalization of ALP. However, in the remaining one-third, PBC may progress to cirrhosis with liver failure and the need for liver transplantation.

Primary Sclerosing Cholangitis

PSC also features signs of autoimmunity but affects both genders in about equal amounts. About 75% of all patients with PSC also have inflammatory bowel disease, 80% of them ulcerative colitis. PBC bears a substantially increased risk of biliary and colorectal malignancies. Predictive markers of progression are lacking, and in Scandinavia, PSC is the major indication for liver transplantation. Pregnancy in women with PSC occurs even less often than in PBC and is associated with prematurity and an increased need for Cesarean section. Fortunately, pregnancy in PSC is not associated with fetal malformation or other complications when pregnancy is not contraindicated [16,17].

Pregnancy after Liver Transplantation

Women of childbearing potential may have healthy children after liver transplantation (similar to the general population) [18–20]. Complications of pregnancies are preeclampsia, preterm delivery, higher rates of cesarean section, and graft rejection.

As fertility following transplantation is restored in the majority of women, as early as 1 month post-transplantation, discussion regarding appropriate contraceptive use is imperative. A year's wait after transplantation is recommended to achieve stable immunosuppression, mainly tacrolimus and/or prednisolone, azathioprine, and cyclosporine. Mycophenolate is associated with congenital abnormalities and should be discontinued with at least a 6-month washout period before conception.

CONCLUSIONS

The most common cholestatic condition in pregnancy is ICP, characterized by pruritus and elevated bile acids, with clinical and biochemical normalization after delivery. Whereas ICP is an established risk factor for the fetus, recent data indicate ICP as a risk condition also for the mother, associated in particular with chronic hepatitis C virus (HCV) and its complications, such as cirrhosis and liver cancer. The mother thus should be tested for HCV (and if positive, treated after delivery) and followed up with liver function tests even without persisting pruritus.

REFERENCES

1. European Association for the Study of the Liver. Management of cholestatic liver diseases. EASL Clinical Practice Guidelines. *J Hepatol*. 2009;51(2):237–67.
2. Geenes V, Williamson C. Intrahepatic cholestasis of pregnancy. *World J Gastroenterol*. 2009;15(17):2049–66.
3. Lammert F, Marschall HU, Glantz A, Matern S. Intrahepatic cholestasis of pregnancy: Molecular pathogenesis, diagnosis and management. *J Hepatol*. 2000;33(6):1012–21.
4. Williamson C, Geenes V. Intrahepatic cholestasis of pregnancy. *Obstet Gynecol*. 2014;124(1):120–33.
5. Marschall HU. Management of intrahepatic cholestasis of pregnancy. *Expert Rev Gastroenterol Hepatol*. 2015;9(10):1273–9.
6. Dixon PH, Wadsworth CA, Chambers J, et al. A comprehensive analysis of common genetic variation around six candidate loci for intrahepatic cholestasis of pregnancy. *Am J Gastroenterol*. 2014;109(1):76–84.
7. Wikstrom Shemer E, Marschall HU, Ludvigsson JF, Stephansson O. Intrahepatic cholestasis of pregnancy and associated adverse pregnancy and fetal outcomes: A 12-year population-based cohort study. *BJOG*. 2013;120(6):717–23.
8. Glantz A, Marschall HU, Mattsson LA. Intrahepatic cholestasis of pregnancy: Relationships between bile acid levels and fetal complication rates. *Hepatology*. 2004;40(2):467–74.
9. Brouwers L, Koster MP, Page-Christiaens GC, et al. Intrahepatic cholestasis of pregnancy: Maternal and fetal outcomes associated with elevated bile acid levels. *Am J Obstet Gynecol*. 2015;212(1):100.e1–7.
10. Geenes V, Chappell LC, Seed PT, Steer PJ, Knight M, Williamson C. Association of severe intrahepatic cholestasis of pregnancy with adverse pregnancy outcomes: A prospective population-based case-control study. *Hepatology*. 2014;59(4):1482–91.
11. Martineau M, Raker C, Powrie R, Williamson C. Intrahepatic cholestasis of pregnancy is associated with an increased risk of gestational diabetes. *Eur J Obstet Gynecol Reprod Biol*. 2014;176:80–85.
12. Ropponen A, Sund R, Riikonen S, Ylikorkala O, Aittomaki K. Intrahepatic cholestasis of pregnancy as an indicator of liver and biliary diseases: A population-based study. *Hepatology*. 2006;43(4):723–8.
13. Marschall HU, Wikstrom Shemer E, Ludvigsson JF, Stephansson O. Intrahepatic cholestasis of pregnancy and associated hepatobiliary disease: A population-based cohort study. *Hepatology*. 2013;58(4):1385–91.
14. Wikstrom Shemer EA, Stephansson O, Thuresson M, Thorsell M, Ludvigsson JF, Marschall HU. Intrahepatic cholestasis of pregnancy and cancer, immune-mediated and cardiovascular diseases: A population-based cohort study. *J Hepatol*. 2015;63(2):456–61.
15. Abu-Hayyeh S, Ovadia C, Lieu T, et al. Prognostic and mechanistic potential of progesterone sulfates in intrahepatic cholestasis of pregnancy and pruritus gravidarum. *Hepatology*. 2015;64(4):1287–98.
16. Ludvigsson JF, Bergquist A, Ajne G, Kane S, Ekbom A, Stephansson O. A population-based cohort study of pregnancy outcomes among women with primary sclerosing cholangitis. *Clin Gastroenterol Hepatol*. 2014;12(1):95–100.e1.
17. Wellge BE, Sterneck M, Teufel A, et al. Pregnancy in primary sclerosing cholangitis. *Gut*. 2011;60(8):1117–21.
18. Blume C, Sensoy A, Gross MM, et al. A comparison of the outcome of pregnancies after liver and kidney transplantation. *Transplantation*. 2013;95(1):222–7.
19. Deshpande NA, James NT, Kucirka LM, et al. Pregnancy outcomes of liver transplant recipients: A systematic review and meta-analysis. *Liver Transpl*. 2012;18(6):621–9.
20. Westbrook RH, Dusheiko G, Williamson C. Pregnancy and liver disease. *J Hepatol*. 2015 ePub.

11

Fertility Treatment and Maternal Cardiovascular Risk

Judah Weiss and Avi Harlev

Introduction

Infertility is a common medical issue and has been reported in approximately 10% of couples [1]. It is defined as a failure of conception after 12 months of unprotected and frequent intercourse [2]. There are many etiologic causes of infertility including both male and female factors. Approximately 26% of infertility can be attributed to male factors. Other causes including ovulatory dysfunction (21%), endometriosis (6%), and cervical and mechanical factors such as tubal occlusions (17%) account for female infertility. Another factor that plays a role is coital failure and accounts for up to 6% of cases. There is also a significant amount of unexplained causes (Figure 11.1) [3,4]. Another factor to consider for the high rates of infertility can be ascribed to increasing maternal age after the first successful delivery [5].

Assisted reproductive technology (ART) describes the techniques used to treat infertility via ovulation induction (OI) followed by timed intercourse, intrauterine insemination, or in vitro fertilization (IVF). These techniques have been used increasingly in recent decades [6]. The first successful birth utilizing IVF was in 1978 [7]. Since then, 1.5% of all births in the United States have been facilitated through IVF [8]. The incidence of multiple births in IVF is particularly high, accounting for 20% of all such cases [6].

Ovulation Induction and IVF

A major part of ART treatment is OI. As explained by Beckmann et al. [2], indications for OI include anovulation and oligoovulation. Before OI is considered, possible causes of anovulation such as polycystic ovarian syndrome, hypothyroidism, anorexia nervosa, and stress should be considered and treated if diagnosed. Normally, the corpus luteum produces estrogen and progesterone, which inhibit the release of luteinizing hormone, follicle-stimulating hormone, and gonadotropin-releasing hormone. If fertilization does not take place, the corpus luteum deteriorates in the absence of human chorionic gonadotropin (hCG).

OI can be achieved by several agents. Clomiphene citrate is a selective estrogen receptor modulator and is a commonly used medication in OI. By competitively inhibiting estrogen receptors in the hypothalamus and pituitary, there is inhibition of the negative feedback of estrogen on gonadotropin release. The timing of clomiphene citrate administration is important. It is started between days 3 to 5 of the menstrual cycle for 5 days. During that time of the menstrual cycle, FSH is increasing and producing follicles, which in turn produce estrogen. Since the negative feedback effect of estrogen on gonadotropin is inhibited by clomiphene, there is an increased GnRH release, which causes an increased release of FSH and LH. The increased FSH leads to an increased production of follicles. If the amount of clomiphene is adequate, ovulation should occur between 5 to 12 days after the last dose. Clomiphene citrate administration has potential adverse outcomes. Risks include a slightly increased risk of ovarian hyperstimulation syndrome (OHSS) and ovarian cyst formation [2].

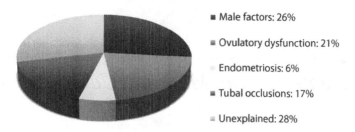

- Male factors: 26%
- Ovulatory dysfunction: 21%
- Endometriosis: 6%
- Tubal occlusions: 17%
- Unexplained: 28%

FIGURE 11.1   Causes of infertility. (Adapted from Hull MG, et al., *Br Med J (Clin Res Ed)*, 291(6510), 1693–7, 1985.)

A different approach to OI involves the use of gonadotropins. There are several protocols that can be used. The long protocol uses a GnRH agonist to control the menstrual cycle and is administered for 2 weeks until LH production from the pituitary is inhibited. A decrease in LH release prevents the LH surge prior to fully mature ovarian follicles. FSH is concurrently administered to trigger follicular growth. The other approach uses a GnRH antagonist, which controls the menstrual cycle by inhibiting LH and FSH. It controls the cycle quicker when compared with the use of a GnRH agonist. It is commonly administered on day 7 of the menstrual cycle and continued daily until maturation of the follicles. Recombinant hCG is then given to elicit ovulation and maintain the corpus luteum. The main potential adverse outcomes of gonadotropin administration include multiple pregnancy, ectopic pregnancy, and OHSS [2].

Ovarian stimulation is one of the first steps involved in IVF. After ovarian stimulation, oocytes are extracted from the ovaries using transvaginal ultrasound-guided follicular aspiration. In cases of good semen parameters, fertilization can be accomplished by inseminating the oocytes with spermatozoa while in a medium culture. In cases of abnormal sperm parameters, spermatozoa can be injected directly to the ovum. After fertilization of the oocyte is confirmed, the embryo is transferred to the uterus [2]. The experience of the person performing the implantation and the type of catheter used has shown to affect implantation success [9–11]. The optimal time to transfer the embryo is debated and is either performed after day 2, 3 or 5, when the blastocyst is formed [12]. Progesterone is administered during the luteal phase to enhance endometrial receptivity and increase the chances of implantation. It can be administered either intramuscularly or vaginally [2].

Maternal Adverse Outcomes after Infertility Treatment

IVF is a relatively new medical technique, and long-term maternal complications are only recently being discovered. With an increasing number of women, particularly older women, who try to conceive by IVF [13], it is important to address its potential short- and long-term adverse outcomes. Most of the short-term complications can be attributed to OHSS, bleeding, infection, or damage to adjacent organs during the ovum harvesting. Hormonal stimulation resulting in increased estrogen levels is a major cause of the long-term complications.

The aim of this chapter is to investigate whether there is an increased risk of long-term maternal cardiovascular morbidity after undergoing fertility treatment, specifically IVF or OI.

Before discussing the potential maternal cardiovascular complications, many other adverse outcomes after receiving infertility treatment have been documented. In the United Kingdom, 25% of maternal mortality from IVF treatment was due to OHSS [13]. Additional complications include abdominal bleeding and ovarian torsion [14,15]. Patients who have undergone fertility treatment were previously reported to have a higher risk of developing obstetric complications including preeclampsia, placental abruption, placenta previa, and the premature rupture of membranes (Table 11.1) [16]. Women who received infertility treatments had a significantly higher perinatal mortality rate when compared with a control group [15,17].

TABLE 11.1

Adverse Perinatal Outcomes following Fertility Treatment (Results from Selected Studies)

Complication	Experimental Group ART (%)	Control Group (%)	p Value	Hazard Ratio	95% CI	Source
Perinatal mortality	3.3 (IVF) 2.1 (OI)	1.3	<.001	N/A	N/A	Silberstein et al. 2014 [17]
Nonreassuring fetal heart rate	4.2 (IVF) 2.1 (OI)	1.8	<.001	N/A	N/A	Silberstein et al. 2014 [17]
Ovarian torsion	0.08	0.01	<0.05	11	5.7–20.0	Kallen et al. 2005 [16]
Maternal hypertension	0.022	0.018	<0.05	1.27	1.13–1.41	Westerlund et al. 2014 [28]
Severe preeclampsia	2.7 (IVF) 1.8 (OI)	1.1	<.001	N/A	N/A	Silberstein et al. 2014 [17]
Placental abruption	2.3 (IVF) 1.0 (OI)	0.7	<.001	N/A	N/A	Silberstein et al. 2014 [17]
Placenta previa	1.3	0.3	<0.05	3.7	3.2–4.2	Kallen et al. 2005 [16]
Premature rupture of membranes	4.4	1.4	<0.05	2.5	2.3–2.8	Kallen et al. 2005 [16]

Long-Term Consequences following Fertility Treatments

Literature on maternal long-term complications following infertility treatment is limited. The data on whether ART increases the risk of maternal malignancies depends on the cancer being discussed. Althuis et al. [18] investigated long-term morbidity in 8422 women (155,527 women-years) evaluated for infertility between the years 1965 and 1988. In this retrospective cohort study, women who received gonadotropins or clomiphene citrate for OI did not have an increased risk of developing melanoma (RR 1.66, 95% CI 0.9–3.1), colon (RR 0.83, 95% CI 0.4–1.9), cervical, (RR 1.61, 95% CI 0.5–4.7), or thyroid cancer (RR 1.42, 95% CI 0.5–3.7).

Salhab et al. [19] investigated the possible association between ART and an increased risk of breast cancer development. The combined analysis of case-control (*n* breast cancer = 11,303, *n* control = 10,930; RR 0.88; *p* = .231) and cohort studies (*n* = 60,050; RR 1.06; *p* = .337) showed that there was no significant association between the two. While this analysis concluded that there was no increased risk of breast cancer after receiving ART treatment, it should be noted that treatment was associated with an increased risk of breast cancer of those with a family history of the illness and also showed higher expected incidence of breast cancer within the first year of ART treatment.

There are conflicting studies regarding whether there is an increased risk of ovarian cancer after IVF. Brinton et al. [20] assessed the long-term effects of ovulation-stimulating drugs on the risk of ovarian cancer. Interestingly, patients following fertility treatments had a significantly elevated ovarian cancer risk compared with the general population (standardized incidence ratio 1.98, 95% CI 1.4–2.6). However, when patient characteristics were controlled for, the rate ratios were nonsignificant. The rate ratios associated with ever usage were 0.82 (95% CI 0.4–1.5) for clomiphene and 1.09 (95% CI 0.4–2.8) for gonadotropins. There were higher, albeit nonsignificant, risks with follow-up time, with the rate ratios after 15 or more years being 1.48 (95% CI 0.7–3.2) for exposure to clomiphene (five exposed cancer patients) and 2.46 (95% CI 0.7–8.3) for gonadotropins (three exposed cancer patients).

While the results of this study were generally reassuring in not confirming a strong link between ovulation-stimulating drugs and ovarian cancer, the study did find a slight elevation in risk associated with drug usage among certain subgroups of users [20].

In contrast, Kessous et al. [21] found in a population-based study of 106,031 women that there was a significantly increased risk of ovarian (HR 3.9, 95% CI 1.2–12.6; *p* = .022) and uterine cancer (HR 4.6,

95% CI 1.4–14.9; $p = .011$) for women who received IVF when compared with women who received OI and women who received no treatment at all.

The effect on future maternal ophthalmic complications after receiving fertility treatment was investigated by Ratson et al. [22] In a cohort-based study of 106,004 women from the years 1988 to 2013, patients with a history of fertility treatments, as a group, did not have a significantly higher incidence of ophthalmic complications. However, women who had undergone IVF treatment were shown to have a significantly higher risk of retinal detachment (0.3% vs. 0.1%; HR 3.4, 95% CI 1.2–9.3; $p = .011$) when compared with a control group and a group of women who received OI.

Risk of Cardiovascular Disease

Cardiovascular disease is one of the leading causes of death in women in the United States [23]. Therefore, it is important to understand the risk factors for developing cardiovascular disease, which allows appropriate counseling for patients.

Long-term cardiovascular complications from obstetric syndromes have only recently been studied. Preeclampsia in previous pregnancies is a significant risk factor for future maternal cardiovascular morbidity [24]. Women with gestational hypertension and placental abruption in a previous pregnancy have a higher risk of developing premature heart failure and dysrhythmias, and this risk is increased in cases of perinatal morbidity [25]. Preterm delivery has also been defined as an independent risk factor for long-term maternal cardiovascular-related complications and higher rates of cardiovascular events [26]. Bonamy et al. [27] concluded that long-term maternal cardiovascular morbidity is increased when mothers have had previous pregnancies with fetal growth restriction.

The link between infertility treatment and an increased risk of cardiovascular disease can be suggested based on the previous studies mentioned. Since there is an increased risk of preeclampsia and placental abruption following infertility treatment [16], and gestational hypertension, preeclampsia, and placental abruption are risk factors for cardiovascular disease [25,26], it is possible that infertility treatments are an independent risk factor for future maternal cardiovascular disease.

Through retrospective studies, possible long-term maternal cardiovascular complications related to infertility treatments have been brought to light. It should be noted that the research regarding these long-term complications following fertility treatment is quite limited. A retrospective cohort study conducted by Westerlund et al. [28] reviewed the incidence of coronary artery disease, stroke, hypertension, and diabetes with regard to women who underwent fertility treatment. Using a group of 23,498 women who received IVF and successfully delivered between 1990 and 2008, the study showed an increased risk of hypertension (HR 1.27, 95% CI 1.13–1.41) and a tendency to stroke (HR 1.27, 95% CI 0.96–1.68) compared with the control group ($n = 116,960$). Incidences of diabetes (HR 0.96, 95% CI 0.81–1.14) and coronary artery disease (HR 0.72, 95% CI 0.44–1.17) were not significantly different between the two groups [28]. Hypertension is a well-established risk factor for cardiovascular disease; therefore, clinicians should take extra precaution when assessing patients who have undergone fertility treatments [29]. Nevertheless, the limitations of this study should be considered as well. The mean age of the cohorts was 33, and the follow-up period was only 8.6 years. This short duration could underestimate cardiovascular morbidity in both groups. A longer follow-up period could be helpful in determining if in fact there is an increased risk of coronary artery disease and diabetes mellitus [28].

Contrary to the conclusion reported by Westerlund et al. [28], in a cohort study in Canada from the years 1993 to 2010 ($n = 1,186,753$), Udell et al. [13] reported that after a median follow-up of 9.7 years, patients who received IVF had a decreased risk of cardiovascular complications such as coronary ischemia (HR 0.56, 95% CI 0.25–1.25; $p = .15$), cerebrovascular events (HR 1.14, 95% CI 0.54–2.44; $p = .73$), and heart failure (HR 0.60, 95% CI 0.30–1.22; $p = .16$) after adjusting for age, baseline cardiovascular risk factors, the number of gestations, and the development of OHSS. Indicators for cardiovascular disease included ischemic heart disease, cardiomyopathy, cerebrovascular disease, thromboembolic disease, and peripheral artery disease. Additionally, there was no significant difference between the groups when assessing the development of cardiovascular risk factors including diabetes, hyperlipidemia, and hypertension (HR 0.86, 95% CI 0.82–0.90; $p < .0001$). Moreover, there was no increased risk of coronary revascularization after receiving IVF (HR 1.18, 95% CI 0.55–2.51; $p = .67$). This was despite the fact that women receiving in vitro fertilization had a higher rate of cardiovascular risk factors at baseline, including hypertension, diabetes, and hyperlipidemia, when compared with the control group. It should be noted that the experimental group had a higher average age than the control group as well. However, there was no significant difference between the two groups in cardiovascular disease at baseline [13].

In another retrospective cohort study, supporting the findings of Udell et al. [13], Djaoui Ben Yakov et al. [30] researched whether patients who had undergone fertility treatments, defined as OI or IVF, were at increased risk of developing long-term cardiovascular morbidity when compared with a group of women who conceived spontaneously, or when compared with each other. Specifically, the incidence of hospitalization, angina pectoris, heart failure, and noninvasive and invasive cardiac diagnostic procedures were investigated for both groups. A noninvasive test was defined as a treadmill stress test and an invasive test was defined as placing a stent. The mean follow-up time for fertility treatments was 11.1 years and 11.2 years for the control group.

During the 25 years of the study period, 99,291 patients met the inclusion criteria; 4.1% ($n = 4153$) occurred in patients with exposure to fertility treatments (1177 following IVF and 2976 following OI). The rate of obesity (2.0% vs. 1.0%; $p = .001$) and pregnancy complications such as recurrent pregnancy loss (6.1% vs. 4.5%; $p = .001$), preeclampsia (9.1% vs. 4.7%; $p = .001$), pregestational diabetes mellitus and gestational diabetes mellitus (14.1% vs. 6.2%; $p = .001$), placental abruption (1.3% vs. 0.7%; $p = .001$), and small size for gestational age (6.7% vs. 4.9%; $p = .001$) were all significantly higher in the group treated with in vitro fertilization.

Hospitalizations due to cardiovascular complications between the OI group, IVF group, and control group were not significantly different (IVF = 3.4%, OI = 2.6%, control = 3.3%; $p = .305$) (Figure 11.2). The group of women who received IVF or OI showed no increased long-term risk of angina pectoris (IVF = 1.2%, OI = 1.0%, control = 1.4%; $p = .14$), heart failure (IVF = 1.8%, OI = 1.3%, control = 1.7%; $p = .319$), cardiac noninvasive diagnostic procedures (IVF = 0.9%, OI = 1.0%, control = 1.0%; $p = .903$), or cardiac invasive diagnostic procedures (IVF = 0.8%, OI = 0.2%, control = 0.4%; $p = .598$) when compared with the control group ($n = 95,138$). Similar results were reported when comparing women who received either OI or IVF with the group of women who conceived spontaneously (Table 11.2).

The authors concluded that in a population of women who delivered later on, and during a mean follow-up period of 11.7 years, results show no increased risk of cardiovascular morbidity in women

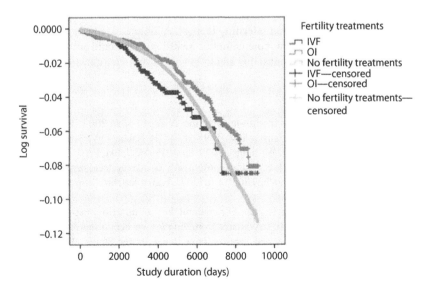

FIGURE 11.2 Kaplan–Meier survival analysis showing the risk of long-term cardiovascular disease in pregnancies following fertility treatments. The graph compares pregnancies conceived following IVF and OI compared with spontaneous pregnancies. (Adapted from Ben-Yaakov RD, Kessous R, Shoham-Vardi I, Sergienko R, Pariente G, Sheiner E. *Am J Perinatol*. 2016. https://www.thieme-connect.com/DOI/DOI?10.1055/s-0036-1582444.)

TABLE 11.2

Incidence of Hospitalizations for Specific and All-Cardiovascular Causes during the Follow-Up Period in Patients Conceiving with and without Fertility Treatments

	Fertility Treatments ($n = 2,976$)	No Fertility Treatment ($n = 95,138$)	OR	95% CI	p Value
Simple cardiovascular events	1.1%	1.4%	0.8	0.6–1.1	.083
Complex cardiovascular events	1.4%	1.7%	0.8	0.6–1.1	.151
Cardiac noninvasive diagnostic procedures	1.0%	1.0%	1.0	0.7–1.3	.959
Cardiac invasive diagnostic procedures	0.4%	0.4%	0.9	0.5–1.5	.709
Total cardiovascular hospitalizations	2.8%	3.3%	0.9	0.7–1.1	.305

Source: Ben-Yaakov RD, Kessous R, Shoham-Vardi I, Sergienko R, Pariente G, Sheiner E. *Am J Perinatol.* 2016 May 9. https://www.thieme-connect.com/DOI/DOI?10.1055/s-0036-1582444.

undergoing fertility treatments, either IVF or OI. Given the high and increased prevalence of these treatments, the results add to physicians' ability to reassure patients regarding the long-term risks of the treatments.

CONCLUSION

The limited and conflicting studies investigating whether fertility treatment increase the risk of long-term maternal cardiovascular morbidity make it difficult to determine if in fact there is an association between the two. Due to the increasing usage of infertility treatments, it is important to determine if there is a correlation between CVD and infertility therapy. Additional studies are required with longer follow-up periods in order to provide a more definite conclusion, and would accordingly assist primary care doctors to delineate the proper counseling and follow-up of women following fertility treatments.

REFERENCES

1. Van Voorhis BJ. Clinical practice: In vitro fertilization. *N Engl J Med.* 2007;356:379 –86.
2. Beckmann CRB, Ling FW, Barzansky BM, Herbert WNP, Laube DW, Smith PR. *Obstetrics and Gynecology.* 2010:497. Lippincott, Williams and Wilkins. Philadelphia, PA.
3. Hull MG, Glazener CM, Kelly NJ, et al. Population study of causes, treatment, and outcome of infertility. *Br Med J (Clin Res Ed).* 1985;291(6510):1693–7. Available from: http://www.ncbi.nlm.nih.gov/pubmed/3935248.
4. Bhattacharya S, Porter M, Amalraj E, et al. The epidemiology of infertility in the north east of Scotland. *Hum Reprod.* 2009;24(12):3096–107. Available from: http://www.ncbi.nlm.nih.gov/pubmed/19684046.
5. Hamilton BE, Ventura SJ. Fertility and abortion rates in the United States, 1960–2002. *Int J Androl.* 2006;29(1):34–45. Available from: http://doi.wiley.com/10.1111/j.1365-2605.2005.00638.x.
6. Sunderam S, Kissin DM, Crawford SB, et al. Assisted reproductive technology surveillance: United States, 2013. *MMWR Surveill Summ.* 2015;64(11):1–25. Available from: http://www.ncbi.nlm.nih.gov/pubmed/26633040.
7. Steptoe PC, Edwards RG. Birth after the reimplantation of a human embryo. *Lancet.* 1978;312(8085):366. Available from: http://www.sciencedirect.com/science/article/pii/S0140673678929574 (accessed March 3, 2016).

8. Ory SJ. The national epidemic of multiple pregnancy and the contribution of assisted reproductive technology. *Fertil Steril.* 2013;100(4):929–30. Available from: http://linkinghub.elsevier.com/retrieve/pii/S0015028213006985.

9. Buckett WM. A review and meta-analysis of prospective trials comparing different catheters used for embryo transfer. *Fertil Steril.* 2006;85(3):728–34. Available from: http://www.ncbi.nlm.nih.gov/pubmed/16500345.

10. Derks RS, Farquhar C, Mol BWJ, Buckingham K, Heineman MJ. Techniques for preparation prior to embryo transfer. *Cochrane Database Syst Rev.* 2009;4:CD007682. Available from: http://www.ncbi.nlm.nih.gov/pubmed/19821435.

11. Brown J, Buckingham K, Abou-Setta AM, Buckett W. Ultrasound versus "clinical touch" for catheter guidance during embryo transfer in women. *Cochrane Database Syst Rev.* 2010;1:CD006107. Available from: http://www.ncbi.nlm.nih.gov/pubmed/20091584.

12. Practice Committee of the American Society for Reproductive Medicine. Blastocyst production and transfer in clinical assisted reproduction. *Fertil Steril.* 2004;82(Suppl 1):S149–50. Available from: http://www.ncbi.nlm.nih.gov/pubmed/15363713.

13. Udell JA, Lu H, Redelmeier DA. Long-term cardiovascular risk in women prescribed fertility therapy. *J Am Coll Cardiol.* 2013;62(18):1704–12.

14. Serour GI, Aboulghar M, Mansour R, Sattar MA, Amin Y, Aboulghar H. Complications of medically assisted conception in 3,500 cycles. *Fertil Steril.* 1998;70(4):638–42. Available from: http://www.ncbi.nlm.nih.gov/pubmed/9797090.

15. Braat DDM, Schutte JM, Bernardus RE, Mooij TM, Van Leeuwen FE. Maternal death related to IVF in the Netherlands 1984–2008. *Hum Reprod.* 2010;25(7):1782–6.

16. Källén B, Finnström O, Nygren KG, Otterblad Olausson P, Wennerholm UB. In vitro fertilisation in Sweden: Obstetric characteristics, maternal morbidity and mortality. *BJOG An Int J Obstet Gynaecol.* 2005;112(11):1529–35.

17. Silberstein T, Levy A, Harlev A, Saphier O, Sheiner E. Perinatal outcome of pregnancies following in vitro fertilization and ovulation induction. *J Matern Fetal Neonatal Med.* 2014;27(13):1316–9. Available from: http://www.ncbi.nlm.nih.gov/pubmed/24175873.

18. Althuis MD, Scoccia B, Lamb EJ, et al. Melanoma, thyroid, cervical, and colon cancer risk after use of fertility drugs. *Am J Obstet Gynecol.* 2005;193(3 Pt 1):668–74. Available from: http://www.ncbi.nlm.nih.gov/pubmed/16150258.

19. Salhab M, Al Sarakbi W, Mokbel K. In vitro fertilization and breast cancer risk: A review. *Int J Fertil Womens Med.* 50(6):259–66. Available from: http://www.ncbi.nlm.nih.gov/pubmed/16526416.

20. Brinton LA, Lamb EJ, Moghissi KS, et al. Ovarian cancer risk after the use of ovulation-stimulating drugs. *Obstet Gynecol.* 2004;103(6):1194–203. Available from: http://www.ncbi.nlm.nih.gov/pubmed/15172852.

21. Kessous R, Davidson E, Meirovitz M, Sergienko R, Sheiner E. The risk of female malignancies after fertility treatments: A cohort study with 25-year follow-up. *J Cancer Res Clin Oncol.* 2016;142(1):287–93. Available from: http://link.springer.com/10.1007/s00432-015-2035-x.

22. Ratson R, Sheiner E, Davidson E, Sergienko R, Beharier O, Kessous R. Fertility treatments and the risk for ophthalmic complications: A cohort study with 25-year follow-up. *J Matern Neonatal Med.* 2015;7058:1–4. Available from: http://www.tandfonline.com/doi/full/10.3109/14767058.2015.1120717 (accessed March 3, 2016).

23. Kochanek KD, Xu J, Murphy SL, Minino AM, Kung HC. National vital statistics reports deaths: Final data for 2009. *Natl Cent Heal Stat.* 2012;60(3):1–117. Available from: http://www.cdc.gov/nchs/data/nvsr/nvsr58/nvsr58_19.pdf.

24. Kessous R, Shoham-Vardi I, Pariente G, Sergienko R, Sheiner E. Long-term maternal atherosclerotic morbidity in women with pre-eclampsia. *Heart.* 2015;101(6):442–6. Available from: http://www.ncbi.nlm.nih.gov/pubmed/25564558.

25. Ray JG, Schull MJ, Kingdom JC, Vermeulen MJ. Heart failure and dysrhythmias after maternal placental syndromes: HAD MPS study. *Heart.* 2012;98(15):1136–41. Available from: http://heart.bmj.com/cgi/doi/10.1136/heartjnl-2011-301548.

26. Kessous R, Shoham-Vardi I, Pariente G, Holcberg G, Sheiner E. An association between preterm delivery and long-term maternal cardiovascular morbidity. *Am J Obstet Gynecol.* 2013;209(4):368.e1–8. Available from: http://linkinghub.elsevier.com/retrieve/pii/S0002937813005309.

27. Bonamy AKE, Parikh NI, Cnattingius S, Ludvigsson JF, Ingelsson E. Birth characteristics and subsequent risks of maternal cardiovascular disease: Effects of gestational age and fetal growth. *Circulation*. 2011;124(25):2839–46. Available from: http://www.ncbi.nlm.nih.gov/pubmed/22124377.

28. Westerlund E, Brandt L, Hovatta O, Wallén H, Ekbom A, Henriksson P. Incidence of hypertension, stroke, coronary heart disease, and diabetes in women who have delivered after in vitro fertilization: A population-based cohort study from Sweden. *Fertil Steril*. 2014;102(4):1096–102.

29. Brown DW, Giles WH, Croft JB. Left ventricular hypertrophy as a predictor of coronary heart disease mortality and the effect of hypertension. *Am Heart J*. 2000;140(6):848–56. Available from: http://www.sciencedirect.com/science/article/pii/S0002870300828112 (accessed March 3, 2016).

30. Ben-Yakov RR, Kessous R, Shoham Vardi I, Sergienko R, Pariente G, Sheiner E. Fertility treatments in women who become pregnant and carried to viability, and the risk for long-term maternal cardiovascular morbidity. *Am J Perinatol*. 2016. https://www.thieme-connect.com/DOI/DOI?10.1055/s-0036-1582444.

12

Pregnancy as an Opportunity for Weight Control and Smoking Cessation

Sharon Davidesko and Asnat Walfisch

Introduction

Pregnancy is a unique time in a woman's life when she is increasingly focused on her health and the impact it has on her growing fetus. This focus can be directed to positively reinforcing healthy life choices and to making drastic changes in regard to unhealthy ones. The pregnant woman is often more motivated to make these positive life changes and the increased number of patient–physician interactions during this time allows for increased support during the critical time of adjustment. This chapter provides a summary of recent evidence pertaining to smoking and weight gain during pregnancy, outlining possible strategies for intervention and long-term health benefits.

Effect of Obesity and Gestational Weight Gain on Pregnancy Outcomes and Long-Term Maternal Health

Close to one-third of women of reproductive age are classified as obese and a further quarter defined as overweight in the United States [1–3]. The relationship between obesity and long-term morbidity such as cardiovascular disease, diabetes, stroke, arthritis, and even some forms of cancer is well known in the general population [4]. Nevertheless, the issue of obesity is often underaddressed when treating pregnant women. As a physician treating pregnant women, one must recognize this window of opportunity to positively affect the long-term health of the pregnant female population and utilize this opportunity by offering support and advice and by promoting healthy lifestyle choices.

It is widely accepted from decades of observation and research that maternal weight prior to pregnancy, maternal BMI, and gestational weight gain have important effects on pregnancy outcome, neonatal morbidity and mortality, and the long-term health of the offspring (Table 12.1) [4]. Obesity is associated with a lower spontaneous pregnancy rate not only due to the association with polycystic ovary syndrome, but also in obese women with regular ovulation [5]. Some congenital anomalies, including congenital heart anomalies and neural tube defects, have been associated with maternal obesity with a possible dose-related relationship [6]. Although the mechanism is unknown it has been suggested that hormonal imbalances such as hyperinsulinemia are responsible. There is also a relationship between maternal obesity and fetal or infant death, and a link to indicated or spontaneous preterm delivery and its associated complications in the newborn. The long-term effects of maternal obesity on the offspring include an increased risk of the future development of diabetes, hypertension, and cardiovascular disease, as having an obese mother is a strong risk factor for obesity in the child [7]. Recent studies have also explored a possible link between maternal obesity and autism spectrum disorders, neurodevelopmental disorders, and asthma [8]. Another well-established association was repeatedly shown between maternal obesity and complications during pregnancy and delivery including hypertensive disorders of pregnancy, gestational diabetes mellitus (GDM), macrosomia, shoulder dystocia, venous thromboembolism, labor

TABLE 12.1

Possible Effects of Maternal Obesity on Fertility, Pregnancy, and the Offspring

- Lower spontaneous pregnancy rate
- Congenital anomalies: congenital heart defects and neural tube defects
- Fetal/neonatal death
- Preterm delivery (and associated complications)
- Long-term effects on the offspring: obesity, diabetes, hypertension, cardiovascular disease
- Autism, neurodevelopmental diseases of the offspring
- Hypertensive disorders of pregnancy: gestational hypertension, preeclampsia, eclampsia, HELLP syndrome
- GDM
- Macrosomia
- Shoulder dystocia
- Venous thromboembolism
- Labor induction
- Cesarean delivery
- Postcesarean surgical site infection

induction, cesarean delivery, and postcesarean surgical site infection [3]. Cesarean delivery in obese women will be discussed fully later in this chapter.

Both weight retention after delivery and excessive weight gain during pregnancy have been found to be important predictors of long-term weight changes and increased body mass index (BMI) [2,9,10], leading to an increased risk of obesity with its associated detrimental effects on health. In a study of 46,688 pregnant women who delivered between the years 1988 and 1999 and were followed for over a decade, patients with obesity (BMI $\geq$ 30 kg/m^2) had higher rates of cardiovascular events and total number of cardiovascular hospitalizations, with a tendency for earlier complications [11].

An important and underemphasized problem is the impact of excessive gestational weight gain on long-term maternal health [2]. A relationship has been found between excessive gestational weight gain and the future risk of obesity, as the retention of additional weight gained during pregnancy is a common problem after childbirth [9]. Increased body weight and fat distribution after the first pregnancy may be persistent, but these changes vary according to race and ethnic background [12], marital status, age, income, education, occupation, working outside the home, physical activity, and smoking. Weight gain exceeding the recommended guidelines during pregnancy can be attributed mostly to an increase in adipose tissue. Progesterone is partially responsible for the fat accumulation during the first and second trimesters and for the mobilization of adipose tissue during the third trimester. There is also a positive correlation between increased leptin levels during pregnancy and body fat content and BMI, which appears to be directly involved in the process of gestational weight gain and postpartum weight retention [13,14]. Excessive weight gain may also be attributed to pathological processes such as edema in preeclamptic women, but these are the minority of cases.

The recommendations regarding weight gain during pregnancy have changed dramatically over the past century. From a universal recommendation to gain no more than 7 kg during pregnancy in the United States in the 1930s regardless of prepregnancy weight, today we are aware of the pregravid body mass index (BMI) as an independent predictor of birth weight (directly linked to pregnancy outcome), and therefore, weight gain recommendations are individualized and are primarily based on the prepregnancy weight status.

The Committee on Nutritional Status during Pregnancy and Lactation of the Institute of Medicine (IOM), published originally in 1990, formulated recommendations for healthy weight gain during pregnancy. Present recommendations, published almost two decades later, are based on the World Health Organization (WHO) criteria for weight categories and include recommendations for weight gain in singleton and twin pregnancies (Table 12.2) [15]. Despite these established recommendations, most women gain too much or too little weight during pregnancy [16]. When converted to average weight gain targets, underweight and normal-weight women should gain around 0.5 kg/week and overweight and obese women should gain 0.25 kg/week during the second and third trimesters.

TABLE 12.2

Weight Gain Recommendations in Singleton and Twin Pregnancies

Prepregnancy BMI (kg/m²)	Singleton Pregnancy Weight Gain Recommendations (kg)	Twin Pregnancy Weight Gain Recommendations (kg)
<18.5 (underweight)	12.5–18.0	Insufficient data
18.5–24.9 (normal weight)	11.5–16.0	16.8–24.5
25.0–29.9 (overweight)	7.0–11.5	14.1–22.7
≥30.0 (obese)	5.0–9.0	11.4–19.1

These guidelines apply to the general obstetric population, independent of age, parity, smoking history, race, and ethnic background. However, various subgroups may benefit from a more customized medical approach. For example, pregnant women under the age of 18 years may require increased weight gain in order to decrease the risk of low–birth weight offspring [17] and women with severe obesity may benefit from even greater weight gain restrictions during pregnancy when compared with women with milder obesity.

Techniques for Weight Control

The importance of weight loss is clear, with a link to decreased mortality and better quality of life. Several methods of weight loss have been proposed, ranging from lifestyle changes to pharmacologic therapy and bariatric surgery. As the patient loses weight her energy expenditure decreases, making it difficult to further or maintain weight loss. Regaining weight lost is a common problem, although frequent self-weighing or other behavioral interventions, such as reduced calorie intake or increased physical activity, may help.

Patients should be selected based on an initial assessment of BMI, abdominal obesity, and cardiovascular risk factors, and goals and expectations should be addressed. Often patients have unrealistic initial weight loss goals. Women seeking to improve fertility and decrease perinatal complications associated with obesity should attempt to lose weight before conception in order to maximize the benefits of weight loss [18].

Initial interventions including lifestyle interventions based on a combination of diet, exercise, and behavior modification should be implemented, leading to an energy deficit. A greater potential for weight loss has been demonstrated with treatments leading to decreased energy intake as opposed to those based on increased energy expenditure through exercise. Comprehensive programs include the self-regulation of energy intake, physical activity, and the monitoring of body weight. The goal of behavioral interventions is to change the patient's response to cues in the environment and modify their attitude to food intake and exercise. This is achieved with the support of psychologists or other trained personnel and self-help groups. Adherence to a set diet often predicts the success of weight loss, irrespective of the type of diet chosen; therefore, the choice of diet should be based on patient preferences. Diet programs based on caloric restriction have been proven to be effective. Despite the expectation that severe caloric restriction will induce more rapid weight loss, a study comparing 400 versus 800 kcal/day diets showed no difference in weight loss; therefore, severe diet restriction is not recommended.

Current recommendations for nonpregnant adults with a BMI ≥ 40 kg/m² who fail with lifestyle interventions and pharmacologic therapy suggest a potential benefit from bariatric surgery. Patients with comorbidities may be offered these options at a lower BMI threshold.

Bariatric surgery is the most extreme intervention for weight loss, but is also the most effective for obese women as many morbidly obese women appear to be resistant to other weight loss techniques [19]. Bariatric surgery appears to be more popular among the female population, who comprise 80% of surgeries performed, with the majority of them at reproductive age [20].

There are two main categories of bariatric surgeries: restrictive or malabsorptive procedures [21]. Restrictive procedures physically reduce stomach volume, limiting the gross amount of food consumed, such as with gastric banding or sleeve gastrectomies. These surgeries are considered easier to perform and less invasive, although without proper dietary education patients may still fail to lose weight by ingesting increased quantities of soft solid or liquid high-calorie foods that easily pass the restricted stomach [22]. An additional disadvantage of the laparoscopic adjustable gastric band (LAGB) procedure is the need for frequent visits to the physician for band adjustment [23]. Procedures leading to a malabsorptive state, such as the Roux-en-Y gastric bypass (RYGB) and biliopancreatic diversion (BPD), are achieved by shortening the effective length of the small bowel [24]. In addition, the manipulation of the proximal duodenum leads to neuroendocrine changes, altering the hormonal signaling related to metabolism [21]. These procedures are associated with a longer period of rapid weight loss when compared with restrictive procedures [25].

Pregnancy should be delayed for 12–24 months following surgery [26] in order to avoid potential nutritional imbalances during the rapid weight loss stage [24], which may be exacerbated by the additional nutritional requirements of the developing fetus [27]. Contraceptive counseling should be offered, although few complications have been proven to be associated with conception less than a year postoperatively, and it is not considered a reason for termination [28]. Despite the theoretical concerns of fetal malnutrition following maternal bariatric surgery, such a relationship has not been demonstrated. Intrauterine growth restriction (IUGR) and malformations are not increased in this population [25].

Bariatric surgery has been shown to be one of the most effective means currently available for preventing GDM in obese women and is capable of reducing the incidence of GDM to a level equivalent to that of the general population [29]. Although some studies found that the reduced risk of GDM after bariatric surgery was still higher than that of the general population, this was not significant when controlled for confounders [30]. The standard methods of GDM screening using a 50 g glucose challenge test should not be used in patients following RYGB, as around 50% of women will develop dumping syndrome [31]. As an alternative, glycated hemoglobin A1C levels or fasting and postprandial blood glucose levels can be monitored. Studies have also shown a significant decrease in the incidence of hypertensive disorders in pregnant women after bariatric surgery [32]. The effect of bariatric surgery on birth weight has been addressed in several studies, with general findings including a decrease in mean birth weight [33,34] and the incidence of macrosomia [33], and an increase in the number of small-for-gestational-age (SGA) neonates [34]. No difference in the incidence of growth-restricted neonates was demonstrated [33]. The increase in SGA and decrease in macrosomic infants may be linked to a reduction in the rate of cesarean section deliveries [29,32], although the effect of bariatric surgery on surgical delivery rates is controversial, with some studies showing increased rates of cesarean delivery in this population [35]. The significant weight loss achieved after surgery may also improve fertility [31], although in some studies an increase in fertility has not been demonstrated [30].

Both types of bariatric surgeries appear to exhibit similar safety and efficacy in reducing fetal and perinatal complications of maternal obesity [28]. Bowel obstruction in pregnant women following bariatric surgery has been reported [36], and women should be monitored for signs and symptoms such as fever, leukocytosis, hyperemesis, esophageal reflux, and abdominal pain. Many of these symptoms are nonspecific and are common in uncomplicated pregnancies. Therefore, a lower threshold of suspicion should be applied in postoperative pregnant women. Changes in nutrient absorption following bariatric surgeries, particularly those utilizing malabsorptive methods, may require micronutrient supplementation—for example, maternal anemia due to decreased vitamin B12 and iron absorption, or a potential increase in neural tube defects due to folic acid deficiency, which has been noted in case reports. Patients following bariatric surgery should be provided with supplementation individually tailored to the type of surgery they have undergone, in addition to obstetric recommendations of nutrient needs during pregnancy.

In conclusion, the benefits of bariatric surgery as a preventative measure for perinatal and long-term maternal health complications seem clear, although no randomized controlled trials or prospective cohort studies have been performed to date, and therefore, this area requires further research.

Cesarean Delivery of the Obese Woman

Many factors increase morbidity in obese women undergoing a cesarean delivery in addition to an increased probability of emergency cesarean section [3,16,37], which of itself leads to increased morbidity [37,38]. Respiratory dysfunction is a major concern. The most common respiratory problems associated with obesity are obstructive sleep apnea (OSA) and obesity hypoventilation syndrome (OHS). Nevertheless, even in the absence of these conditions, respiratory dysfunction due to obesity-related functional changes may complicate ventilation during surgery. Central venous access may be required due to subcutaneous adiposity complicating the placement of peripheral lines, and specialized equipment (lifts, long instruments, high–weight capacity operating tables, and large blood pressure cuffs) may be required. Epidural or spinal catheter placement may require more attempts, although the rate of successful neuraxial anesthesia is similar for obese women and nonobese women. An additional anesthetic consideration includes altered pharmacodynamics, leading to both subtherapeutic and toxic responses in some cases. Surgery is often longer, with increased incision-to-delivery time and increased blood loss. Wound infection and disruption, endometritis, and thromboembolism complicate postoperative recuperation at higher rates in obese women.

In order to address these issues, current recommendations include preoperative consultation in the early to mid-third trimester (in the case of preterm delivery). Assessment should include history, physical examination, and selective testing to identify patients with comorbidities such as OSA, diabetes mellitus, and cardiovascular disease.

Studies have shown that regional anesthesia is safer than general anesthesia in this patient population [39] and is therefore recommended despite the need for an increased number of attempts at initial catheter placement or replacement, which is characteristic of obese patients [40].

When making the abdominal wall incision it is imperative to be aware of the atypical location of soft-tissue landmarks—for example, caudal displacement of the umbilicus. Reliable landmarks include the pubic symphysis and iliac crests [41]. The choice of incision is a controversial issue. Suprapubic incisions made two finger breadths cephalad to the pubic symphysis with retraction of the panniculus include low transverse Pfannenstiel or low midline vertical incisions. Some studies have reported a higher incidence of wound infection when midline vertical incisions are used [42], while others have reported fewer wound complications, and additional studies have observed no difference in outcome [43]. Placement of the surgical wound under the panniculus, a warm, moist environment with high bacterial colonization, potentially increases the risk of infection. Supraumbilical incisions for morbidly obese women, particularly those over 180 kg, may be advantageous. The wound is not buried under the panniculus and abdominal exposure is excellent, although transverse supraumbilical incision has not been proven to lead to fewer complications than the Pfannenstiel incision [44]. Suboptimal exposure of the lower uterine segment in supraumbilical incisions may necessitate vertical hysterotomy in the mid-portion of the uterus, a major disadvantage associated with a higher risk of uterine rupture in subsequent pregnancies. The Smead–Jones interrupted technique or continuous closure of the fascia are equally effective in reducing the risk of hernia formation or wound dehiscence. Closure of the subcutaneous adipose layer is recommended when ≥2 cm thick in order to decrease the risk of subsequent wound disruption [45]. The use of subcutaneous drains does not decrease the risk of wound complications in obese women [42], as has been observed in multiple randomized trials, and may even be associated with an increase in wound complication rates in cases with ≥4 cm subcutaneous thickness [46].

A number of interventions have been suggested to reduce the risk of postoperative complications, including thromboembolism and infections specifically in the obese population. In the United States, mechanical thromboprophylaxis in the form of pneumatic compression devices is standard procedure for all women undergoing cesarean section using a device sized to accommodate the diameter of the legs of obese women. Pharmacological prophylaxis may be given as an alternative or adjunctive therapy, although the dose and duration of postpartum continuation of the prophylactic treatment must be individualized according to patient-specific factors. Many interventions to reduce the incidence of postoperative surgical site infection have been proposed, including the minimization of the duration of surgery, the optimal glycemic control of diabetic patients, and antibiotic prophylaxis [47]. Perioperative antibiotic prophylaxis has been proven to reduce the incidence of wound infection, although the altered pharmacodynamics in obese patients leads to low serum and tissue levels [48], particularly of cephalosporins [48], and therefore, higher doses of the antimicrobial agent should be administered [49]. Current recommendations use cephazolin 2 g for women < 120 kg and 3 g for women ≥ 120 kg. For penicillin-allergic patients recommendations include combination therapy of clindamycin 900 mg with gentamycin 5 mg/kg [50].

The postoperative monitoring of all patients should include the regular assessment of respiratory function and the level of sedation, as this population is at increased risk of perioperative respiratory complications. Euvolemia should be maintained by monitoring fluid intake and output in order to minimize cardiopulmonary complications. Early ambulation and respiratory physiotherapy can help prevent venous thrombosis and respiratory complications, respectively. All patients should be monitored for wound complications both during hospitalization and following discharge as diagnosis of wound disruption may occur after patient release in up to 86% of cases [42].

Effects of Smoking on Pregnancy and the Importance of Smoking Cessation

The detrimental effects of smoking on long-term health are well known. For decades, smoking has been considered the most important modifiable risk factor associated with adverse pregnancy outcomes [51]. The most commonly reported adverse outcomes associated with maternal smoking include spontaneous pregnancy loss, placental abruption, preterm premature rupture of membranes (PPROM), placenta previa, preterm labor and delivery, low birth weight (LBW), and ectopic pregnancy [52]. In addition, smoking has a significant negative impact on long-term maternal health. Thus, smoking status should be assessed in all maternity care settings. Despite evidence that women who smoke cigarettes have a significantly lower risk of preeclampsia, the multiple risks of smoking on both maternal and fetal health greatly outweigh this potential benefit [53].

Tobacco may be smoked or absorbed through the buccal mucosal membranes in dissolvable products. More recently, electronic nicotine delivery systems (ENDS) have become fashionable, allowing aerosolized nicotine to be inhaled as with traditional smoking, but with fewer of the multiple potential toxins found in cigarettes. All of these products expose the pregnant woman and fetus to potentially harmful substances associated with an increased incidence of maternal and fetal obstetric complications and long-term health detriments. Despite the well-publicized health risks of tobacco smoking, studies in the United States show that roughly 30% of females and 35% of males of reproductive age smoke [52]. It is difficult to discern the true prevalence of smoking, especially in a population of pregnant women, as most studies rely on the self-reporting techniques of smoking behavior, which are well known for underreporting. Decreased disclosure of true smoking status by some women is a possible result of social pressures [54]. This has been proven in studies that compare self-reported smoking status with measured cotinine levels, a metabolite of nicotine, which remains detectable in the urine, blood, and saliva, for approximately 5 days following exposure [55,56]. In one study, 21.7% of self-reported nonsmokers had increased urine cotinine concentrations, which leads to the conclusion that self-reporting may result in underrepresentation of smoking in the pregnant population [54,56]. The routine biochemical verification of self-reported quitting may therefore be essential to evaluate smoking cessation [57]. Cotinine levels may be increased to a lesser degree in women exposed to secondhand smoke [55].

Data from the Pregnancy Risk Assessment Monitoring System (PRAMS), a surveillance study collecting population-based data regarding attitudes and experiences before, during, and after pregnancy, show that around one in five women (20%) report smoking before their pregnancy. This statistic has remained generally unchanged during the decade of the study [58]. Nevertheless, a statistically significant decrease in the percentage of women who reported smoking during and following pregnancy was reported. Recent data from the United Kingdom show that 11% of pregnant women smoke, an all-time low [59]. Additional encouraging data come from another study, which combined information from both surveys and birth certificate data, demonstrating that 35%–43% of women who smoked prior to pregnancy had quit by the end of pregnancy [60]. In another even more optimistic study, 50% of women quit. However, at follow-up after 4 years, only one-third of these continued to abstain [61]. Table 12.3 details predictive characteristics for long-term abstinence, risk factors for continued smoking, and reasons cited by women for not quitting [61–63]. Many of these factors are related, obscuring to some extent the independent effect of each factor [64].

TABLE 12.3

Risk Factors for Continued Smoking, Predictive Characteristics for Long-Term Abstinence, and Reasons Cited by Women for Not Quitting

Risk Factors for Continued Maternal Smoking	Predictors of Long-Term Abstinence	Reasons for Not Quitting
• Heavy smokers (>10–20 cigarettes per day) • Younger women • Less-educated women (lower than high school level) • Unmarried women • Women with low-income status claiming health benefits	• Older maternal age • Primiparas • Light smokers • Women living with partners • Women who become pregnant again • Women who breastfed over 52 weeks • Women whose child has been diagnosed with asthma or rhinitis	• Poor awareness • Skepticism regarding the detrimental effects of maternal smoking on the offspring • Smoking behavior of family members or partners • Psychological and/or physiological dependence on nicotine

Smoking Cessation Techniques

The smoking cessation techniques addressed in this section include behavioral interventions as well as pharmacotherapy.

The Five As [65] can be utilized as a tool for physicians who undertake the task of assisting patients to quit smoking in a systematic way (Figure 12.1).

1. *Ask*: All patients should be asked about tobacco use [66]. A full assessment of smoking patients includes an evaluation of the frequency of use, products used, the degree of dependence, a history of previous attempts to abstain, and the readiness of the patient to quit at this point in time [67]. Various tools to assess nicotine dependence, including subjective methods such as the self-reporting of smoking habits or objective methods such as quantitative cotinine levels in body fluids, are important, as the balance between dependence and motivation to quit may determine the success of interventions. In addition, highly dependent patients, such as those who report smoking from a young age and for many years, heavy smokers, and patients whose first cigarette is smoked within the first 30 minutes after waking up, may benefit from more intensive methods of intervention [67,68]. Enquiries regarding exposure to secondhand smoke can include asking if the patient lives with any smokers, or if smoking is allowed in the home, car, or workplace. Obstetricians should continue to ask about smoking status for the duration of pregnancy and the postpartum period.

2. *Advise*: Studies have shown that short sessions of counseling provided by the physician at each follow-up, advising the patient to quit smoking, can increase quit rates [69], although some studies have concluded that advice alone has a negligent effect on cessation [70]. Patients have also reported greater satisfaction with their care when regularly advised to quit smoking, regardless of their readiness at the time to attempt abstinence [71]. Complete cessation is always preferable to a decrease in the number of cigarettes smoked, as no evidence has proven that a recommendation to reduce smoking has lead to clear health benefits. In addition, studies have shown that women advised to reduce the number of cigarettes smoked per day are less likely to cease smoking than those advised to quit completely [72].

3. *Assess*: With each visit the patient's readiness to quit smoking should be assessed. The physician must understand that change is a gradual process; therefore, some stage-based help interventions, such as the Stages of Change model [73], may be helpful, although the validity of such models is debatable. Regardless of the patient's decision, the physician should remain nonjudgmental and continue to offer encouragement and assistance in future visits.

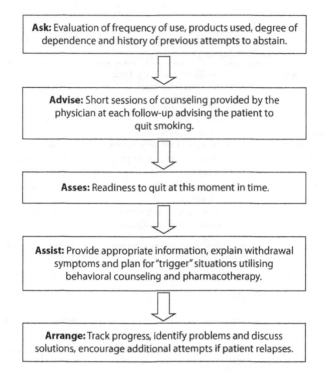

FIGURE 12.1   A diagram detailing the five As systematic approach of assisting patients to quit smoking.

4. *Assist*: If a patient is ready to quit, the appropriate information should be provided to assist. This includes an explanation of possible withdrawal symptoms and a plan of how to respond to such effects. Nicotine is a compound known for causing physical tolerance [74], and the sudden cessation of smoking may lead to nicotine withdrawal syndrome, characterized by increased appetite, weight gain, negative changes in mood, insomnia, irritability, difficulty concentrating, and restlessness. Psychological dependence, especially in certain *trigger* environments, such as after a meal, when drinking alcohol, or in social situations, should also be discussed along with methods for coping in these situations.

   A number of methods have been suggested to ready the patient to quit smoking.

   a. *Behavioral counseling*, such as structured support, is available in several formats, such as written material, computer programs and web-based interventions, phone apps, phone calls, and one-on-one or group counseling sessions, and should be pregnancy specific when possible [75]. Direct referral to a smoker's quit line can provide ongoing support from any location as a supplement to brief physician interventions. Patients may also be referred to a smoking cessation counselor or health educator [75]. Providing financial incentives increases the odds of quitting [76].

   b. *Pharmacotherapy* has proven efficacy for smoking cessation [77], but its use in the pregnant population remains controversial and requires further study.

   c. *Alternative therapies* such as acupuncture and hypnosis have not proven efficient, but some studies show potential benefits and, therefore, these methods should be further studied.

   If the patient is not ready to quit the physician should try to understand the patient's perspective on smoking, the reasons she is not ready to utilize the available resources for quitting, as well as any concerns related to smoking cessation. The health risks of secondhand smoke exposure to other household members should be emphasized, and patients should be urged to commit to keeping a smoke-free home or car, especially if children are present.

5. *Arrange*: Follow-up visits tracking the progress of the patient's quit attempts should include congratulating the patient for success, encouraging the patient to continue to abstain, identifying problems encountered, such as withdrawal symptoms and the side effects of medication, and anticipating future challenges. If the patient was unable to quit, the physician should try to understand why and address the problems identified. Solutions should be explored for future implementation in the next attempt—for example, addressing comorbid psychiatric illness or suboptimal dosing of pharmacotherapy. Long-term follow-up for months or even years after cessation may be beneficial as relapse rates are high and successful quitters remain at high risk of relapse for several years. Patients who relapse should be encouraged to attempt to quit again, as most patients typically require multiple attempts before permanently quitting.

Behavioral Interventions

Current recommendations encourage physicians to ask all adults, including pregnant women, about their past and current use of tobacco products [66]. Data published in 2015 by the US Preventive Services Task Force (USPSTF) recommend asking pregnant women about tobacco use, advising patients to cease using tobacco products, and providing behavioral interventions to assist adults who currently use these products [66]. In addition to current smoking status, it is important to ascertain smoking status at conception and, with women who currently smoke, the number of cigarettes smoked per day. A dose-dependent relationship between tobacco exposure and the prevalence of adverse complications is reported for most known smoking-related adverse pregnancy outcomes [78].

Behavioral interventions include providing information regarding the risks of continued smoking, frequent follow-up to assess the progress of smoking cessation, pregnancy-specific self-help manuals, one-off or multiple sessions with a trained health-care educator, and media, such as films depicting the risks of smoking and the benefits of smoking cessation.

Several studies have demonstrated that health care–initiated interventions encouraging smoking cessation in pregnancy lead to a reduction in the proportion of pregnant women still smoking at the end of the pregnancy and in some cases decrease the incidence of known complications of maternal smoking, such as low birth weight [79,80]. One study that set out to determine the extent to which tobacco exposure assessment and patient education methods could be provided, and then documented the behavioral impact of these interventions, found that 17.3% of women reported quitting as opposed to only 8.8% of the control group. This finding was validated with biochemical testing [65]. However, findings are not consistent; in one meta-analysis only a small percentage of biochemically validated continued abstinence was documented at a 6-month period following behavioral interventions, including counseling alone [75]. It is unclear which combination of interventions is the most effective, but the single most successful technique seems to be providing incentives such as vouchers for shopping, especially if the reward is received only after biochemical validation of abstinence, as proven by exhaled carbon monoxide or cotinine [76,80]. This technique is clearly unfeasible on a large scale and, therefore, a more a cost-effective approach should be sought.

Despite the evidence provided and many other studies proving a link between behavioral interventions and decreased maternal smoking, one study found that over half (51%) of obstetricians fail to utilize the given opportunity to advise about smoking cessation and do not provide follow-up to assess progress [62]. The same study found that only 28% of physicians discuss specific techniques for quitting.

There is insufficient evidence to recommend the use of electronic cigarettes as an alternative to traditional tobacco products [66], although in the United States approximately 3% of female adults use alternative tobacco products [81] and, therefore, this area requires further research.

Pharmacotherapy

Pharmacotherapy significantly increases quit rates when compared with placebo, as proven in randomized controlled trials in the nonpregnant population. However, concern regarding the potential adverse effects on the fetus leads to underutilization of these medications in pregnant women. The use of pharmacotherapy is controversial and the guidelines are unclear, with some agencies advocating use for all smokers unless contraindicated [65] and others stating that at present there is insufficient evidence to evaluate the benefits of pharmacotherapy as opposed to the risks of these treatments in the pregnant subpopulation [66]. One meta-analysis concluded that there may be clinical evidence to support the use of pharmacotherapy for smoking cessation in pregnant women, as few minor or major adverse effects were reported, but further randomized controlled trials are needed [77]. Patients who are unlikely to cease smoking, such as heavy smokers, women continuing to smoke late in pregnancy, and those with several failed attempts to quit, may benefit from pharmacotherapy. Medications should be given at the lowest efficient dose and treatment should be delayed until the second trimester if possible to avoid possible teratogenic effects of medications on the developing embryo.

Nicotine replacement can be used as an adjunct to behavioral interventions [82], as a first- or second-line option for pregnant patients with a high motivation to quit. Advocates of this treatment state that when compared with cigarette smoking, blood levels of nicotine are lower and exposure to other potentially toxic compounds is eliminated. In addition, treatment is temporary and is therefore preferable to the continuation of smoking. At present there are few data documenting the increased risk of adverse perinatal and fetal outcomes in pregnant women who received nicotine replacement compared with women who did not but continued to smoke [83], including studies comparing development outcomes [84] and major congenital anomalies [85]. Although effective in the nonpregnant population, there is a lack of research proving efficiency in the pregnant population [86]. One possible explanation is the rapid metabolism of nicotine in pregnancy, leading to underdosing.

Bupropion is an atypical antidepressant whose mechanism of action is only partly understood. This treatment may be used as a first- or second-line drug for smoking cessation in pregnant women and may be advantageous to nicotine treatment, as higher abstinence rates have been demonstrated with bupropion use when compared with placebo or nicotine patches alone [87]. Pregnant women not receiving bupropion have also been shown to be less likely to quit than those receiving treatment [88]. However, concerns regarding the safety of this medication exist as it crosses the placenta and has been linked to some adverse pregnancy outcomes (miscarriage and congenital anomalies such as left ventricular outflow obstruction) [89,90]. These studies were based on small numbers of cases and thus a clear association cannot be proven, but delaying treatment to the second trimester may be warranted.

Varenicline is a nicotinic receptor partial agonist leading to the reduction of both the withdrawal and pleasurable effects of nicotine, and its utilization in the nonpregnant smoking population is well founded. However, there is no information regarding the safety of its use in pregnant women and, therefore, should probably be avoided.

In breastfeeding women, nicotine replacement is preferable to bupropion despite its known transfer into breast milk, as available data on bupropion are limited [91,92]. Both methods are preferable to continued smoking.

Postpartum relapse is common and there are no proven interventions for prevention [93]. Relapse may be attributed to postpartum blues (reported in up to 70% of women after delivery), the continued smoking of family members, or a lack of social support, making parturients vulnerable in this time [93]. In addition, the increased motivation to quit during pregnancy "for the baby's sake" is no longer a factor, and many women may consider smoking cessation temporary during pregnancy and relapse during the postpartum period [94].

CONCLUSIONS

Maternal smoking is associated with adverse pregnancy outcomes, including spontaneous pregnancy loss, placental abruption, preterm premature rupture of membranes, placenta previa, preterm labor and delivery, LBW, and ectopic pregnancy. Additionally, smoking has a significant negative impact on long-term maternal health. Smoking status should be assessed in all maternity care settings, and smoking cessation should be recommended to all smokers. Around one-third of women of reproductive age smoke, although this number may be higher as smoking behavior is notoriously underreported by pregnant women; therefore, biochemical verification of quitting is warranted if available. Current data suggest that smoking during pregnancy is at an all-time low, but long-term follow-up studies show that only a minority of women continue to abstain long term. The Five As can be utilized as a tool to assist physicians who undertake the task of assisting patients to quit smoking in a systematic way. Behavioral interventions include providing information regarding the risks of continued smoking, frequent follow-up to assess the progress of smoking cessation, pregnancy-specific self-help manuals, one-off or multiple sessions with a trained health-care educator, and media, such as films depicting the risks of smoking and the benefits of smoking cessation. It is unclear which combination of interventions is the most effective, but the single most successful technique seems to be providing financial incentives, especially if the reward is received only after biochemical validation of abstinence. Pharmacotherapy significantly increases quit rates when compared with placebo. Nicotine replacement or bupropion can be used as adjunctive agents to behavioral therapy as first- or second-line agents, although varenicline should be avoided as there is no information regarding the safety of its use in pregnant women.

REFERENCES

1. Hedley AA, Ogden CL, Johnson CL, et al. Prevalence of overweight and obesity among U.S. children, adolescents, and adults, 1999–2002. *JAMA*. 2004;291:2847–50.
2. Sarwer DB, Allison KC, Gibbons LM, et al. Pregnancy and obesity: A review and agenda for future research. *J Womens Health (Larchmt)*. 2006;15:720–33.
3. Aviram A, Hod M, Yegev Y. Maternal obesity: Implications for pregnancy outcome and long term risks: A link to maternal nutrition. *Int J Gynaecol Obstet*. 2011;115:S6–10.
4. Must A, Spadano J, Coakley EH, et al. The disease burden associated with overweight and obesity. *JAMA*. 1999;282:1523–9.
5. van deer Steeg JW, Steures P, Eijkemans MJ, et al. Obesity affects spontaneous pregnancy chances in subfertile, ovulatory women. *Hum Reprod*. 2008;23:324.
6. Cai GJ, Sun XX, Zhang L, Hong Q, et al. Association between maternal body mass index and congenital heart defects in offspring: A systematic review. *Am J Obstet Gynecol*. 2014;211:91.
7. Whitaker RC. Predicting preschooler obesity at birth: The role of maternal obesity in early pregnancy. *Pediatrics*. 2004;114:e29–36.
8. Krakowiak P, Walker CK, Bremer AA, et al. Maternal metabolic conditions and risk for autism and other neurodevelopmental disorders. *Pediatrics*. 2012;129:e1121.
9. Luoto R, Mannisto S, Raintanen J. Ten-year change in the association between obesity and parity: Results from the National FINRISK Population Study. *Gend* Med. 2011;8:399–406.
10. Linne Y, Dye L, Barkeling B, Rossner S. Long-term weight development in women: A 15-year follow-up of the effects of pregnancy. *Obes* Res. 2004;12:1166–78.
11. Yaniv-Salem S, Shoham Vardi I, Kessous R, Pariente G, Sergienko R, Sheiner E. Obesity in pregnancy: What's next? Long-term cardiovascular morbidity in a follow-up period of more than a decade. *J Mat-Fetal Neonat* Med. 2016;29(4):619–23.
12. Smith DE, Lewis CE, Caveny JL, et al. Longitudinal changes in adiposity associated with pregnancy: The CARDIA Study. *JAMA*. 1994;271:1747.
13. Butte NF, Hopkinson JM, Nicolson MA. Leptin in human reproduction: Serum leptin levels in pregnant and lactating women. *J Clin Endocrinol Metab*. 1997;82:585.
14. Stein TP, Scholl TO, Schluter MD, Schroeder CM. Plasma leptin influences gestational weight gain and postpartum weight retention. *Am J Clin Nutr*. 1998;68:1236.
15. Institute of Medicine. *Weight Gain during Pregnancy: Re-examining the Guidelines*. Washington, DC: National Academy Press; 2009.
16. Chung JG, Taylor RS, Thompson JM, et al. Gestational weight gain and adverse pregnancy outcomes in a nulliparous cohort. *Eur J Obstet Gynecol Reprod Biol*. 2013;167:149.
17. Harper LM, Chang JJ, Macones GA. Adolescent pregnancy and gestational weight gain: Do the Institute of Medicine recommendations apply? *Am J Obstet Gyencol*. 2011;205:140.e1.
18. American College of Obstetricians and Gynecologists. Obesity in pregnancy. ACOG Committee Opinion no. 549. *Obstet Gynecol*. 2013;121:213.
19. Davis MM, Slish K, Chao C, Cabana MD. National trends in bariatric surgery, 1996–2002. *Arch Surg*. 2006;141:71–4, discussion 75.

20. Maggard MA, Shugerman LR, Suttorp M, et al. Meta-analysis: Surgical treatment of obesity. *Ann Intern Med.* 2005;142:547–59.

21. Akkary E. Bariatric surgery evolution from the malabsorptive to the hormonal era. *Obes Surg.* 2012;22:827–31.

22. Dixon JB, Dixon ME, O-Brien PE. Birth outcomes in women after laparoscopic adjustable gastric banding. *Obstet Gynecol.* 2005;106:965–72.

23. Facchiano E, Ianelli A, Santulli P, Mandelbrot L, Msika S. Pregnancy after laparascopic bariatric surgery: Comparative study of adjustable gastric banding and Roex-en-Y gastric bypass. *Surg Obes Relat Dis.* 2012;8:429–33.

24. Wax JR, Pinette MG, Cartin A, Blackstone J. Female reproductive issues following bariatric surgery. *Obstet Gynecol Surv.* 2007;62:595–604.

25. Kral KG, Kava RA, Catalano PM, Moore BJ. Severe obesity: The neglected epidemic. *Obes Facts.* 2012;5:254–69.

26. Sheiner E, Edri A, Balaban E, Levi I, Aricha-Tamir B. Pregnancy outcome of patients who conceive during or after the first year following bariatric surgery. *Am J Obstet Gynecol.* 2011;204:50.e1–6.

27. Iavazzo C, Ntziora F, Rousos I, Paschalinopoulos D. Complications in pregnancy after bariatric surgery. *Arch Gynecol Obstet.* 2010;282:225–7.

28. Willis K, Sheiner E. Bariatric surgery and pregnancy: The magical solution? *J Perinat Med.* 2013;41:133–40.

29. Burke AE, Bennet WL, Jamshidi RM, et al. Reduced incidence of gestational diabetes with bariatric surgery. *J Am Coll Surg.* 2010;211:169–75.

30. Sheiner E, Levy A, Silverberg D, et al. Pregnancy after bariatric surgery is not associated with adverse perinatal outcome. *Am J Obstet Gynecol.* 2004;190:1335–40.

31. Maggard MA, Yermilov I, Li Z, et al. Pregnancy and fertility following bariatric surgery: A systematic review. *J Am Med Assoc.* 2008;300:2286–96.

32. Aricha-Tamir B, Weintraub AY, Levi I, Sheiner E. Downsizing pregnancy complications: A study of paired pregnancy outcomes before and after bariatric surgery. *Surg Obes Relat Dis.* 2012;8:434–9.

33. Weintraub AY, Levy A, Levi I, Mazor M, Witnitzer A, Sheiner E. Effect of bariatric surgery on pregnancy outcome. *Int J Gynecol Obstet.* 2008;103:246–51.

34. Lesko J, Peaceman A. Pregnancy outcomes in women after bariatric surgery compared with obese and morbidly obese controls. *Obstet Gynecol.* 2012;119:547–54.

35. Dell'Agnolo CM, Carvalho MD de B, Pelloso SM. Pregnancy after bariatric surgery: Implications for mother and newborn. *Obes Surg.* 2011;21:699–706.

36. Moore KA, Ouyang DW, Whang EE. Maternal and fetal deaths after gastric bypass surgery for morbid obesity. *N Eng J Med.* 2004;351:721.

37. Alexander CI, Liston WA. Operating on the obese women: A review. *BJOG.* 2006;113:1167.

38. Gunatilake RP, Perlow JH. Obesity and pregnancy: Clinical management of the obese gravid. *Am J Obstet Gynecol.* 2011;204:106.

39. Roofthooft E. Anaesthesia for the morbidly obese parturient. *Curr Opin Anaesthesiol.* 2009;22:341.

40. Vricella LK, Louis JM, Mercer BM, Bolden N. Anaesthesia complications during scheduled caesarean delivery for morbidly obese women. *Am J Obstet Gynecol.* 2010;203:276.e1.

41. Tixier H, Thouvenot S, Coulange L, et al. Caesarean section in morbidly obese women: Supra or sub-umbilical transverse incision? *Acta Obstet Gynecol Scand.* 2009;88:1049.

42. Alanis MC, Villers MS, Law TL, et al. Complications of caesarean delivery in the massively obese parturient. *Am J Obstet Gynecol.* 2010;203:271.e1.

43. Wolfe HM, Gross TL, Sokol RJ, et al. Determinants of morbidity in obese women delivered by caesarean. *Obstet Gynecol.* 1988;71:691.

44. Houston MC, Raynor BP. Postoperative morbidity in the morbidly obese parturient woman: Supraumbilical and low transverse abdominal approaches. *Am J Obstet Gynecol.* 2000;182:1033.

45. Chelmow D, Rodrigez EJ, Sabatini MM. Suture closure of subcutaneous fat and wound disruption after caesarean delivery: A meta-analysis. *Am J Obstet Gynecol.* 2007;197:229.

46. Ramsey PS, White AM, Guinn DA, et al. Subcutaneous tissue reapproximation, alone or in combination with drain, in obese women undergoing caesarean delivery. *Obstet Gynecol.* 2005;105:967.

47. Dronge AS, Perkal MF, Kancir S, et al. Long-term glycemic control and postoperative infectious complications. *Arch Surg.* 2006;141:375.

48. Pevzner L, Swank M, Krepel C, et al. Effects of maternal obesity on tissue concentrations of prophylactic cefazolin during caesarean delivery. *Obstet Gynecol*. 2011;117:877.

49. Chopra T, Zhao JJ, Alangaden G, et al. Preventing surgical site infections after bariatric surgery: Value of perioperative antibiotic regimens. *Exp Rev Pharmacoecon Outcomes* Res. 2010;10:317.

50. Bratzler DW, Dellinger EP, Olsen KM, et al. Clinical practice guidelines for antimicrobial prophylaxis in surgery. *Am J Health Sys Pharm*. 2013;70:195.

51. Heffner LJ, Sherman CB, Speizer FE, Weiss ST. Clinical and environmental predictors of preterm labor. *Obstet Gynecol*. 1993;81:750.

52. Practice Committee of the American Society for Reproductive Medicine. Smoking and infertility: A committee opinion. *Fertil Steril*. 2012;98:1400.

53. Castles A, Adams EK, Melvin CL, et al. Effects of smoking during pregnancy. Five meta-analyses. *Am J Prev* Med. 1999;16:208.

54. Spencer K, Cowans NJ. Accuracy of self-reported smoking status in the first trimester aneuploidy screening. *Prenat Diagn*. 2013;33:245.

55. Swamy GK, Reddick KL, Brouwer RJ, et al. Smoking prevalence in early pregnancy: A comparison of self-report and anonymous urine cotinine testing. *J Matern Fetal Neonat* Med. 2011;24:86.

56. Moore L, Campbell R, Whelan A, et al. Self help smoking cessation in pregnancy: Cluster randomised controlled trial. *BMJ*. 2002;325:1383.

57. Kendrick JS, Zahniser SC, Miller N, et al. Integrating smoking cessation into routine public prenatal care: The Smoking Cessation in Pregnancy project. *Am J Public Health*. 1995;85:217.

58. Tong VT, Dietz PM, Morrow B, et al. Trends in smoking before, during and after pregnancy: Pregnancy risk assessment monitoring system, United States, 40 sites 2000–2010. Available from: http://www.cdc.gov.myaccess.library.utoronto.ca/mmwr/preview/mmwrhtml/ss6206a1.htm?s_cid=ss6206a1_e (accessed November 8, 2013).

59. Kmietowicz Z. Smoking rates among pregnant women fall to all time low of 11%. *BMJ*. 2015;350:h3335.

60. Tong VT, Dietz PM, Farr SL, et al. Estimates of smoking before and during pregnancy, and smoking cessation during pregnancy: Comparing two population-based data sources. *Pub Health* Rep. 2013;128:179.

61. Alves E, Azevedo A, Correia S, Barros H. Long-term maintenance of smoking cessation in pregnancy: An analysis of the birth cohort generation XXI. *Nicotine Tob Res*. 2013;15:1598.

62. Orleans CT, Barker DC, Kaufman NJ, Marx JF. Helping pregnant smokers quit: Meeting the challenge in the next decade. *Tob Control*. 2000;9(Suppl 3): III6.

63. Mas R, Escriba V, Colomer C. Who quits smoking during pregnancy? *Scand J Soc Med*. 1996;24:102.

64. Wewers ME, Salsberry PJ, Ferketich AK, et al. Risk factors for smoking in rural women. *J Womens Health (Larchmt)*. 2012;21:548.

65. Windsor RA, Woodcy LL, Miller TM, et al. Effectiveness of Agency for Health Care Policy and Research clinical practise guideline and patient education methods for pregnancy smokers in Medicaid maternity care. *Am J Obstet Gynecol*. 2000;182:68.

66. Siu AL. Behavioural and pharmacotherapy interventions for tobacco smoking cessation in adults, including pregnant women: U.S. Preventive Services Task Force recommendation statement. *Ann Intern Med*. 2015; 163(8):622–34.

67. West R. Assessment of dependence and motivation to stop smoking. *BMJ*. 2004;328:338.

68. Heatherton TF, Kozlowski LT, Frecker RC, Fagerstrom KO. The Fagerstrom test for nicotine dependence: A revision of the Fagerstrom tolerance questionnaire. *Br J Addict*. 1991;86:1119.

69. Agency for Health Care Policy and Research. Smoking cessation: Information for specialists. *Clin Pract Guidel Quick Ref Guide Clin* 1996;18B;1.

70. Stead LF, Buitrago D, Preciado N, et al. Physician advise for smoking cessation. *Cochrane Database Syst* Rev. 2013;5:CD000165.

71. Solberg LI, Boyle RG, Davidson G, et al. Patient satisfaction and discussion of smoking cessation during clinical visits. *Mayo Clin Proc*. 2001;76:138.

72. National Institute for Health and Care Excellence. Quitting smoking in pregnancy and following childbirth (PH26). Available from: http://nice.org.uk/PH26 (accessed June 3, 2013).

73. DiClemente CC, Prochaska JO, Fairhurst SK, et al. The process of smoking cessation: An analysis of precontemplation, contemplation and preparation stages of change. *J Consult Clin Physcol*. 1991;59:295.

74. Henningfield JE, Miyasato K, Jasinski DR. Abuse liability and pharmacodynamic characteristics of intravenous and inhaled nicotine. *J Pharmacol Exp Ther*. 1985;234:1.

75. Filion KB, Abenhaim HA, Mottillo S, et al. The effect of smoking cessation counselling in pregnant women: A meta-analysis of randomised controlled trials. *BJOG*. 2011;118:1422.
76. Higgins ST, Washio Y, Heil SH, et al. Financial incentives for smoking cessation among pregnant and newly post-partum women. *Prev Med*. 2012;55(Suppl):S33.
77. Myung SK, Ju W, Jung HS, et al. Efficacy and safety of pharmacotherapy for smoking cessation among pregnant smokers: A meta-analysis. *BJOG*. 2012;119:1029.
78. Mei-Dan E, Walfisch A, Weisz B, Hallak M, Brown R, Shrim A. The unborn smoker: Association between smoking during pregnancy and adverse perinatal outcomes. *J Perinat Med*. 2015;43(5):553–8.
79. Lumley J, Chamberlain C, Dowswell T, et al. Interventions for promoting smoking cessation during pregnancy. *Cochrane Database Syst Rev*. 2009;4:CD01055.
80. Chamberlain C, O'Mara-Eves A, Oliver S, et al. Psychosocial interventions for supporting women to stop smoking in pregnancy. *Cochrane Database Syst Rev*. 2013;10:CD001055.
81. Tobacco product use among adults: United States, 2012–2013. Available from: http://www.cdc.gov.myaccess.library.utoronto.ca/mmwr/preview/mmwrhtml/mm63e06241a1.htm?s_cid=mm63e06241a1_e (accessed June 24, 2014).
82. Pollak KI, Oncken CA, Lipkus IM, et al. Nicotine replacement and behavioural therapy for smoking cessation in pregnancy. *Am J Prev Med*. 2007; 33:297.
83. Swamy GK, Roelands JJ, Peterson BL, et al. Predictors of adverse events among pregnant smokers exposed in a nicotine replacement trial. *Am J Obstet Gynecol*. 2009;201:354.e1.
84. Cooper S, Taggar J, Lewis S, et al. Effect of nicotine patches in pregnancy on infant and maternal outcomes at 2 years: Follow-up from the randomised, double-blind, placebo controlled SNAP trial. *Lancet Respir Med*. 2014;2:728.
85. Dhalwani NN, Szatkowski L, Coleman T, et al. Nicotine replacement therapy in pregnancy and major congenital anomalies in offspring. *Pediatrics*. 2015;135:859.
86. Coleman T, Chamberlain C, Davey MA, et al. Pharmacological interventions for promoting smoking cessation during pregnancy. *Cochrane Database Syst Rev*. 2012;9:CD010078.
87. Jorenby DE, Leischow SJ, Nides MA, et al. A controlled trial of sustained release bupropion, a nicotine patch, or both for smoking cessation. *N Engl J Med*. 1999;340;685.
88. Chen YF, Madan J, Welton N, et al. Effectiveness and cost-effectiveness of computer and other electronic aids for smoking cessation: A systematic review and network meta-analysis. *Health Technol Assess*. 2012;16:1.
89. Chun-Fai-Chan B, Koren G, Fayez I, et al. Pregnancy outcome of women exposed to buproprion during pregnancy: A prospective comparative study. *Am J Obstet Gynecol*. 2005;192:932.
90. Alwan S, Reefhuis J, Botto LD, et al. Maternal use of bupropion and risk for congenital heart defects. *Am J Obstet Gynecol*. 2010;203:52.e1.
91. Sachs HC, Comittee on Drugs. *Transfer of drugs and therapeutics into human breast milk: An update on selected topics. Pediatrics*. 2013;132:e796.
92. Truven Health Analytics: Micromedix Solutions. Available from: http://www.micromedex.com (accessed October 7, 2013).
93. Van't Hof SM, Wall MA, Dowler DW, Stark MJ. Randomised controlled trial of a postpartum relapse prevention intervention. *Tob Control*. 2000;9(Suppl 3):III64.
94. DiClemente CC, Dolan-Mullen P, Windsor RA. The process of pregnancy smoking cessation: Implications for interventions. *Tob Control*. 2000;9(Suppl 3):III16.

13

Preeclampsia and Long-Term Risk for the Offspring

Kira Nahum Sacks and Eyal Sheiner

Introduction

Preeclampsia is a disease characterized by gestational hypertension and proteinuria that effects 2%–8% of pregnancies worldwide [1]. In 2010, the rate of preeclampsia in the United States was 3.8%: an increase from 2.5% in 1987 [2]. This increase is disturbing since preeclampsia has a substantial impact on the intrauterine environment and is a leading cause of maternal and fetal mortality and morbidity [3,4]. It is well established that preeclampsia might have long-term consequences on the mother [5,6]. Regarding the offspring, previous studies have mainly addressed the increased risk of short-term outcomes such as cerebral palsy, encephalopathy, and febrile seizures [7]. This chapter will discuss what is currently known about the long-term morbidity associated with in utero exposure to preeclampsia.

Placental and Maternal Preeclampsia

When addressing morbidity in offspring exposed in utero to preeclampsia we must remember that preeclampsia is now viewed as an heterogeneous condition, composed of two different entities with different etiologies that simply manifest with the same symptoms of hypertension and proteinuria [8]. *Placental preeclampsia*, characterized by preeclampsia with onset before 34 gestational weeks, occurs predominantly in response to inadequate placentation, while *maternal preeclampsia*, characterized by preeclampsia with onset at or near term, occurs predominantly as a result of preexisting maternal conditions [9,10]. With this said, there will be women who will develop a blended form of preeclampsia on the basis of both placental and maternal factors [9]. Research in the field attempting to predict the later development of preeclampsia has recently proposed that preeclampsia can usefully be subclassified on the basis of biomarkers reflecting placental versus maternal preeclampsia [11,12].

Many of the studies that will be mentioned in the following chapter did not address this difference in onset week, primarily because this differentiation had not yet been made. With this said, all studies addressed gestational week at delivery, and although many cases of mild early-onset preeclampsia would be managed conservatively and ultimately reach a delivery near term, cases of early-onset severe preeclampsia or eclampsia would necessitate an early delivery. Therefore, until studies in the field of preeclampsia begin using the week of onset routinely, one might be able to extrapolate that findings unique to preterm preeclamptic deliveries may actually be attributed to early-onset preeclampsia.

Biochemical Mechanisms of Long-Term Offspring Morbidity

Another differentiation that needs to be made is between two dichotomous theories regarding the potential biochemical mechanisms underlying the association between preeclampsia and long-term offspring morbidity. One theory explains that adaptive responses to the preeclampsia intrauterine environment may result in epigenetic changes that affect disease susceptibility later in life [13]. This theory is strengthened by the notion that the pathophysiology of preeclampsia begins well before 20 weeks [14], and recently, imbalances in angiogenic biomarkers have been detected as early as 10 weeks in women who later developed preeclampsia [15]. Another acceptable theory is that genetic and environmental factors that predispose both the mother and the fetus to both pregnancy-related disorders and disorders later in life are inherited by the offspring [16]. These theories will be discussed further throughout the chapter, but as we review the emerging morbidity patterns in offspring exposed in utero to preeclampsia, there is a possibility that these patterns will shed light on the biochemical mechanisms underlying preeclampsia.

Long-Term Cardiovascular Morbidity

Already at birth, children born to preeclamptic mothers demonstrate a higher incidence of congenital heart defects [17]. Early-onset preeclampsia (before 34 weeks) is a significant risk factor for several heart defects, ranging from atrial and ventricle septal defects to common ventricle and endocardial cushions. Late-onset preeclampsia was also found to be associated with heart defects, but this association was far weaker, and aside from an association with tetralogy of Fallot, the association was primarily with non-critical heart defects such as atrial and ventricular septal defects [17].

Beyond this very early risk of congenital heart defects, prepubertal children who were prenatally exposed to preeclampsia have already been documented to have an increased incidence of various cardiovascular risk factors [16–26]. Fugelseth et al. found that in a group of 60 children as young as 5–8 years old, those exposed to preeclampsia in utero had smaller hearts, increased heart rate, and increased late diastolic velocity through the mitral valve [18]. Recently, Jayet et al. studied 48 children and found that pulmonary artery pressure was roughly 30% higher in the offspring of mothers with preeclampsia [19].

Children exposed in utero to preeclampsia have an increased BMI, but show no significant increase before the age of 10 years old [20–22] and increased total cholesterol and low-density lipoprotein [23,24], which is highest in children born small for gestational age (SGA).

There are scarce data regarding endpoint cardiovascular morbidity (Table 13.1), and the only endpoint morbidities that have been found to be associated with in utero exposure to preeclampsia have been hypertension [20,23,25–28], arrhythmias, cardiomyopathy, and heart failure [29]. While the association with hypertension has been proven and reproduced in multiple studies, other associations were found in a recent study [29]. Because in the majority of cases these conditions take many years to develop, the lack of data probably results from a lack of sufficient follow-up time. Figure 13.1 demonstrates that, by age 18, children prenatally exposed to eclampsia who later on developed a cardiovascular condition did so at a younger age than children unexposed to preeclampsia. An even longer follow-up time might help to reach a conclusion regarding children exposed to mild or severe preeclampsia as well.

Several theories have attempted to explain this association between preeclampsia and long-term cardiovascular morbidity in the offspring. Many of these theories are built on the understanding that preeclampsia and cardiovascular disease share common angiogenic pathways. It is already known that both conditions share common imbalances in proangiogenic signaling proteins such as vascular endothelial growth factor and placental growth factor, and in antiangiogenic proteins such as soluble endoglin and fms-like tyrosine kinase 1.

TABLE 13.1

Incidence Rates for Disease-Specific Cardiovascular Morbidity

Pediatric Morbidity	No Preeclampsia ($n = 243,701$)	Mild Preeclampsia ($n = 7,660$)	Severe Preeclampsia ($n = 2,366$)	Eclampsia ($n = 81$)	p Value[a]
Total cardiovascular morbidity ($n = 615$)	0.2%	0.3%	0.5%	0.3%	.001
Hypertension ($n = 158$)	0.1%	0.1%	0.1%	1.2%	.005
Arrhythmias ($n = 324$)	0.1%	0.2%	0.2%	0.2%	.093
Cardiomyopathy ($n = 42$)	0.0%	0.1%	0.0%	0.0%	.021
Heart failure ($n = 81$)	0.0%	0.0%	0.2%	0.0%	.011

Source: Sacks KDN, et al., *Am J Obstet Gynecol*, 214, S260, 2016.

[a] Data evaluated with χ^2 test for trends.

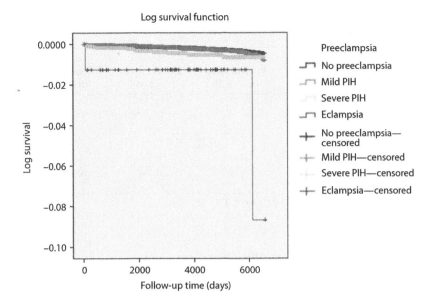

FIGURE 13.1 Kaplan–Meier survival curve demonstrating survival until the development of cardiovascular morbidity in children exposed to varying degrees of preeclampsia.

One theory says that either genetic or environmental factors that affect these pathways predispose both the mother and the fetus to both pregnancy-related disorders and cardiovascular disorders later in life. This theory is supported both by the fact that women born to preeclamptic mothers have a higher incidence of preeclampsia [30], and also by the fact that women who had preeclampsia have a higher incidence of cardiovascular morbidity [5].

Another theory is that this imbalance originates in maternal pathology, and the preeclampsia intrauterine environment of imbalanced proangiogenic and antiangiogenic proteins affects the development of a healthy cardiovascular system. Consistent with this theory, studies have shown imbalances in angiogenic biomarkers as early as 10 weeks in women who later developed preeclampsia, early enough to affect fetal heart morphogenesis [17]. An interesting finding that might contradict this theory is that in multiple gestations, even though fms-like tyrosine kinase is elevated, there is no association between preeclampsia and heart defects in the offspring. This finding supports the notion that it is not the in utero exposure to elevated antiangiogenic proteins that predisposes children to future cardiovascular morbidity.

Long-Term Endocrinological Morbidity

Studies have found that children exposed in utero to preeclampsia have increased fasting glucose level beyond age 12, but this association was found only in children born preterm [23,27]. Obesity, on the other hand, has been found to be strongly associated to in utero exposure to preeclampsia (Table 13.2) regardless of gestational week at birth [29]. The rate of childhood obesity (until the age of 18 years) is 0.4% in children born to preeclamptic patients versus 0.2% in children born to mothers without preeclampsia ($p < .001$).

These finding may represent the early stages in the development of diabetes mellitus, but it is unclear at what age these predispositions may, if at all, manifest into a full-blown disease. Currently, the longest follow-up documented is a study that followed offspring until age 18 [29], and at least in that study there was no significant statistical association between preeclampsia and diabetes mellitus of the offspring (the rate was 0.1% in the preeclampsia group vs. 0.1% in the comparison group; $p = .809$).

It is very likely that a longer follow-up is needed, since according to the Centers for Disease Control (CDC) most new cases of type 2 diabetes mellitus are diagnosed in the age group between 45 and 64 [31], and therefore a significant difference might be detectable only later on in life. With this said, the

TABLE 13.2

Incidence Rates for Disease-Specific Endocrine Morbidity

Pediatric Morbidity	No Preeclampsia ($n = 243,701$)	Mild Preeclampsia ($n = 7,660$)	Severe Preeclampsia ($n = 2,366$)	Eclampsia ($n = 81$)	p Value[a]
Total endocrinological morbidity ($n = 1,084$)	0.4%	0.7%	0.7%	1.2%	.002
Obesity ($n = 473$)	0.2%	0.4%	0.3%	1.2%	.001
Diabetes mellitus ($n = 233$)	0.1%	0.1%	0.2%	0.0%	.546

Source: Sacks KDN, et al., *Am J Obstet Gynecol*, 214, S260, 2016.

[a]   Data evaluated with x^2 test for trends.

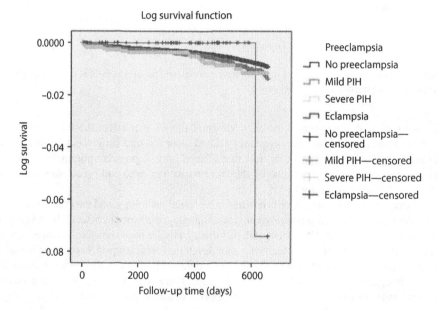

FIGURE 13.2   Kaplan–Meier survival curve demonstrating survival until the development of endocrine morbidity in children exposed to varying degrees of preeclampsia.

same study used Kaplan–Meier survival curves to see if children prenatally exposed to preeclampsia that developed endocrine morbidity did so at a younger age than their unexposed counterparts, and found no significant difference in the rates at which children exposed or unexposed in utero to preeclampsia developed endocrine morbidity (Figure 13.2).

Long-Term Neuropsychiatric Morbidity

In utero exposure to preeclampsia has been found to be associated with an increased risk of obstructive sleep apnea (OSA) [29], autistic spectrum disorder [32], epilepsy in children born at term [7], and cerebral palsy in children born at term [13] (Table 13.3). In a recent study, children exposed in utero to preeclampsia had a significantly higher incidence of OSA, and the incidence of OSA increased linearly with the severity of preeclampsia [29]. Undoubtedly, this finding must be reproduced in order to improve generalizability and in order to be addressed adequately. An important disclaimer is that the

TABLE 13.3

Incidence Rates for Disease-Specific Neurological Morbidity

Pediatric Morbidity	No Preeclampsia ($n = 243{,}701$)	Mild Preeclampsia ($n = 7{,}660$)	Severe Preeclampsia ($n = 2{,}366$)	Eclampsia ($n = 81$)	p Value[a]
Total neurological morbidity ($n = 2{,}532$)	1.0%	1.2%	1.9%	1.2%	<.001
OSA[b] ($n = 1{,}404$)	0.5%	0.6%	1.1%	0.0%	.002
Epilepsy ($n = 466$)	0.2%	0.2%	0.4%	1.2%	.005
CP[b] ($n = 233$)	0.1%	0.1%	0.2%	0.0%	.450

Source: Sacks KDN, et al., *Am J Obstet Gynecol*, 214, S260, 2016.

[a] Data evaluated with x^2 test for trends.

[b] OSA: obstructive sleep apnea; CP: cerebral palsy.

pathophysiology of OSA is unclear and is currently being treated by otolaryngologists, pulmonologists, and neurologists. We have included OSA, a condition resulting from a combination of narrow airways, insufficient neuromuscular activity, and impaired ventilator control [33] under neurologic morbidity, in the same way that it is classified in the Ninth Revision of the *International Classification of Diseases* (ICD), respiratory morbidities have not been associated with in utero exposure to preeclampsia (ours), and therefore, it seems more likely that the predisposition should be attributed to the neurological system.

The association between in utero exposure to preeclampsia and epilepsy or infantile spasms in the offspring has been demonstrated and reproduced in a number of papers. While one study found this association significant only in children born at term [7], another found preeclampsia to be an independent risk factor for epilepsy in the offspring regardless of gestational week at delivery [29].

There is clashing evidence regarding all other neurologic morbidity. In a study by Walker et al. they found that in utero exposure to preeclampsia is associated with an increased risk of autistic spectrum disorder [32], but another study found no such association [29]. A study by Wu et al. found that singletons exposed prenatally to preeclampsia were at increased risk of cerebral palsy in children born at term and a decreased risk of cerebral palsy in children born preterm [16,34]. This association was found statistically insignificant in other research [29]. Despite these inconsistencies, when the incidence rate of neurological morbidity is analyzed as a group of neuropsychiatric conditions, neurological morbidity has been found to be associated to in utero exposure to preeclampsia (the rate was 1.0% in the preeclampsia group vs. 1.3% in the comparison group; $p < .01$) [29]. Furthermore, the Kaplan–Meier curve in Figure 13.3 demonstrates that children prenatally exposed to severe preeclampsia that developed neurologic morbidity later on in life developed their condition at a younger age than children unexposed to preeclampsia.

Unclassified Morbidities

One of the biggest studies in the field was conducted in Denmark by Wu et al., who performed a population-based cohort study of 1,618,481 singletons with up to 27 years follow-up. The findings unique to this research were an increased risk of anemia and purpura and an increased risk of urogenital malformations [13]. Figure 13.4 demonstrates that children prenatally exposed to eclampsia who later on developed hematological disease did so at a younger age than children exposed to mild preeclampsia. Figure 13.5 demonstrates that children prenatally exposed to eclampsia who later on developed urinary disease did so at a younger age than children exposed to any milder form of preeclampsia. Since hematopoiesis and cardiac morphogenesis share common embryonic pathways, it is possible that these disturbances in the hematological system may be explained by the same mechanisms as cardiovascular morbidities. Regarding urogenital malformations, it is unclear what might be the underlying mechanism.

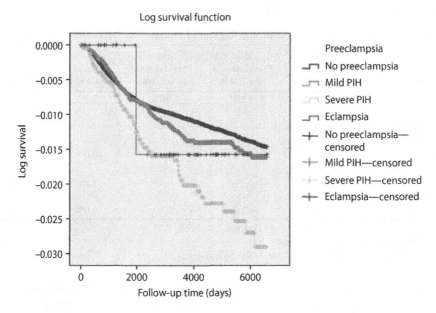

FIGURE 13.3   Kaplan–Meier survival curve demonstrating survival until the development of neurological morbidity in children exposed to varying degrees of preeclampsia.

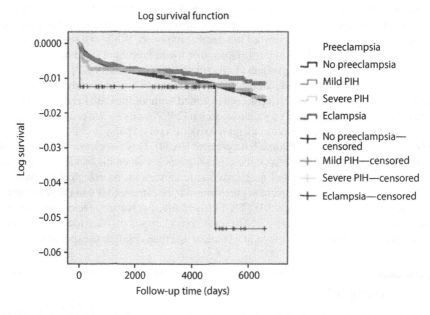

FIGURE 13.4   Kaplan–Meier survival curve demonstrating survival until the development of hematological morbidity in children exposed to varying degrees of preeclampsia.

FUTURE IMPLICATIONS

It seems that the immediate and obvious implication of identifying and characterizing the morbidities associated with in utero exposure to preeclampsia is in the field of pediatrics. In a world where we begin medically treating cardiovascular risks already in early adulthood, we should understand which in utero environment constitutes a cardiovascular risk factor. In addition, characterizing the morbidities

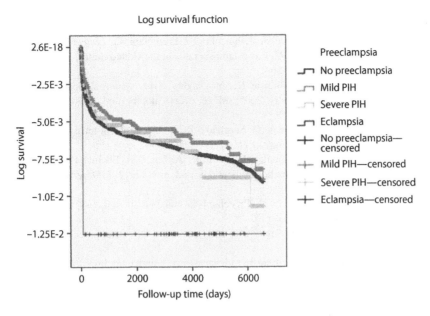

FIGURE 13.5 Kaplan–Meier survival curve demonstrating survival until the development of urinary morbidity in children exposed to varying degrees of preeclampsia.

TABLE 13.4

Risk of Pediatric Morbidity in Children Prenatally Exposed to Preeclampsia, by Category of Pediatric Health

Pediatric Morbidity	Odds Ratio[a,b]	95% CI[c]	p Value
Cardiovascular	1.59	1.14–2.23	.006
Endocrine	1.42	1.11–1.84	.006
Neurologic	1.36	1.14–1.64	.001
Respiratory	1.32	1.21–1.45	.001
Hematological	1.62	0.76–1.16	.570
Urinary	1.13	0.88–1.45	.326

Source: Sacks KDN, et al., *Am J Obstet Gynecol*, 214, S260, 2016.
[a] Data evaluated with a generalized estimating equation (GEE) logistic regression model analysis.
[b] Adjusted for maternal age and gestational week at delivery, maternal diabetes mellitus, and offspring age at first hospitalization.
[c] CI: confidence interval.

associated with preeclampsia exposure might also help make difficult pediatric diagnoses. In the arena of basic science, the morbidity patterns emerging among preeclampsia offspring may help navigate researchers toward possible pathophysiology, as was discussed previously.

As for the primary prevention of pediatric morbidity, there is still much to learn before obstetricians can make clinical decisions based on the long-term impact on the offspring. This chapter describes a clear *association* between prenatal exposure to preeclampsia and long-term pediatric morbidity (Table 13.4), but these findings are insufficient to conclude *causation*. This association may be due to common genetic pathways or impaired in utero environments, but it may also be due to the treatment preeclamptic women are receiving to lower blood pressure or prevent seizures. Further research should assess how varying clinical management impacts this association between preeclampsia and future fetal health.

REFERENCES

1. Steegers EA, von Dadelszen P, Duvekot JJ, Pijnenborg R. Pre-eclampsia. *Lancet*. 2010;376(9741):631–44.
2. Ananth CV, Keyes KM, Wapner RJ. Pre-eclampsia rates in the United States, 1980–2010: Age-period-cohort analysis. *BMJ*. 2013;347:f6564.
3. Roberts JM, Gammill HS. Preeclampsia: Recent insights. *Hypertension*. 2005;46(6):1243–9.
4. Matthews Z. World health report 2005: Make every mother and child count. *World Health*. 2005;33(6):409–11.
5. Kessous R, Shoham-Vardi I, Pariente G, Sergienko R, Sheiner E. Long-term maternal atherosclerotic morbidity in women with pre-eclampsia. *Heart*. 2015;101(6):442–6.
6. Shalom G, Shoham-Vardi I, Sergienko R, Wiznitzer A, Sherf M, Sheiner E. Is preeclampsia a significant risk factor for long-term hospitalizations and morbidity? *J Matern Fetal Neonatal Med*. 2013;26(1):13–15.
7. Wu CS, Sun Y, Vestergaard M, et al. Preeclampsia and risk for epilepsy in offspring. *Pediatrics*. 2008;122(5):1072–8.
8. Raymond D, Peterson E. A critical review of early-onset and late-onset preeclampsia. *Obstet Gynecol Surv*. 2011;66(8):497–506.
9. Redman CW, Sargent IL. Latest advances in understanding preeclampsia. *Science*. 2005;308(5728):1592–4.
10. von Dadelszen P, Magee LA, Roberts JM. Subclassification of preeclampsia. *Hypertens Pregnancy*. 2003;22(2):143–8.
11. Chappell LC, Duckworth S, Seed PT, et al. Diagnostic accuracy of placental growth factor in women with suspected preeclampsia: A prospective multicenter study. *Circulation*. 2013;128(19):2121–31.
12. Staff AC, Benton SJ, von Dadelszen P, et al. Redefining preeclampsia using placenta-derived biomarkers. *Hypertension*. 2013;61(5):932–42.
13. Gluckman PD, Hanson MA, Cooper C, Thornburg KL. Effect of in utero and early-life conditions on adult health and disease. *N Engl J Med*. 2014;359(1):61–73.
14. Roberts JM, Bell MJ. If we know so much about preeclampsia, why haven't we cured the disease? *J Reprod Immunol*. 2013;99(1–2):1–9.
15. Noori M, Donald AE, Angelakopoulou A, Hingorani AD, Williams DJ. Prospective study of placental angiogenic factors and maternal vascular function before and after preeclampsia and gestational hypertension. *Circulation*. 2010;122(5):478–87.
16. Wu CS, Nohr EA, Bech BH, Vestergaard M, Catov JM, Olsen J. Health of children born to mothers who had preeclampsia: A population-based cohort study. *Am J Obstet Gynecol*. 2009;201(3):269. e1–10.
17. Auger N, Fraser WD, Healy-Profitós J, Arbour L. Association between preeclampsia and congenital heart defects. *JAMA*. 2015;314(15):1588.
18. Fugelseth D, Ramstad HB, Kvehaugen AS, Nestaas E, Støylen A, Staff AC. Myocardial function in offspring 5–8 years after pregnancy complicated by preeclampsia. *Early Hum Dev*. 2011;87(8):531–5.
19. Xiang AH, Wang X, Martinez MP, et al. Association of maternal diabetes with autism in offspring. *JAMA*. 2015;313(14):1425.
20. Davis EF, Lazdam M, Lewandowski AJ, et al. Cardiovascular risk factors in children and young adults born to preeclamptic pregnancies: A systematic review. *Pediatrics*. 2012;129(6):e1552–61.
21. Seidman DS, Laor A, Gale R, Stevenson DK, Mashiach S, Danon YL. Pre-eclampsia and offspring's blood pressure, cognitive ability and physical development at 17-years-of-age. *Br J Obstet Gynaecol*. 1991;98(10):1009–14.
22. Ogland B, Vatten LJ, Romundstad PR, Nilsen ST, Forman MR. Pubertal anthropometry in sons and daughters of women with preeclamptic or normotensive pregnancies. *Arch Dis Child*. 2009;94(11):855–9.
23. Lazdam M, De La Horra A, Pitcher A, et al. Elevated blood pressure in offspring born premature to hypertensive pregnancy: Is endothelial dysfunction the underlying vascular mechanism? *Hypertension*. 2010;56:159–65.
24. Kvehaugen AS, Dechend R, Ramstad HB, Troisi R, Fugelseth D, Staff AC. Endothelial function and circulating biomarkers are disturbed in women and children after preeclampsia. *Hypertension*. 2011;58(1):63–9.

25. Vatten LJ, Romundstad PR, Holmen TL, Hsieh CC, Trichopoulos D, Stuver SO. Intrauterine exposure to preeclampsia and adolescent blood pressure, body size, and age at menarche in female offspring. *Obstet Gynecol*. 2003;101(3):529–33.
26. Palti H, Rothschild E. Blood pressure and growth at 6 years of age among offsprings of mothers with hypertension of pregnancy. *Early Hum Dev*. 1989;19(4):263–9.
27. Tenhola S, Rahiala E. Blood pressure, serum lipids, fasting insulin, and adrenal hormones in 12-year-old children born with maternal preeclampsia. *J Clin Endocrinol Metab*. 2003;88(3):1217–22.
28. Lazdam M, De La Horra A, Diesch J, et al. Unique blood pressure characteristics in mother and offspring after early onset preeclampsia. *Hypertension*. 2012;60(5):1338–45.
29. Sacks KDN, Friger M, Spiegel E, et al. Prenatal exposure to preeclampsia as an independent risk factor for long-term pediatric morbidity of the offspring. *Am J Obstet Gynecol*. 2016;214(1):S260.
30. Sherf Y, Sheiner E, Shoham Vardi I, Bilenko N. Like mother like daughter; Low birthweight and preeclampsia tend to re-occur at the next generation. *Am J Obstet Gynecol*. 2015;212(1):S34.
31. US Centers for Disease Control and Prevention. National diabetes fact sheet: National estimates and general information on diabetes and prediabetes in the United States, 2011. *US Dep Heal Hum Serv Centers Dis Control Prev*. 2011;3:1–12.
32. Walker CK, Krakowiak P, Baker A, Hansen RL, Ozonoff S, Hertz-Picciotto I. Preeclampsia, placental insufficiency, and autism spectrum disorder or developmental delay. *JAMA Pediatr*. 2014;95817:1–9.
33. Katz ES, D'Ambrosio CM. Pathophysiology of pediatric obstructive sleep apnea. *Proc Am Thorac Soc*. 2008;5(2):253–62.
34. Thorngren-Jerneck K, Herbst A. Perinatal factors associated with cerebral palsy in children born in Sweden. *Obs Gynecol*. 2006;108(6):1499–505.

14

Life Course Outcomes for the Child of the Diabetic Mother

Jonah Susser Kreniske, Ron Charach, and Eyal Sheiner

Introduction

In the early twenty-first century, diabetes mellitus has developed into a global epidemic. The burden of disease is expanding at an alarming rate, particularly in the developing world [1]. While diabetes strikes in all social strata, a great tragedy of this disease is its proclivity to preferentially impact those with the least resources to manage its complications [2]. Given the high prevalence of diabetes, it should come as no surprise that diabetes in pregnancy has become an epidemic in its own right, affecting an estimated 16% of pregnancies worldwide, 90% of which are in low- or middle-income countries [3]. As the condition becomes increasingly common, it is ever more necessary to understand its mechanisms and its sequelae.

Perinatal and Life Course Outcomes

Perinatal Complications in the Child of the Diabetic Mother

The fetal complications of diabetes mellitus in pregnancy are significant and diverse. Both short- and long-term sequelae have been reported in the offspring of diabetic mothers, and each has implications for the life course of the child. The nature and frequency of these complications varies depending whether the mother has pregestational (type 1 or 2 diabetes) or gestational diabetes mellitus (PGDM/GDM). Table 14.1 summarizes the common perinatal outcomes associated with each. A common underlying mechanism influencing many of these outcomes seems to involve maternal hyperglycemia (and possibly abnormalities in circulating lipids and amino acids), which characterizes both PGDM and GDM. Because glucose can cross the placenta but insulin cannot, maternal hyperglycemia induces a sugar-rich intrauterine environment, the fetal response to which involves both insulin hypersecretion and potentially long-lasting insulin resistance [4]. The consequences of this imbalance, and other abnormalities, on perinatal outcomes for the child of the diabetic mother are discussed in this section.

PGDM mothers, both type 1 and type 2, experience a dramatically increased incidence of congenital malformations in their offspring, with odds ratios ranging from 1.9 to 10 times the risk in the general population. By contrast, the risk of congenital malformation in GDM is far less significant. Though GDM may represent a risk factor for congenital malformation, odds ratios range between 1.1 and 1.3, and may be accounted for by previously undiagnosed type 2 diabetes [1–3,8,9].

The manifestations of the congenital malformations associated with PGDM are varied and involve nearly every organ system, including cardiac malformations (transposition of the great vessels, atrial septal defects, ventriculoseptal defects, coarctation of the aorta), gastrointestinal malformations (duodenal or rectal atresia, hypoplasia of the colon), CNS and spinal malformations (neural tube defects, caudal regression syndrome), as well as urogenital abnormalities. The mechanism of teratogenicity may be associated with maternal hyperglycemia in the first trimester, the primary window of organogenesis. This early hyperglycemic state may expose the fetus to oxidative stresses, perhaps leading to a disturbance in

TABLE 14.1

Prenatal Outcomes of GDM and PGDM

Perinatal Outcome	Association with Gestational Diabetes Mellitus	Association with Pregestational Diabetes Mellitus
Congenital malformation	Weak	Strong
Perinatal death	Weak	Strong

organ development and apoptosis [10]. The later onset of hyperglycemia in GDM as opposed to PGDM may account for the difference in congenital anomalies, with second- and third-trimester hyperglycemia more frequently resulting in fetal hyperglycemia, hyperinsulinemia, and macrosomia [11].

In part, though not entirely, due to the congenital malformations discussed previously, both types of PGDM mothers are at greater risk of giving birth to children who are either stillborn or die within the first month of life. The risk is comparable in these two groups, at three to five times that of the general population [12,13]. While glycemic control in PGDM mothers has been proposed as the most important factor for minimizing the risk of perinatal mortality in this population, it is interesting to note that, even with improved glycemic control, type 2 diabetic mothers are at higher risk of these complications than are type 1 diabetic mothers with comparable hemoglobin A1C levels [14,15]. This disparity may suggest the influence of other risk factors associated with type 2 diabetes such as obesity, ethnicity, and low socioeconomic status [16].

Perinatal infant mortality in GDM is much lower than in PGDM and, as with the risk of congenital malformation, the minor correlation between perinatal mortality and GDM may be attributable to previously undiagnosed type 2 diabetes [7,17–19].

Preterm birth is the leading cause of infant morbidity and mortality in the general population, and women with pregestational diabetes have been found to demonstrate up to a 25% greater risk of premature delivery [20]. In type 2 diabetic mothers, the risk of preterm delivery is predicted by third-trimester glycemic control, whereas in type 1 mothers pregestational hypertension is a more reliable predictor [21]. GDM has also been found to be an independent risk factor for early delivery [22]. There is a significant body of evidence establishing the far-reaching life course implications of being born preterm.

Long-Term Complications in the Child of the Diabetic Mother

The long-term impact of maternal diabetes on the life course of the child ranges from an increased susceptibility to early-onset insulin insensitivity to a maladaptive cardiovascular risk profile throughout life. The specifics of these various conditions and their relationship to diabetes in the mother are discussed in this section.

A significant body of evidence suggests the diabetic intrauterine environment predisposes offspring to the development of insulin resistance and type 2 diabetes, regardless of the etiology of the mother's diabetic state [23]. This relationship is further supported by the observation that siblings born to diabetic mothers before and after the onset of disease show discordance in their proclivity to develop insulin resistance [24].

The association between the diabetic intrauterine environment and obesity is more tenuous. There is a significant risk of the children of diabetic mothers developing macrosomia, and higher BMIs at all ages [25]. Establishing a causal relationship, however, between maternal diabetes and obesity in offspring has been challenging. One difficulty in ascertaining the nature of the relationship lies in the confounding variable represented by maternal BMI; thus, it remains unclear whether maternal diabetes or maternal obesity play a more significant role in the development of obesity in the next generation [26]. A recent review has cast significant doubt on the association, with the suggestion that confounders such as parental BMI have not been adequately accounted for in the analysis of the relationship between diabetes during gestation and offspring obesity [27].

Children exposed to the diabetic environment in utero have been shown to develop worse cardiovascular risk profiles than their peers gestated in the nondiabetic womb [28]. Indeed, maternal GDM has been demonstrated as an independent risk factor for long-term cardiovascular complications and hospitalizations in the next generation [29].

In addition to exhibiting an increased risk of cardiovascular disease, children exposed to diabetes in utero have been found to be more vulnerable not only to the renal developmental malformations discussed previously, but also to developing renal function abnormalities in adulthood, including proteinuria and reduced renal functional reserve [30].

The increased risk of prematurity documented in children born to diabetic mothers has far-reaching and well-evidenced implications for long-term health. Preterm birth is an independent risk factor for the development of type 2 diabetes later in life, which compounds the association between the diabetic intrauterine environment and the development of type 2 diabetes [31–34]. In addition to reduced insulin sensitivity, young adults born preterm also appear to have an increased risk of developing hypertension [34].

The relationship between maternal diabetes and autism was recently examined by Xiang et al. in a large cohort study. The authors found that while preexisting diabetes had no influence on the development of autism in the next generation, GDM diagnosed at 26 weeks was associated with autism spectrum disorders in the next generation [35]. While the study did not include potential confounders such as paternal weight or preexisting comorbidities, the nature of this relationship warrants further investigation [36]. In particular, the effect of glycemic control during pregnancy on the risk of autism represents an important next step for research. Recent evidence has also emerged linking GDM to long-term cumulative neurologic morbidity [37]. This finding is illustrated in Figure 14.1.

Further studies demonstrating a relationship between GDM and a variety of other conditions have also appeared. Among these, several morbidities including respiratory and cardiovascular disease and endocrine dysfunction have been correlated with GDM in large cohort analyses [38–40]. Figures 14.2 and 14.3 demonstrate these findings.

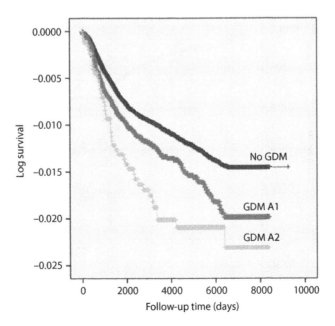

FIGURE 14.1 The results of a retrospective population-based cohort study comparing neurological morbidity among children exposed to prenatal GDM and those unexposed. The exposure variables were diet-controlled GDM (GDM1) and treated GDM (GDM2). A multivariable generalized estimating equation (GEE) logistic regression model analysis was used to control for confounders and for maternal clusters.

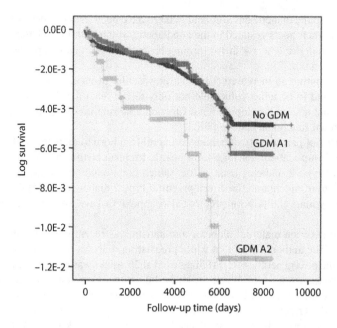

FIGURE 14.2 Long-term cardiovascular outcomes of children prenatally exposed and unexposed to GDM. The exposure variables were diet-controlled GDM (GDM1) and treated GDM (GDM2). A multivariate generalized estimating equation (GEE) logistic regression model analysis was used to control for confounders and for maternal clusters.

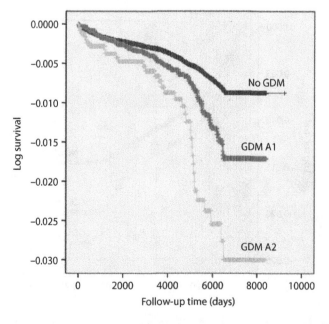

FIGURE 14.3 Long-term outcomes of children prenatally exposed and unexposed to GDM. The exposure variables were diet-controlled GDM (GDM 1) and treated GDM (GDM2). A multivariate generalized estimating equation (GEE) logistic regression model analysis was used to control for confounders and for maternal clusters.

Mechanisms

The Big Picture

The influence of the intrauterine environment on fetal metabolic development has been suggested by epidemiological studies and supported by investigations into the epigenetics of the relationship between mother and fetus. Changes in the developmental makeup of the fetus are induced by alterations in the intrauterine metabolic or nutritional environment, and are also precipitated by maternal hormonal fluctuations. This *programming* or *metabolic imprinting* may permanently alter the course of development and pose a major risk of the development of morbidity in adulthood [41–43].

The intrauterine environment of the diabetic mother has serious implications for fetal metabolic programming independent of classical genetic factors, particularly in the development of the pancreas and insulin-dependent target tissues, which may ultimately have a permanent effect on the risk of obesity and diabetes [44]. This functional influence of the diabetic intrauterine environment may be mediated by epigenetic factors [45].

The effect of nutrition on the indices of fetal and infant health has been established for at least half a century [46]. Epigenetic transmission of diabetes mellitus from mother to child was suggested almost as long ago, dating back to Dorner, Mohnike, and Steindel [47]. This hypothesis has gained traction since, with extensive observational and basic science research, supporting both the process of transmission and its epigenetic mechanism [7,45].

Before delving deeper into the potential functional and epigenetic mechanisms of offspring pathology associated with maternal diabetes, we will turn our attention back to an epidemiological framework in which to contextualize this discussion. A substantial body of research has demonstrated an association between maternal diabetes and offspring insulin insensitivity [24,48–50]. A number of these studies are summarized in Table 14.2. We will focus on two major epidemiological cohorts that have been prospectively examined to elucidate the relationship between the diabetic intrauterine environment and the development of diabetes in the child, as well as obesity and cardiovascular risk factors later in life [23]. Both of these studies—the Pima Indian study and the Diabetes in Pregnancy Study at Northwestern University—were conducted in the United States. The Northwestern study involved a population with a diverse ethnic composition, while the Pima Indian study relied on data from a single American indigenous group with an exceptionally high rate of type 2 diabetes.

The Northwestern study compared long-term glucose tolerance in children born to diabetic mothers (PGDM or GDM) with children born to normoglycemic mothers. The study found a strong correlation between increased insulin concentration in the amniotic fluid and impaired glucose tolerance in the children when they reached adolescence (10–16 years of age). Indeed, in those children whose mothers were diabetic, but in whom insulin levels in the amniotic fluid reflected the control population, the risk of impaired glucose tolerance at adolescence was no higher than that in the control population [51,52].

A series of widely discussed studies conducted among the Pima people of Southern Arizona also suggested a relationship between insulin insensitivity in mother and child. The Arizona Pima people have experienced a substantial social and economic transformation over the past century, and in the process have developed an incidence and prevalence of type 2 diabetes that is among the highest recorded [53,54]. In the process of elucidating parental factors in the development of diabetes among the Pima, Dabelea and Pettitt examined the role of both paternal and maternal diabetes on the susceptibility of offspring to type 2 diabetes in childhood and adolescence. In this analysis, a significant risk was associated with maternal diabetes, but no relationship was found with regard to paternal diabetes [55]. The findings of Silverman et al. and Dablea and Pettitt with regard to offspring diabetes in adolescence are summarized in Figure 14.4.

In order to control for genetic and environmental factors, the authors went on to compare siblings born to the same mother before and after she developed diabetes. In this case, those siblings born after their mother's development of diabetes demonstrated a risk nearly four times that of their siblings born before the mother's diabetes developed [24]. These findings in discordant sibships are suggestive of an influence mediated, in part, by epigenetic factors.

TABLE 14.2

Studies Implicating the Role of Maternal Diabetes in Offspring Risk

Method	Study	Year	Conclusions	*p* value
Retrospective parental and offspring phenotypes	Dorner et al. [47]	1975	Maternal diabetes, not paternal, associated with diabetes in the offspring.	<.001
	Alcolado JC, Alcolado R [48]	1991	Maternal diabetes associated with diabetes in offspring. No association with paternal diabetes.	<.001
	Thomas et al. [49]	1994	Maternal diabetes twice as likely to be associated with offspring diabetes when compared with paternal diabetes.	<.001
Longitudinal study comparing diabetes rates in offspring of prediabetic, nondiabetic, and diabetic mothers during pregnancy	Pettitt et al. [50]	1985	Offspring of diabetic women are far more likely to develop type 2 diabetes at all ages than are offspring of prediabetic or nondiabetic women.	<.05
Prospective measurement of amniotic fluid insulin at 32–38 weeks of gestation and postnatal glucose and insulin measurements	Silverman et al. [52]	1995	Excess fetal insulin secretion in utero predicts insulin resistance in adolescence.	<.001
Longitudinal study measuring the prevalence of diabetes in siblings born before and after their mother was recognized as having diabetes	Dabelea et al. [24]	2000	In discordant sibships, offspring born to mothers after the development of diabetes show an increased risk of type 2 diabetes when compared with siblings born before.	<.05

The risk of obesity and hypertension in children born to diabetic mothers was also examined in both these studies and their subsequent follow-ups. In the Pima people, one analysis of over one thousand children found that the offspring of diabetic mothers were twice as likely to be obese. By adolescence, 58% of children born to diabetic mothers were overweight or obese, compared with 25% of those born

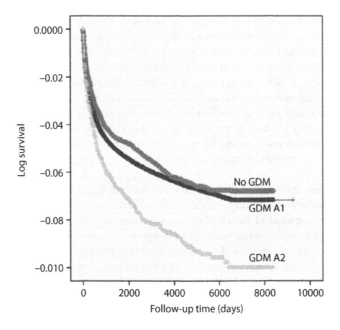

FIGURE 14.4 Long-term respiratory outcomes of children prenatally exposed and unexposed to GDM. The exposure variables were diet-controlled GDM (GDM1) and treated GDM (GDM2). A multivariable generalized estimating equation (GEE) logistic regression model was used to control for confounders and for maternal clusters.

to prediabetic mothers and 17% of those born to nondiabetic women ($p < .001$) [56]. The results from Chicago corroborated these findings [23]. With regard to hypertension, follow-up analysis of the Pima study and the Northwestern study once again yielded consistent results. In both data sets, it was found that offspring exposed to diabetes in utero showed elevated systolic blood pressure during childhood compared with their nonexposed peers [51,57].

Physiology

In the following section, a summary of some of the most current understandings of the functional abnormalities that may underlie the consequences of diabetic pregnancy and their influence on the life course of the child is presented.

The predisposition to hypertension observed in the offspring of diabetic mothers may be related in part to anomalies in renal development. Nephrogenesis, the development of the functional units of the human kidney, occurs during fetal life and is complete by the time birth takes place [58]. Given that nephrons do not multiply after birth, any reduction in their number could have grave implications for kidney and cardiovascular health [59]. A number of animal models have suggested that maternal hyperglycemia precipitates a reduction in fetal nephrogenesis, leading to a relative nephron deficiency, which may play a role in the predisposition of offspring to hypertension [60]. Some models also provide support for the hypothesis that diabetic offspring are less capable of increasing salt excretion upon exposure to high-salt diets, rendering them more susceptible to salt-induced hypertension [59].

Diabetic offspring have been found to have cardiovascular abnormalities independent of the renal impairments discussed previously. Intracellular adhesion molecules are key mediators of the human inflammatory response. Their soluble plasma concentration has been associated with an increased risk of myocardial infarction in healthy men, suggesting that they may play a role in atherogenesis [61]. Perhaps significantly, intrauterine exposure to diabetes has been associated with an increase in the plasma concentration of soluble intracellular adhesion molecules. The proinflammatory state indicated by these findings has been suggested as a potential mediator for adult-onset cardiovascular disease in diabetic offspring [62]. Additional mediators, the levels of which correlate with the extent of maternal hyperglycemia, are also thought to play an atherogenic role in the offspring of diabetic mothers, including endothelial dysfunction, nitric oxide abnormalities, and oxidative stress [63].

The abnormalities in insulin-sensitivity observed consistently in the offspring of diabetic mothers could be associated with alterations in the development of the endocrine pancreas [64]. The differentiation and proliferation of islet cells is highly dependent on metabolic factors, such as fluctuations in the concentration of intrauterine glucose and amino acids. Maternal hyperglycemia may also induce a reduction in fetal pancreatic angiogenesis, which could exacerbate the insult to the developing pancreas [65]. While diabetic offspring have a tendency to develop insulin insensitivity later in life, they also demonstrate a baseline reduction in insulin secretion, which may be related to these functional and mechanical deficits in the genesis of the endocrine pancreas [66]. This potential mechanism is illustrated in Figure 14.5.

Obesity is a complex, multifactorial phenomenon. Cerebral signaling pathways are fundamental to the regulation of appetite and adiposity. Previous research has found abnormalities in both the cortical and hypothalamic development of the child of the diabetic mother [65,67,68]. The hypothalamus is an important regulator of appetite, which likely plays a significant role in the pathogenesis of weight gain [69]. As previously discussed, amniotic fluid insulin levels are elevated in the diabetic pregnancy. Given that the hypothalamus is sensitive to the metabolic environment of both fetus and mother, and may be permanently altered by these influences, it is likely that gestational hyperglycemia influences the development of this key regulator [67,70,71]. Insulin is also an important factor in the signaling of hypothalamic development, and abnormalities in insulin concentrations during gestation alter the function of the hypothalamus [72]. Animal models suggest that anomalies in cerebral development precipitated by hyperinsulinemia may be reversible, if the fetal environment is rectified before the third trimester [73]. Recent studies suggest additional mechanisms for the communication of a predisposition to obesity in the child of the diabetic mother. Both increased cerebral neuropeptide Y levels and decreased leptin sensitivity are well-known mediators of obesity and uncontrollable appetite, and both have also been associated with the reduced insulin sensitivity found in diabetic offspring [74,75].

Epigenetics

Since Dorner et al. first suggested the possibility of an epigenetic mechanism for the influence of the intrauterine environment on life course outcomes in the child of the diabetic mother, the field has expanded precipitously [47]. Where classical genetics takes the nucleotide sequence itself as the currency of inheritance, epigenetics is the passage of traits from one generation to the next, which are transmitted without

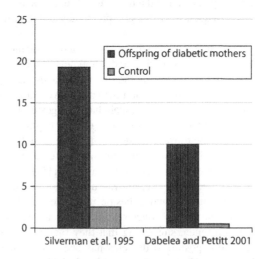

FIGURE 14.5   The cumulative prevalence of type 2 diabetes in the adolescent offspring of diabetic mothers from two major prospective studies. The prevalence from the cohort studies by Silverman et al. 1995 was aged 10–16 years, while the prevalence from Dabelea and Pettitt's 2001 analysis of a Pima Indian cohort was aged 10–14 years.

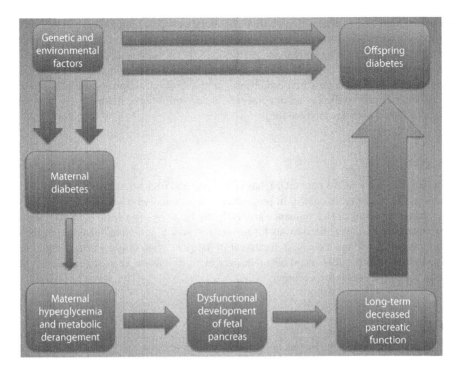

FIGURE 14.6   A potential mechanism for the transmission of insulin resistance from mother to fetus.

alterations this sequence [45]. The alterations may be communicated by DNA methylation, histone modification, and the regulation of microRNA, which targets specific messenger RNA for destruction [76]. The sum of these effects is known as the *epigenome*, which may be influenced by various metabolic factors, including a diabetic intrauterine environment [67]. Although these mechanisms remain an emerging and somewhat enigmatic field, they represent a substantial new focus of research [77].

A number of promising candidate genes have been identified as potential sites of the intrauterine epigenetic modifications elicited by diabetes in pregnancy. Leptin is one such candidate; in diabetic mothers, the leptin gene is preferentially methylated, in a manner that correlates with maternal blood glucose levels [78]. It is speculated that the fetus experiences the inverse effect and the leptin gene is demethylated. This may lead to higher leptin levels, possibly promoting leptin resistance and obesity development.

A second candidate gene examined by the same team codes for adiponectin, a regulator of glucose metabolism and fatty-acid breakdown as well as a factor in insulin sensitization. In this case as well, maternal glucose concentrations correlated with methylation patterns on the fetal gene [79]. A number of other genes have also been implicated in a similar manner. However, it has not been established that any of these alterations are responsible for long-term determination of metabolic function. At least two studies have demonstrated that the concept of intrauterine epigenetic modifications leading to large-scale phenotypic differences in metabolic outcome later in life is a valid one; however, a great deal more work is needed to establish the key players in the epigenetics of transgenerational metabolic influence [80–82].

Treatment

While previous research has demonstrated the efficacy of maternal glycemic control on reducing maternal and fetal morbidity and mortality, no randomized controlled trial has addressed the effect of lowering maternal blood sugar on the probability of offspring insulin resistance in the long term [83]. Previous research has demonstrated the efficacy of maternal glycemic control on reducing maternal and fetal morbidity and mortality [84]. Recently, Casey et al. found in a randomized controlled trial that the reduction of maternal blood sugar with glyburide and dietary modification did not reduce birth weight or improve fetal outcomes versus dietary modification alone, despite a demonstrable improvement in glycemic profile in the pharmacologically managed group [85]. The authors suggest that below a threshold value, the control of maternal hyperglycemia may have diminishing marginal returns, thus rendering it an "imperfect" target. Further research establishing a reduction in offspring insulin insensitivity with maternal glycemic control will play an integral role in determining the nature of the intergenerational transmission of type 2 diabetes mellitus [86].

SUMMARY

GDM, whether pregestational or pure GDM, has significant and lifelong implications for the child of the diabetic mother. Poor glycemic control in pregnancy is associated with significant fetal morbidity and mortality. The mechanisms of this influence are likely mediated by epigenetic modifications, leading to gross organ alterations. A great need exists for further research to establish the nature of these changes and to more thoroughly define the role of treatment in the prevention of long-term complications in the child of the diabetic mother. This need becomes ever more dire as the diabetes epidemic continues its global expansion in the twenty-first century.

REFERENCES

1. Guariguata L, Whiting DR, Hambleton I, Beagley J, Linnenkamp U, Shaw JE. Global estimates of diabetes prevalence for 2013 and projections for 2035. *Diabetes Res Clin Pract*. 2014;103(2):137–49.
2. Gaskin DJ, Thorpe RJ, McGinty EE, et al. Disparities in diabetes: The nexus of race, poverty, and place. *Am J Public Health*. 2013;104(11):2147–55.
3. Guariguata L, Linnenkamp U, Beagley J, Whiting DR, Cho NH. Global estimates of the prevalence of hyperglycaemia in pregnancy. *Diabetes Res Clin Pract*. 2014;103(2):176–85.
4. Plagemann A, Harder T, Kohlhoff R, Rohde W, Dörner G. Glucose tolerance and insulin secretion in children of mothers with pregestational IDDM or gestational diabetes. *Diabetologia*. 1997;40(9):1094–100.
5. Balsells M, García-Patterson A, Gich I, Corcoy R. Major congenital malformations in women with gestational diabetes mellitus: A systematic review and meta-analysis. *Diabetes Metab Res Rev*. 2012;28(3):252–7.
6. Macintosh MCM, Fleming KM, Bailey JA, et al. Perinatal mortality and congenital anomalies in babies of women with type 1 or type 2 diabetes in England, Wales, and Northern Ireland: Population based study. *BMJ*. 2006;333(7560):177.
7. Mitanchez D, Yzydorczyk C, Siddeek B, Boubred F, Benahmed M, Simeoni U. The offspring of the diabetic mother: Short- and long-term implications. *Best Pract Res Clin Obstet Gynaecol*. 2015;29(2):256–69.
8. Farrell T, Neale L, Cundy T. Congenital anomalies in the offspring of women with type 1, type 2 and gestational diabetes. *Diabet Med J Br Diabet Assoc*. 2002;19(4):322–6.
9. Aberg A, Westbom L, Källén B. Congenital malformations among infants whose mothers had gestational diabetes or preexisting diabetes. *Early Hum Dev*. 2001;61(2):85–95.
10. Corrigan N, Brazil DP, McAuliffe F. Fetal cardiac effects of maternal hyperglycemia during pregnancy. *Birth Defects Res A Clin Mol Teratol*. 2009;85(6):523–30.
11. Buchanan TA, Xiang AH, Page KA. Gestational diabetes mellitus: Risks and management during and after pregnancy. *Nat Rev Endocrinol*. 2012;8(11):639–49.
12. Eidem I, Vangen S, Hanssen KF, et al. Perinatal and infant mortality in term and preterm births among women with type 1 diabetes. *Diabetologia*. 2011;54(11):2771–8.
13. Mathiesen ER, Ringholm L, Damm P. Stillbirth in diabetic pregnancies. *Best Pract Res Clin Obstet Gynaecol*. 2011;25(1):105–11.
14. Temple R, Murphy H. Type 2 diabetes in pregnancy: An increasing problem. *Best Pract Res Clin Endocrinol Metab*. 2010;24(4):591–603.
15. Jovanovic LG. Using meal-based self-monitoring of blood glucose as a tool to improve outcomes in pregnancy complicated by diabetes. *Endocr Pract*. 2008;14(2):239–47.

16. Balsells M, García-Patterson A, Gich I, Corcoy R. Maternal and fetal outcome in women with type 2 versus type 1 diabetes mellitus: A systematic review and metaanalysis. *J Clin Endocrinol Metab*. 2009;94(11):4284–91.

17. Karmon A, Levy A, Holcberg G, Wiznitzer A, Mazor M, Sheiner E. Decreased perinatal mortality among women with diet-controlled gestational diabetes mellitus. *Int J Gynaecol Obstet*. 2009;104(3):199–202.

18. Lapolla A, Dalfrà MG, Bonomo M, et al. Gestational diabetes mellitus in Italy: A multicenter study. *Eur J Obstet Gynecol Reprod Biol*. 2009;145(2):149–53.

19. Rosenstein MG, Cheng YW, Snowden JM, Nicholson JA, Doss AE, Caughey AB. The risk of stillbirth and infant death stratified by gestational age in women with gestational diabetes. *Am J Obstet Gynecol*. 2012;206(4):309.e1–7.

20. Yang J, Cummings EA, O'Connell C, Jangaard K. Fetal and neonatal outcomes of diabetic pregnancies. *Obstet Gynecol*. 2006;108(3, Part 1):644–50.

21. Gonzalez-Gonzalez NL, Ramirez O, Mozas J, et al. Factors influencing pregnancy outcome in women with type 2 versus type 1 diabetes mellitus. *Acta Obstet Gynecol Scand*. 2008;87(1):43–9.

22. Hedderson MM, Ferrara A, Sacks DA. Gestational diabetes mellitus and lesser degrees of pregnancy hyperglycemia: Association with increased risk of spontaneous preterm birth. *Obstet Gynecol*. 2003;102(4):850–56.

23. Dabelea D. The predisposition to obesity and diabetes in offspring of diabetic mothers. *Diabetes Care*. 2007;30(Suppl 2):S169–74.

24. Dabelea D, Hanson RL, Lindsay RS, et al. Intrauterine exposure to diabetes conveys risks for type 2 diabetes and obesity: A study of discordant sibships. *Diabetes*. 2000;49(12):2208–11.

25. Monasta L, Batty GD, Cattaneo A, et al. Early-life determinants of overweight and obesity: A review of systematic reviews. *Obes Rev*. 2010;11(10):695–708.

26. Philipps LH, Santhakumaran S, Gale C, et al. The diabetic pregnancy and offspring BMI in childhood: A systematic review and meta-analysis. *Diabetologia*. 2011;54(8):1957–66.

27. Donovan LE, Cundy T. Does exposure to hyperglycaemia in utero increase the risk of obesity and diabetes in the offspring? A critical reappraisal. *Diabet Med*. 2015;32(3):295–304.

28. West NA, Crume TL, Maligie MA, Dabelea D. Cardiovascular risk factors in children exposed to maternal diabetes in utero. *Diabetologia*. 2010;54(3):504–7.

29. Kessous R, Shoham-Vardi I, Pariente G, Sherf M, Sheiner E. An association between gestational diabetes mellitus and long-term maternal cardiovascular morbidity. *Heart Br Card Soc*. 2013;99(15):1118–21.

30. Luyckx VA, Bertram JF, Brenner BM, et al. Effect of fetal and child health on kidney development and long-term risk of hypertension and kidney disease. *Lancet*. 2013;382(9888):273–83.

31. Hovi P, Andersson S, Eriksson JG, et al. Glucose regulation in young adults with very low birth weight. *N Engl J Med*. 2007;356(20):2053–63.

32. Hofman PL, Regan F, Jackson WE, et al. Premature birth and later insulin resistance. *N Engl J Med*. 2004;351(21):2179–86.

33. Crump C, Winkleby MA, Sundquist K, Sundquist J. Risk of diabetes among young adults born preterm in Sweden. *Diabetes Care*. 2011;34(5):1109–13.

34. Rotteveel J, Weissenbruch MM van, Twisk JWR, Waal HADV de. Infant and childhood growth patterns, insulin sensitivity, and blood pressure in prematurely born young adults. *Pediatrics*. 2008;122(2):313–21.

35. Xiang AH, Wang X, Martinez MP, et al. Association of maternal diabetes with autism in offspring. *JAMA*. 2015;313(14):1425–34.

36. Zitser B. Maternal diabetes and autism in offspring. *JAMA*. 2015;314(4):407.

37. Sacks KDN, Friger M, Spiegel E, Abokaf H, Sergienko R, Landau D, Sheiner E. 68: Prenatal exposure to gestational diabetes mellitus as an independent risk factor for long-term neurologic morbidity of the offspring. *Am J Obstet Gynecol*. 2016;214(1):S48–9.

38. Abokaf H, Shoham-Vardi I, Sergeinko R, Spiegel E, Landau D, Sheiner E. 136: Gestational diabetes mellitus: An independent risk factor for long-term pediatric endocrine morbidity of the offspring. *Am J Obstet Gynecol*. 2016;214(1):S91–2.

39. Abokaf H, Shoham-Vardi I, Sergeinko R, Spiegel E, Landau D, Sheiner E. 435: Gestational diabetes mellitus as an independent risk factor for long-term pediatric cardiovascular morbidity of the offspring. *Am J Obstet Gynecol*. 2016;214(1):S239–40.

40. Spiegel E, Shoham-Vardi I, Sergienko R, Landau D, Sheiner E. 383: Gestational diabetes mellitus: An independent risk factor for long-term respiratory morbidity of the offspring. *Am J Obstet Gynecol.* 2016;214(1):S212–3.

41. Seckl JR, Holmes MC. Mechanisms of disease: Glucocorticoids, their placental metabolism and fetal "programming" of adult pathophysiology. *Nat Rev Endocrinol.* 2007;3(6):479–88.

42. Loeken MR. Advances in understanding the molecular causes of diabetes-induced birth defects. *J Soc Gynecol Investig.* 2006;13(1):2–10.

43. Waterland RA, Garza C. Potential mechanisms of metabolic imprinting that lead to chronic disease. *Am J Clin Nutr.* 1999;69(2):179–97.

44. Holness MJ, Langdown ML, Sugden MC. Early-life programming of susceptibility to dysregulation of glucose metabolism and the development of type 2 diabetes mellitus. *Biochem J.* 2000;349(Pt 3):657–65.

45. Ma RCW, Tutino GE, Lillycrop KA, Hanson MA, Tam WH. Maternal diabetes, gestational diabetes and the role of epigenetics in their long term effects on offspring. *Prog Biophys Mol Biol.* 2015;118(1–2):55–68.

46. Stein Z, Susser M. The Dutch Famine, 1944–1945, and the reproductive process: I. Effects on six indices at birth. *Pediatr Res.* 1975;9(2):70–76.

47. Dörner G, Mohnike A, Steindel E. On possible genetic and epigenetic modes of diabetes transmission. *Endokrinologie.* 1975;66(2):225–7.

48. Alcolado JC, Alcolado R. Importance of maternal history of non-insulin dependent diabetic patients. *BMJ.* 1991;302(6786):1178–80.

49. Thomas F, Balkau B, Vauzelle-Kervroedan F, Papoz L. Maternal effect and familial aggregation in NIDDM: The CODIAB Study. *Diabetes.* 1994;43(1):63–7.

50. Pettitt DJ, Bennett PH, Knowler WC, Baird HR, Aleck KA. Gestational diabetes mellitus and impaired glucose tolerance during pregnancy: Long-term effects on obesity and glucose tolerance in the offspring. *Diabetes.* 1985;34(Suppl 2):119–22.

51. Silverman BL, Rizzo T, Green OC, et al. Long-term prospective evaluation of offspring of diabetic mothers. *Diabetes.* 1991;40(Suppl 2):121–5.

52. Silverman BL, Metzger BE, Cho NH, Loeb CA. Impaired glucose tolerance in adolescent offspring of diabetic mothers: Relationship to fetal hyperinsulinism. *Diabetes Care.* 1995;18(5):611–17.

53. Ravussin E, Valencia ME, Esparza J, Bennett PH, Schulz LO. Effects of a traditional lifestyle on obesity in Pima Indians. *Diabetes Care.* 1994;17(9):1067–74.

54. Pearson ER. Dissecting the etiology of type 2 diabetes in the Pima Indian population. *Diabetes.* 2015;64(12):3993–5.

55. Dabelea D, Pettitt DJ. Intrauterine diabetic environment confers risks for type 2 diabetes mellitus and obesity in the offspring, in addition to genetic susceptibility. *J Pediatr Endocrinol Metab.* 2001;14(8):1085–91.

56. Pettitt DJ, Baird HR, Aleck KA, Bennett PH, Knowler WC. Excessive obesity in offspring of Pima Indian women with diabetes during pregnancy. *N Engl J Med.* 1983;308(5):242–5.

57. Bunt JC, Tataranni PA, Salbe AD. Intrauterine exposure to diabetes is a determinant of hemoglobin A(1)c and systolic blood pressure in Pima Indian children. *J Clin Endocrinol Metab.* 2005;90(6):3225–9.

58. Amri K, Freund N, Vilar J, Merlet-Bénichou C, Lelièvre-Pégorier M. Adverse effects of hyperglycemia on kidney development in rats: In vivo and in vitro studies. *Diabetes.* 1999;48(11):2240–5.

59. Nehiri T, Van Huyen JPD, Viltard M, et al. Exposure to maternal diabetes induces salt-sensitive hypertension and impairs renal function in adult rat offspring. *Diabetes.* 2008;57(8):2167–75.

60. Gomes GN, Gil FZ. Prenatally programmed hypertension: Role of maternal diabetes. *Braz J Med Biol Res Rev Bras Pesqui Médicas E Biológicas Soc Bras Biofísica Al.* 2011;44(9):899–904.

61. Ridker PM, Hennekens CH, Roitman-Johnson B, Stampfer MJ, Allen J. Plasma concentration of soluble intercellular adhesion molecule 1 and risks of future myocardial infarction in apparently healthy men. *Lancet.* 1998;351(9096):88–92.

62. Manderson JG, Mullan B, Patterson CC, Hadden DR, Traub AI, McCance DR. Cardiovascular and metabolic abnormalities in the offspring of diabetic pregnancy. *Diabetologia.* 2002;45(7):991–6.

63. Vrachnis N, Antonakopoulos N, Iliodromiti Z, et al. Impact of maternal diabetes on epigenetic modifications leading to diseases in the offspring. *J Diabetes Res J Diabetes Res.* 2012;2012:e538474.

64. Fowden AL, Hill DJ. Intra-uterine programming of the endocrine pancreas. *Br Med Bull.* 2001;60:123–42.

65. Fetita LS, Sobngwi E, Serradas P, Calvo F, Gautier JF. Consequences of fetal exposure to maternal diabetes in offspring. *J Clin Endocrinol Metab*. 2006;91(10):3718–24.

66. Sobngwi E, Boudou P, Mauvais-Jarvis F, et al. Effect of a diabetic environment in utero on predisposition to type 2 diabetes. *Lancet*. 2003;361(9372):1861–5.

67. Ornoy A. Prenatal origin of obesity and their complications: Gestational diabetes, maternal overweight and the paradoxical effects of fetal growth restriction and macrosomia. *Reprod Toxicol*. 2011;32(2):205–12.

68. Ornoy A, Ratzon N, Greenbaum C, Peretz E, Soriano D, Dulitzky M. Neurobehaviour of school age children born to diabetic mothers. *Arch Dis Child Fetal Neonatal Ed*. 1998;79(2):F94–9.

69. Williams LM. Hypothalamic dysfunction in obesity. *Proc Nutr Soc*. 2012;71(4):521–33.

70. HAPO Study Cooperative Research Group. Hyperglycemia and Adverse Pregnancy Outcome (HAPO) Study. *Diabetes*. 2009;58(2):453–9.

71. Weiss PA, Scholz HS, Haas J, Tamussino KF, Seissler J, Borkenstein MH. Long-term follow-up of infants of mothers with type 1 diabetes: Evidence for hereditary and nonhereditary transmission of diabetes and precursors. *Diabetes Care*. 2000;23(7):905–11.

72. Steculorum SM, Vogt MC, Brüning JC. Perinatal programming of metabolic diseases: Role of insulin in the development of hypothalamic neurocircuits. *Endocrinol Metab Clin North Am*. 2013;42(1):149–64.

73. Rkhzay-Jaf J, O'Dowd JF, Stocker CJ. Maternal obesity and the fetal origins of the metabolic syndrome. *Curr Cardiovasc Risk Rep*. 2012;6(5):487–95.

74. Luo ZC, Nuyt AM, Delvin E, et al. Maternal and fetal leptin, adiponectin levels and associations with fetal insulin sensitivity. *Obesity*. 2013;21(1):210–6.

75. Plagemann A. "Fetal programming" and "functional teratogenesis": On epigenetic mechanisms and prevention of perinatally acquired lasting health risks. *J Perinat Med*. 2004;32(4):297–305.

76. Wahid F, Shehzad A, Khan T, Kim YY. MicroRNAs: Synthesis, mechanism, function, and recent clinical trials. *Biochim Biophys Acta*. 2010;1803(11):1231–43.

77. Heard E, Martienssen RA. Transgenerational epigenetic inheritance: Myths and mechanisms. *Cell*. 2014;157(1):95–109.

78. Bouchard L, Thibault S, Guay SP, et al. Leptin gene epigenetic adaptation to impaired glucose metabolism during pregnancy. *Diabetes Care*. 2010;33(11):2436–41.

79. Bouchard L, Hivert M-F, Guay S-P, St-Pierre J, Perron P, Brisson D. Placental adiponectin gene DNA methylation levels are associated with mothers' blood glucose concentration. *Diabetes*. 2012;61(5):1272–80.

80. Clarke-Harris R, Wilkin TJ, Hosking J, et al. PGC1α promoter methylation in blood at 5–7 years predicts adiposity from 9 to 14 years (EarlyBird 50). *Diabetes*. 2014;63(7):2528–37.

81. Godfrey KM, Sheppard A, Gluckman PD, et al. Epigenetic gene promoter methylation at birth is associated with child's later adiposity. *Diabetes*. 2011;60(5):1528–34.

82. El Hajj N, Schneider E, Lehnen H, Haaf T. Epigenetics and life-long consequences of an adverse nutritional and diabetic intrauterine environment. *Reproduction*. 2014;148(6):R111–R120.

83. Ornoy A, Reece EA, Pavlinkova G, Kappen C, Miller RK. Effect of maternal diabetes on the embryo, fetus, and children: Congenital anomalies, genetic and epigenetic changes and developmental outcomes. *Birth Defects Res Part C Embryo Today Rev*. 2015;105(1):53–72.

84. Crowther CA, Hiller JE, Moss JR, McPhee AJ, Jeffries WS, Robinson JS. Effect of treatment of gestational diabetes mellitus on pregnancy outcomes. *N Engl J Med*. 2005;352(24):2477–86.

85. Casey BM, Duryea EL, Abbassi-Ghanavati M, et al. Glyburide in women with mild gestational diabetes: A randomized controlled trial. *Obstet Gynecol*. 2015;126(2):303–9.

86. Poston L. Intergenerational transmission of insulin resistance and type 2 diabetes. *Prog Biophys Mol Biol*. 2011;106(1):315–22.

15

Intrauterine Growth Restriction and Long-Term Disease of the Offspring

Tal Biron-Shental and Hannah Glinter

Introduction

Intrauterine environmental conditions during fetal development affect long-term health and morbidity in later life. Epidemiological observations as well as animal and molecular studies have revealed data supporting the theory that adult diseases originate during the fetal period.

Suboptimal uterine conditions such as hypoxia, vascular and abnormal placental invasion, or malnutrition may lead to placental insufficiency, clinically reflected by intrauterine growth restriction (IUGR), and consequently increase the risk of later-onset cardiovascular morbidity and metabolic syndrome (obesity, hypertension, and hyperlipidemia).

Pregnancies complicated by IUGR also express specific genomic and proteomic modulations in placental trophoblasts, which reflect intrauterine programming and may be the origin of later-onset diseases.

Intrauterine Growth Restriction

The most common definition of IUGR refers to fetuses with an estimated weight below the 10th percentile for gestational age [1].

IUGR can be related to a combination of maternal, fetal, and placental factors.

In general, symmetric growth restriction (shortened femur length and shortened head and abdominal circumferences) is associated with intrauterine infections, chromosomal genetic abnormalities, and vulnerability to toxic insult, while asymmetric growth restriction (the sparing of head growth relative to femur length) is related to placental insufficiency, leading to maternal conditions such as preeclampsia or hypertension. Significant overlap between symmetric and asymmetric IUGR make these definitions less determinant. Whether IUGR onset is early or late during the pregnancy is implicated by its etiology as well, with placental insufficiency tending to cause later-onset IUGR. Abnormal placentation leading to placental insufficiency is one of the most prominent etiologies for IUGR, with subsequent effects on the fetus [1]. It is characterized by accompanying oligohydramnios and abnormal Doppler of the umbilical and other fetal vessels [2,3].

There are two axes of placental growth: length (major) and breadth (minor). Placental growth and outcomes due to placental compromise are partially dependent on the mothers' nutritional status. Malnourished mothers tend to have smaller placentas, while nourished mothers can compensate for placental insufficiency by placental overgrowth. Sex-specific response to maternal undernutrition reveals that boys respond rapidly to the current diet, while girls are more responsive to the mother's lifetime nutritional status. Therefore, while birth weight is a marker for fetal nutrition, placental size can be incorporated as an epidemiological marker for birth weight and long-term health consequences [4]. Generally, low placental weight at birth is typical for IUGR, and hypertensive diseases of pregnancy, including preeclampsia, are shown to predict hypertension and coronary artery disease later in life.

Placental insufficiency results in altered transport capacity and placental growth, elevated apoptosis and autophagy, as well as increased glucocorticoid action in utero [5]. Morphometric and microscopic differences are evident between normal placentas and those of IUGR secondary to placental insufficiency. Gross findings in IUGR placentas include low weight, thin umbilical cord, and parenchymal loss (infarcts). Histological changes in the terminal chorionic villi can be observed, including accelerated villous maturation as a result of chronic placental ischemia due to maternal vascular malperfusion, as well as fetal thrombotic vasculopathy due to fetal vascular malperfusion [6]. Likewise, on a genomic level, abnormal implantation of the placenta, causing uteroplacental insufficiency, has been associated with the differential imprinting of numerous genes [7].

Since the placenta has a significant role in fetal development, all these changes have a tremendous influence on the short- and long-term outcomes of IUGR [8].

IUGR increases the risk of intrauterine death, as well as perinatal morbidity and mortality [9]. Growth restriction is in itself a risk of premature delivery, and therefore, IUGR infants are at greater risk of the complications of prematurity, including lung compromise and necrotizing enterocolitis [10,11]. IUGR infants demonstrate increased rates of perinatal asphyxia, hypothermia, hypoglycemia, compromised immune systems, coagulation dysfunction, and hepatocellular abnormalities [10].

There are also numerous data regarding the long-term implications of IUGR, which will be thoroughly discussed in this chapter.

Some IUGR infants demonstrate early catch-up, referring to fast weight gain in the postnatal period. Postnatal catch-up is additive to intrauterine insult in setting the stage for detrimental effects on long-term disease development and progression [12].

IUGR as a Window for Future Health: The Barker and Thrifty Phenotype Hypotheses

The *developmental origins* hypothesis proposes that the development of chronic diseases such as coronary heart disease, type 2 diabetes, and hypertension begins from early development, by which stresses such as malnutrition or hypoxia in utero cause IUGR and fetal adaptations, leading to long-term effects [13].

The fetal life is a critical period of time, when the systems and organs are sensitive to environmental changes. The placenta, as a mediator of all the communications between the mother and the fetus, has an important influence on the physiological pathways of fetal development [14]. Intrauterine insults may cause permanent structural and functional changes that can disrupt fetal development. Indeed, low birth weight, as a marker of fetal development presents an increased risk of morbidity in adult life [9].

The relationship between low birth weight and developing diseases such as type 2 diabetes, cardiovascular disease, hypertension, and metabolic syndrome in later life has been proposed by Barker and colleagues [15,16]. Barker and colleagues' investigations over many years have revealed data supporting the theory that there are critical periods during development when the fetus adapts to its in utero surroundings and adjusts its development to the environment. The fetus's phenotype is established in this period of time [17]. Table 15.1 presents a list of chronic diseases associated with IUGR.

The *thrifty phenotype* hypothesis theorizes that deficits in the intrauterine environment encountered by the fetus are strongly associated with a number of chronic conditions later in life [18]. This increased susceptibility to chronic disease results from adaptations made by the fetus in an environment limited in its supply of nutrients. If resources are limited, the economical allocation of nutritional and metabolic components is the mechanism by which the fetus adapts to its intrauterine environment [19].

The time period of intrauterine insult affects the vast interplay between different organ systems during their maturation. In utero insults such as maternal malnutrition and uteroplacental insufficiency trigger adaptive changes during organogenesis in the fetus [20].

TABLE 15.1

Chronic Diseases with Correlation
to Intrauterine Growth Restriction

Type 2 diabetes mellitus
Hypertension
Dyslipidemia
Obesity
Cardiovascular diseases
Metabolic syndrome

Epidemiological Data That Support the Theory

The first major epidemiological study examining the relationship between early development and long-term disease outcome took place in Hertfordshire, United Kingdom. The findings in 10,636 men born between 1911 and 1930 revealed that the hazard ratios for coronary heart disease fell with increasing birth weight. Studies have also been performed that revealed the same outcome in females [21]. The populations identified from Hertfordshire and Sheffield who had their birth weight documented showed that those with low birth weight due to growth restriction, rather than due to premature birth, were at greater risk of coronary heart disease, and the pattern persisted with hypertension and insulin-resistant diabetes [17].

The Helsinki Birth Cohort, which comprised 13,345 men and women born in the city during 1934–1944, found that chronic heart failure was associated with a smaller placental surface area, mostly in mothers who were malnourished. This was modified by those taking medications for type 2 diabetes. The risk of chronic heart disease was further increased by rapid growth after the first 2 years [22].

Famine situations such as wartime were studied by examining the Dutch Famine Birth Cohort. These studies revealed that babies born between 1943 and 1947 in Amsterdam to mothers eating roughly a quarter of the daily recommended intake exhibited an increased risk of cardiovascular and metabolic/endocrine diseases later in life due to the hypomethylation of the imprinted IGF2-H19 locus [23].

Another epidemiologic study examined a low-income cohort of patients in South Africa. Obesity rates in adults as measured by BMI at 18 years correlated with IUGR and an early weight catch-up during the first year of life, as well as earlier menarche in females. Females with earlier menarche were more likely to be overweight prepubertal, and also showed a greater likelihood of developing adult-onset diabetes [24].

Both historical records and modern studies show significant associations between birth weight and adult height and blood pressure [25].

In a recent population-based cohort study, the authors investigated whether being delivered small for gestational age (SGA) at term poses an increased risk of long-term pediatric morbidity. The authors compared the incidence of long-term pediatric hospitalizations due to cardiovascular, hematologic, and respiratory morbidity of children born SGA (birth weight below the fifth percentile for gestational age) at term (37–42 weeks gestation) between the years 1991 and 2014 in a tertiary medical center. Congenital malformations as well as multiple pregnancies were excluded. During the study period 236,504 deliveries met the inclusion criteria, of which 4.8% were SGA neonates ($n = 11,319$). During the follow-up period, children born SGA at term had a significantly higher rate of long-term cardiovascular (Figure 15.1), hematologic (Figure 15.2), and respiratory morbidity (Figure 15.3). Using a multivariable generalized estimating equation (GEE) logistic regression model, controlling for the time to event, maternal age, and diabetes mellitus, being born SGA at term was found to be an independent risk factor for long-term cardiovascular, hematologic, and respiratory disease during childhood. The authors concluded that being delivered SGA at term is an independent risk factor for long-term cardiovascular, hematologic, and respiratory morbidity of the offspring [26].

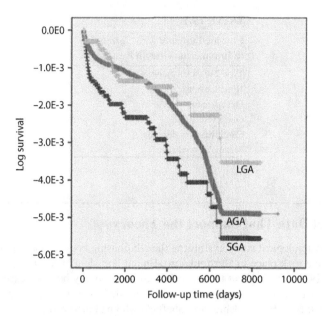

FIGURE 15.1 Cardiovascular morbidity until the age of 18 years according to small- (SGA) vs. appropriate- (AGA) and large-for-gestational-age (LGA) newborns (survival curve).

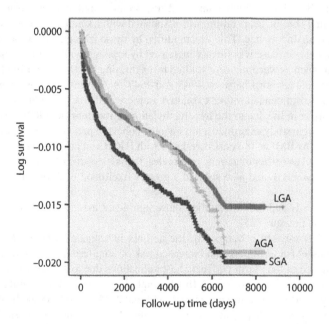

FIGURE 15.2 Hematological morbidity until the age of 18 years according to SGA vs. AGA and LGA newborns (survival curve).

Criticism about epidemiological studies is related to their methodology. These are all long-term retrospective historical cohort studies with inaccuracies of data. However, the consistent results, based on different studies that included different populations, imply that the conclusions should be taken seriously despite the studies' weaknesses. Furthermore, because of the major future risks, diagnosis and clinical management strategies of IUGR represent a key issue for public health.

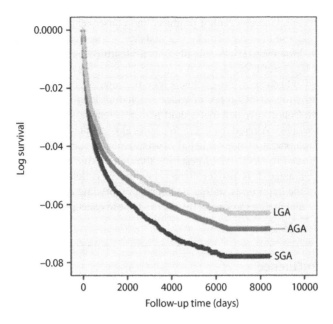

FIGURE 15.3 Respiratory morbidity until the age of 18 years according to SGA vs. AGA and LGA newborns (survival curve).

Examples from Clinical Data Supporting Barker's Theory

Barker and colleagues showed that malnutrition in fetal and early life might be responsible for the initiation of cardiovascular disease through intrauterine programming [19]. IUGR due to placental insufficiency is characterized by low placental surface area. An association has been established between a small placenta and the later onset of chronic heart failure [22].

The long-term effects of placental insult persist into adulthood, and also correlate with a higher incidence of coronary artery disease and stroke [27].

There is evidence that people whose weight at birth was low tend to have higher blood pressure and an increased risk of death from cardiovascular disease as adults. These observations might be related to the impaired synthesis of elastin in the walls of the large arteries of IUGR fetuses [28].

Echocardiography was used to assess the cardiac function of IUGR fetuses at the age of 6 months after delivery. Markers of heart dysfunction were shown in the uterus and remained constant postnatally. Controlling for maternal characteristics, the changes in IUGR included larger atria and thicker myocardial walls in order to compensate for pressure changes and volume overload due to chronic hypoxia and placental hypertension. Vascular evaluation was obtained through blood pressure readings and was also shown to be disrupted with a correlation to increased blood pressures. This population is considered at higher risk of cardiovascular disease later in life [29].

A genetic basis for type 2 diabetes is widely accepted based on the variance of the disease in populations, familial aggregation, and high twin concordance. Environmental influences play a role too, primarily lifestyle in adult life. Likewise, in utero environmental influences serve as major causative factors in the development of the disease [30]. Malnutrition in fetal and early life may be detrimental to the development of the beta cells of the endocrine pancreas, leading to the in utero initiation of diabetes [19]. The rapid growth of beta cells during fetal life is crucial for normal pancreatic function. Intrauterine hypoxia or malnutrition may insult the pancreatic beta cells and impair their growth and future function. These pancreatic abnormalities contribute to the in utero origins of impaired glucose tolerance. The effects of the placental insult may persist and correlate with a higher incidence of type 2 diabetes mellitus and metabolic syndrome [27].

It has been demonstrated that the effects of placental changes caused by intrauterine insults are more problematic once proper nutrition is introduced postnatally. There is a greater need for effective insulin release, which the affected pancreas cannot produce, and consequently diabetes occurs [31]. It is also known that impaired glucose tolerance and type 2 diabetes are associated with ischemic heart disease and hypertension [31]. Moreover, IUGR has also been identified as a risk factor for neurocognitive impairment and lower IQ scores [32].

Malignancies have also been shown to correlate with intrauterine alterations. Smaller placentas were shown to be associated with various types of cancer, including lung cancers [33]. Moreover, evidence from the Helsinki Birth Cohort revealed that a short placental length is associated with the development of Hodgkin's lymphoma [34]. Altered exposure to perinatal hormones and preterm birth may be a risk factor for the later development of nonepithelial ovarian and sex cord–stromal tumors [35]. Placental shape is determined around weeks 8–12 of gestation through uterine artery plugs, a protective mechanism against oxidative damage. It is also a critical time point of cellular differentiation and organogenesis. This concurs with the hypothesis stating that during embryonic development, stem cells are more vulnerable to stressors, and their exposure to insults predispose cancer development later in life [36].

Early Catch-Up Influence

Several studies, including those from the Helsinki cohort, have shown that the highest death rates from coronary heart disease occurred in boys who were thin at birth but had catch-up resulting in average or above-average body mass from 7 years old [12]. This pattern has also been demonstrated in populations of Indian children who were born with low birth weight and who demonstrated a high growth velocity before 8 years of age [37]. One explanation is the fact that babies with small birth weight and fast-paced catch-up growth may cause disproportionately high levels of fat accumulation, leading to detrimental effects in adulthood [12].

IUGR is well known as a precursor of cardiovascular remodeling in childhood, leading to lower left-ventricular cardiac function and increased blood pressures. Based on cohort data of children born following IUGR, breastfeeding and healthy-fat dietary intake improved while increased BMI worsened cardiovascular function. These results support the influence of catch-up and postnatal nutrition on later health [38].

Placental levels of corticotrophin-releasing hormone (CRH) have been identified as a risk factor for early catch-up growth in the first 2 years of life. Therefore, in utero CRH exposure may contribute to the fetal outcomes that lead to obesity and metabolic disease [39].

Animal Models

The advantage of animal models is the ability to mimic natural epidemiological phenomena in a controlled environment in a shorter time frame.

Data from animal models support the epidemiological studies regarding the intrauterine origins of adult diseases in fetuses that suffered from IUGR. The mechanisms underlying these observations are not fully understood. Using animal models enables one to determine the involved mechanisms and signaling pathways.

Rabbit models may be considered useful in the analysis of IUGR on fetal development. Pregnant rabbits were restricted to 50% of the daily nutritional requirement, but this did not affect maternal body weight or fetal mortality rate. Offspring size was measured by ultrasonography, and hemodynamic features by Doppler ultrasonography, both valuable tools in assessing human fetal development. Underfeeding rabbits in order to induce IUGR fetuses showed compensatory blood flow perfusion indicating a *brain-sparing effect* [40]. Rodents have also served as models for the deleterious effects of IUGR on organogenesis. Late-gestation uterine vessel ligation in rats resulted in growth restriction, mimicking human growth restriction due to uteroplacental insufficiency, independent of nutrient intake. This procedure caused a decrease in nephron numbers, with an increase in glomerular volume, a likely compensatory mechanism to maintain an adequate glomerular filtration rate [20].

In another rat model, effects on placental nutrient transporters were examined by various stresses. Uteroplacental insufficiency was demonstrated through bilateral uterine artery and vein ligation. Fatty-acid transporters were increased post stressors, a potential compensatory mechanism for brain development with effects on energy metabolism, while protein and carbohydrate transporters were greatly reduced. The placenta reacts to the insults by modulating the transport activity of nutrients to the growing fetus. This adaptation reduces fetal (and postnatal) demand and alters the expression of receptors for maximal usage [41].

As in humans, mice models of IUGR developed obesity and glucose intolerance with aging in response to undernutrition during fetal life [42].

Rat models of IUGR, induced by bilateral uterine artery ligation, showed pancreatic beta cell loss as well as methylated DNA distribution in pancreatic beta cells. These findings may explain the increased risk of diabetes in those who suffered from IUGR [43]. Another study revealed that rat fetuses that were exposed to a low-protein diet during pregnancy had reduced pancreatic beta cell mass and islet vascularization with increased corticosterone levels. These findings are concordant with intrauterine stress and an increased risk of diabetes [44].

In low-protein diet–induced rats, female IUGR offspring showed significant impairment in renal function compared with non-IUGR counterparts, while male rats showed no significant difference in age-related renal function decline between IUGR and non-IUGR. Females were also found to be more vulnerable to vascular compromise when subjected to IUGR conditions in utero, associated with an increase in arterial pressure in later ages [45].

Adult mice that were exposed to malnutrition in utero revealed decreased cardiac respiration, which may be an indicator for decreased cardiac function and the development of long-term cardiovascular disease. Changes in myocardial energy metabolism influence disease risk in the offspring [46]. In sheep, glucose homeostasis was affected by undernutrition, particularly during late gestation, and revealed adverse effects in adult offspring. Disturbed glucose homeostasis appeared to be tissue specific, however, with adipose affected and not muscle [47].

Studies in sheep, regarding changes in maternal food intake and postnatal nutrition, support kidney and cardiac remodeling in the uterus and an adverse metabolic effect of the early catch-up phenomenon of postnatal overnutrition [48].

The intrauterine environment influences epigenetic regulation for the rest of life and, therefore, is prone to later metabolism impairment and associated diseases [49–52].

As illustrated in rat models, inducing gestational protein deficiency with the aim to identify epigenetic alterations in IUGR placentas leads to eventual disease susceptibility and pathogenesis in adulthood through differential expression of genes, including those responsible for the vascularization of placenta and transmembrane glycoproteins [53].

IUGR leads to intrauterine programming as part of the adjustment to the insulted environment. The altered energy metabolism created by intrauterine starvation leads to enhanced fat synthesis and obesity, especially with exposure to a rich postnatal diet and early catch-up. The catch-up influence was demonstrated in animal models to be similar to humans. These observations were demonstrated in rodents and also in pigs [54,55].

In a maternal protein-restricted rat model, low birth weight followed by accelerated postnatal growth led to adipose dysregulation and consequently insulin resistance, an elevated risk of type 2 diabetes, and other components of metabolic syndrome [55].

The effect of birth weight on reproductive performance was assessed in male pigs. The findings suggest that growth restriction affects sperm production via reproductive organ development and epigenetic regulation [56].

Cellular Models and Data from Placental Studies

Cells cultured under starvation or hypoxic conditions mimic the intrauterine environment of IUGR and therefore are considered as acceptable research models for IUGR. Experiments with cell lines or with primary human trophoblasts cultured in hypoxic conditions or with malnourished media reveal genetic and epigenetic modifications, which allow them to survive in a similar way to intrauterine programming allowing IUGR fetuses to thrive. Interestingly, changes in those cells are similar to previously described intrauterine programming in humans and in animal models. Furthermore, those changes are associated with cellular alterations found in cases of obesity, metabolic syndrome, and aging-related diseases.

Primary human trophoblasts cultured in hypoxic conditions expressed increased lipid droplets and the enhanced expression of fatty acid–binding proteins, suggesting cellular fat accumulation in hypoxic conditions [57]. Hypoxia also activates transcriptional regulators of cellular metabolism that promote cholesterol efflux and lipogenesis in primary human trophoblasts [58]. Furthermore, primary human trophoblasts cultured under hypoxic conditions expressed upregulated hypoxia-inducible factor 1 alpha (HIF1α) and vascular endothelial growth factor (VEGF) and reduced concentrations of leptin. These changes imply fetal programming of endothelium as well as leptin resistance and adiposity in later life [59].

Telomeres are nucleoprotein structures located at the termini of chromosomes. They are essential for chromosome stability. Telomeres become shorter due to mitotic cycles and environmental factors. When telomeres are shortened and therefore dysfunctional, cellular senescence occurs and organ dysfunction might develop. During pregnancy, fetal growth restriction secondary to placental insufficiency has been linked to impaired telomere homeostasis, in which telomeres are shorter, telomerase is decreased, and the compensatory mechanisms of telomere capture are enhanced. These characteristics, along with increased signs of senescence, indicate telomere dysfunction in trophoblasts from placentas affected by IUGR. Impaired telomere homeostasis might play a role in the pathophysiology of IUGR and might affect intrauterine programming related to the origin of some diseases that arise in adults [50–62]. It has been proposed that shortened telomeres are also related to energy-saving mechanisms during compromised conditions. It is associated with adaptations of the immune system that might result in chronic infections, inflammatory stress, and premature aging [63].

The placental production and utilization of amino acids plays an active role in fetal development. The syncytiotrophoblast is the key structure in regulating transplacental amino acid passage. The concentration of most amino acids is significantly decreased both in the placenta and in the umbilical vessels of IUGR pregnancies compared with normally grown controls, with correlation to the severity of the IUGR. Decreased placental and fetal levels of amino acids disrupt fetal development and organ function and maturation, causing a predisposition for adult-onset diseases and the early aging of those who were IUGR [64,65].

Epigenetic Modifications

Epigenetic modification is the interplay of several mechanisms resulting in heritable changes in gene expression without accompanying alterations in DNA sequence. Environmental cues trigger persistent epigenetic modifications that lead to alterations in gene regulation, including DNA methylation and histone modification. Epigenetic changes have been proposed to play a role as an adaptive mechanism to a changing environment, particularly in early life. Maternal malnutrition leading to fetal hypoglycemia raises nonesterified fatty acid and ketone body concentrations that can regulate DNA stability and phenotypic adaptation [66,67]. The impairment of DNA methylation as an epigenetic mechanism affects placental development—one etiology for fetal growth retardation [53]. In addition, placental methylation patterns of 22 loci have been found as potential predictors of fetal growth restriction [68]. Early uterine environments such as poor maternal nutrition during gestation can lead to IUGR and also can impact the neonatal epigenome, rendering disease susceptibility in adulthood.

Tissues and organs that control metabolic homeostasis (hypothalamus, adipose tissue, stomach, skeletal muscle, and heart) respond to nutritional restriction or to induced hypoxia by epigenetic modulations including DNA methylation, histone acetylation, and protein expression and function, all of which trigger the development of the metabolic syndrome. IUGR fetuses adapt for energy saving by remodeling the hypothalamic–pituitary–adrenal axis. Their cortisol levels are increased to facilitate organ and tissue maturation [69–71].

Cues that trigger epigenetic modifications leading to the consequences of IUGR include fetal overnutrition, maternal diabetes, and maternal obesity, which contribute to metabolic disease in the offspring.

Interestingly, both overnutrition and undernutrition states in fetal life lead to differential methylation patterns of specific genes implicated in diabetes, obesity, and cardiovascular disease.

However, very few epigenetic markers have been demonstrated after birth in the implication of the long-term morbidity of the offspring. Therefore, if the modulation of the epigenome can reduce the risk of metabolic syndrome later on, interventions should be geared toward the time period of conception to birth [23].

While epigenetic markers are normally erased or reprogrammed in the germline and early embryo, errors in reprogramming result in the retention of epigenetic modifications, leading to the preservation of traits in subsequent generations [72]. Adverse effects due to poor fetal nutrition may have intergenerational effects, as was shown in undernourished mothers who gave birth to babies of normal birth weight who then gave birth to lower birth weight offspring in the next generation [73]. In utero nutritional status leading to developmental epigenetic modification is also believed to play a role in the phenomenon of the intergenerational development of type 2 diabetes, cardiovascular disease, and obesity [42].

CONCLUSIONS AND CLINICAL CONSIDERATIONS

The accumulating data from epidemiological studies, animal models, and cellular experiments reveal consistent results regarding the correlation between IUGR caused by placental insufficiency and adult morbidities, among which are cardiovascular diseases, endocrine abnormalities, metabolic syndrome, and more. It is postulated that the unfavorable intrauterine environment that causes IUGR (or SGA birth weight) initiates modifications that are termed *intrauterine programming*. These adaptations to the hostile environment enable fetal survival under poor conditions, insult the developing organs, and lead to a predisposition to later-onset diseases. Furthermore, early catch-up by overnutrition of those newborns accelerates their susceptibility to the metabolic syndrome and other adult diseases (Figure 15.4).

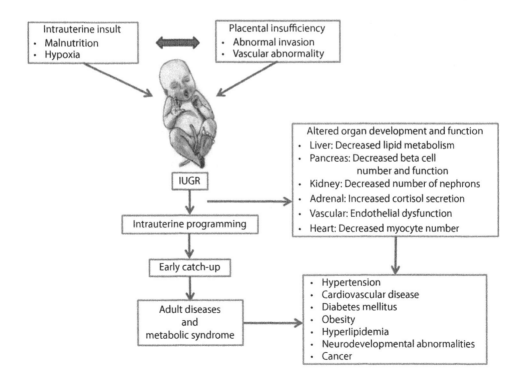

FIGURE 15.4 Catch-up by overnutrition of IUGR newborns accelerates their susceptibility to metabolic syndrome and other adult diseases.

There is a vicious cycle of IUGR fetuses, which turn into adults with obesity and metabolic syndrome then get pregnant, carrying all these risk factors and transferring them to the next generation. By breaking this cycle through awareness, education, better nutrition, and some preventive measures, the burden of disease may be reduced and morbidity and mortality alleviated. Prevention is based on personal lifestyle modification and medication, especially in Western countries, where lifestyle plays a major role in the development of cardiovascular disease and metabolic syndrome [74]. With evidence through longitudinal studies, the prediction in utero of increased risk for adult development of disease may provide a basis for the prevention of cardiovascular disease.

REFERENCES

1. American College of Obstetricians and Gynecologists. Fetal growth restriction. ACOG Practice Bulletin no. 134. *Obstet Gynecol*. 2013;121(5):1122–33.
2. Vayssière C, Sentilhes L, Ego A, et al. Fetal growth restriction and intra-uterine growth restriction: Guidelines for clinical practice from the French College of Gynaecologists and Obstetricians. *Eur J Obstet Gynecol Reprod Biol*. 2015;193:10–18.
3. Royal College of Obstetricians and Gynecologists. *The Investigation and Management of the Small-for-Gestational-Age Fetus*. Guideline no. 31. London: RCOG; 2002.
4. Barker DJ, Thornburg KL, Osmond C, Kajantie E, Eriksson JG. Beyond birthweight: The maternal and placental origins of chronic disease. *J Dev Orig Health Dis*. 2010;1(6):360–64.
5. Zhang S, Regnault TR, Barker PL, et al. Placental adaptations in growth restriction. *Nutrients*. 2015;7(1):360–89.
6. Redline RW. Classification of placental lesions. *Am J Obstet Gynecol*. 2015;213(4 Suppl):S21–8.
7. Diplas AI, Lambertini L, Lee MJ, et al. Differential expression of imprinted genes in normal and IUGR human placentas. *Epigenetics*. 2009;4(4):235–40.
8. Thornburg KL, Marshall N. The placenta is the center of the chronic disease universe. *Am J Obstet Gynecol*. 2015;213(4 Suppl):S14–20.
9. McIntire DD, Bloom SL, Casey BM, Leveno KJ. Birth weight in relation to morbidity and mortality among newborn infants. *N Engl J Med*. 1999;340(16):1234–8.
10. Pallotto EK, Kilbride HW. Perinatal outcome and later implications of intrauterine growth restriction. *Clin Obstet Gynecol*. 2006;49(2):257–69.
11. Sasi A, Abraham V, Davies-Tuck M, et al. Impact of intrauterine growth restriction on preterm lung disease. *Acta Paediatr*. 2015;104(12):e552–6.
12. Eriksson JG, Forsén T, Tuomilehto J, Winter PD, Osmond C, Barker DJ. Catch-up growth in childhood and death from coronary heart disease: Longitudinal study. *BMJ*. 1999;318(7181):427–31.
13. Barker DJ. Adult consequences of fetal growth restriction. *Clin Obstet Gynecol*. 2006;49(2):270–83.
14. Entringer S, Buss C, Wadhwa PD. Prenatal stress, telomere biology, and fetal programming of health and disease risk. *Sci Signal*. 2012;5(248):pt12.
15. Barker DJ, Osmond C, Golding J, Kuh D, Wadsworth ME. Growth in utero, blood pressure in childhood and adult life, and mortality from cardiovascular disease. *BMJ*. 1989;298(6673):564–7.
16. Barker DJ, Bull AR, Osmond C, Simmonds SJ. Fetal and placental size and risk of hypertension in adult life. *BMJ*. 1990;301(6746):259–62.
17. Barker DJ. Fetal origins of coronary heart disease. *BMJ*. 1995;311(6998):171–4.
18. Hales CN, Barker DJ. The thrifty phenotype hypothesis. *Br Med Bull*. 2001;60:5–20.
19. Barker DJ, Lampl M. Commentary: The meaning of thrift. *Int J Epidemiol*. 2013;42(5):1229–30.
20. Richter V, Briffa JF, Moritz KM, Wlodek ME, Hryciw DH. The role of maternal nutrition, metabolic function and the placenta in developmental programming of renal dysfunction. *Clin Exp Pharmacol Physiol*. 2016;43(1):135–41.
21. Barker DJ, Osmond C, Kajantie E, Eriksson JG. Growth and chronic disease: Findings in the Helsinki Birth Cohort. *Ann Hum Biol*. 2009;36(5):445–58.
22. Barker DJ, Gelow J, Thornburg K, Osmond C, Kajantie E, Eriksson JG. The early origins of chronic heart failure: Impaired placental growth and initiation of insulin resistance in childhood. *Eur J Heart Fail*. 2010;12(8):819–25.

23. El Hajj N, Schneider E, Lehnen H, Haaf T. Epigenetics and life-long consequences of an adverse nutritional and diabetic intrauterine environment. *Reproduction*. 2014;148(6):R111–20.
24. Salgin B, Norris SA, Prentice P, et al. Even transient rapid infancy weight gain is associated with higher BMI in young adults and earlier menarche. *Int J Obes (Lond)*. 2015;39(6):939–44.
25. Roberts E, Wood P. Birth weight and adult health in historical perspective: Evidence from a New Zealand cohort, 1907–1922. *Soc Sci Med*. 2014;107:154–61.
26. Spigel E, Shoham-Vardi I, Sergienko R, Landau D, Sheiner E. Small for gestational age at term: An independent risk factor for long-term pediatric morbidity. *Am J Obstet Gynecol*. 2016;214:S250.
27. Smith CJ, Ryckman KK. Epigenetic and developmental influences on the risk of obesity, diabetes, and metabolic syndrome. *Diabetes Metab Syndr Obes*. 2015;8:295–302.
28. Martyn CN, Greenwald SE. A hypothesis about a mechanism for the programming of blood pressure and vascular disease in early life. *Clin Exp Pharmacol Physiol*. 2001;28(11):948–51.
29. Cruz-Lemini M, Crispi F, Valenzuela-Alcaraz B, et al. Fetal cardiovascular remodelling persists at 6 months of life in infants with intrauterine growth restriction. *Ultrasound Obstet Gynecol*. 2015;48(3):349–56.
30. Hales CN, Desai M, Ozanne SE. The thrifty phenotype hypothesis: How does it look after 5 years? *Diabet Med*. 1997;14(3):189–95.
31. Hales CN, Barker DJ. Type 2 (non-insulin-dependent) diabetes mellitus: The thrifty phenotype hypothesis. *Diabetologia*. 1992;35(7):595–601.
32. Løhaugen GC, Østgård HF, Andreassen S, et al. Small for gestational age and intrauterine growth restriction decreases cognitive function in young adults. *J Pediatr*. 2013;163(2):447–53.
33. Barker DJ. Sir Richard Doll Lecture: Developmental origins of chronic disease. *Public Health*. 2012;126(3):185–9.
34. Barker DJ, Osmond C, Thornburg KL, Kajantie E, Eriksson JG. The intrauterine origins of Hodgkin's lymphoma. *Cancer Epidemiol*. 2013;37(3):321-3.
35. Sieh W, Sundquist K, Sundquist J, Winkleby MA, Crump C. Intrauterine factors and risk of nonepithelial ovarian cancers. *Gynecol Oncol*. 2014;133(2):293–7.
36. Barker DJ, Thornburg KL. Placental programming of chronic diseases, cancer and lifespan: A review. *Placenta*. 2013;34(10):841–5.
37. Yajnik C. Interactions of perturbations in intrauterine growth and growth during childhood on the risk of adult-onset disease. *Proc Nutr Soc*. 2000;59(2):257–65.
38. Rodriguez-Lopez M, Osorio L, Acosta-Rojas R, et al. Influence of breastfeeding and postnatal nutrition on cardiovascular remodeling induced by fetal growth restriction. *Pediatr Res*. 2016; 79 (1-1): 100–106.
39. Stout SA, Espel EV, Sandman CA, Glynn LM, Davis EP. Fetal programming of children's obesity risk. *Psychoneuroendocrinology*. 2015;53:29–39.
40. López-Tello J, Barbero A, González-Bulnes A, et al. Characterization of early changes in fetoplacental hemodynamics in a diet-induced rabbit model of IUGR. *J Dev Orig Health Dis*. 2015;6(5):454–61.
41. Nüsken E, Gellhaus A, Kühnel E, et al. Increased rat placental fatty acid, but decreased amino acid and glucose transporters potentially modify intrauterine programming. *J Cell Biochem*. 2015;117(7):1594–603..
42. Jimenez-Chillaron JC, Ramon-Krauel M, Ribo S, Diaz R. Transgenerational epigenetic inheritance of diabetes risk as a consequence of early nutritional imbalances. *Proc Nutr Soc*. 2016;75(1):78–89.
43. Thompson RF, Fazzari MJ, Niu H, Barzilai N, Simmons RA, Greally JM. Experimental intrauterine growth restriction induces alterations in DNA methylation and gene expression in pancreatic islets of rats. *J Biol Chem*. 2010;285(20):15111–8.
44. Dumortier O, Blondeau B, Duvillie B, Reusens B, Breant B, Remacle C. Different mechanisms operating during different critical time-windows reduce rat fetal beta cell mass due to a maternal low-protein or low-energy diet. *Diabetologia*. 2007;50:2495–503.
45. Black MJ, Lim K, Zimanyi MA, et al. Accelerated age-related decline in renal and vascular function in female rats following early-life growth restriction. *Am J Physiol Regul Integr Comp Physiol*. 2015;309(9):R1153–61.
46. Beauchamp B, Thrush AB, Quizi J, et al. Undernutrition during pregnancy in mice leads to dysfunctional cardiac muscle respiration in adult offspring. *Biosci Rep*. 2015;35(3):e00200.
47. Gardner DS, Tingey K, Van Bon BW, et al. Programming of glucose–insulin metabolism in adult sheep after maternal undernutrition. *Am J Physiol Regul Integr Comp Physiol*. 2005;289(4):R947–54.
48. Sébert SP, Hyatt MA, Chan LL, et al. Maternal nutrient restriction between early and midgestation and its impact upon appetite regulation after juvenile obesity. *Endocrinology*. 2009;150(2):634–41.

49. Waterland RA, Michels KB. Epigenetic epidemiology of the developmental origins hypothesis. *Annu Rev Nutr*. 2007;27:363–88.

50. Strakovsky RS, Zhou D, Pan YX. A low-protein diet during gestation in rats activates the placental mammalian amino acid response pathway and programs the growth capacity of offspring. *J Nutr*. 2010;140(12):2116–20.

51. Coan PM, Vaughan OR, Sekita Y, et al. Adaptations in placental phenotype support fetal growth during undernutrition of pregnant mice. *J Physiol*. 2010;588(Pt 3):527–38.

52. Solomons NW. Developmental origins of health and disease: Concepts, caveats, and consequences for public health nutrition. *Nutr Rev*. 2009;67(Suppl 1):S12–16.

53. Reamon-Buettner SM, Buschmann J, Lewin G. Identifying placental epigenetic alterations in an intra-uterine growth restriction (IUGR) rat model induced by gestational protein deficiency. *Reprod Toxicol*. 2014;45:117–24.

54. Krueger R, Derno M, Goers S, et al. Higher body fatness in intrauterine growth retarded juvenile pigs is associated with lower fat and higher carbohydrate oxidation during ad libitum and restricted feeding. *Eur J Nutr*. 2014;53(2):583–97.

55. Berends LM, Fernandez-Twinn DS, Martin-Gronert MS, Cripps RL, Ozanne SE. Catch-up growth following intra-uterine growth-restriction programmes an insulin-resistant phenotype in adipose tissue. *Int J Obes (Lond)*. 2013;37(8):1051–7.

56. Lin Y, Cheng X, Sutovsky P, et al. Effect of intra-uterine growth restriction on long-term fertility in boars. *Reprod Fertil Dev*. 2015 [Epub ahead of print].

57. Biron-Shental T, Schaiff WT, Ratajczak CK, Bildirici I, Nelson DM, Sadovsky Y. Hypoxia regulates the expression of fatty acid–binding proteins in primary term human trophoblasts. *Am J Obstet Gynecol*. 2007;197(5):516.e1–6.

58. Larkin JC, Sears SB, Sadovsky Y. The influence of ligand-activated LXR on primary human trophoblasts. *Placenta*. 2014;35(11):919–24.

59. Nüsken E, Herrmann Y, Wohlfarth M, et al. Strong hypoxia reduces leptin synthesis in purified primary human trophoblasts. *Placenta*. 2015;36(4):427–32.

60. Biron-Shental T, Sadeh-Mestechkin D, Amiel A. Telomere homeostasis in IUGR placentas: A review. *Placenta*. 2016;39:21e23.

61. Biron-Shental T, Sukenik-Halevy R, Sharon Y, Laish I, Fejgin MD, Amiel A. Telomere shortening in intra uterine growth restriction placentas. *Early Hum Dev*. 2014;90(9):465–9.

62. Toutain J, Prochazkova-Carlotti M, Cappellen D, et al. Reduced placental telomere length during pregnancies complicated by intrauterine growth restriction. *PLoS One*. 2013;8(1):e54013.

63. Eisenberg DT. An evolutionary review of human telomere biology: The thrifty telomere hypothesis and notes on potential adaptive paternal effects. *Am J Hum Biol*. 2011;23(2):149–67.

64. Jansson T, Powell TL. Human placental transport in altered fetal growth: Does the placenta function as a nutrient sensor? A review. *Placenta*. 2006;27:91–7.

65. Cetin I, Ronzoni S, Marconi AM, et al. Maternal concentrations and fetal-maternal concentration differences of plasma amino acids in normal and intrauterine growth-restricted pregnancies. *Am J Obstet Gynecol*. 1996;174(5):1575–83.

66. Herrera E, Amusquivar E. Lipid metabolism in the fetus and the newborn. *Diabetes Metab Res Rev*. 2000;16(3):202–10.

67. Morgan HD, Sutherland HG, Martin DI, Whitelaw E. Epigenetic inheritance at the agouti locus in the mouse. *Nat Genet*. 1999;23(3):314–18.

68. Januar V, Desoye G, Novakovic B, Cvitic S, Saffery R. Epigenetic regulation of human placental function and pregnancy outcome: Considerations for causal inference. *Am J Obstet Gynecol*. 2015;213(4 Suppl):S182–96.

69. Gardner DS, Hosking J, Metcalf BS, Jeffery AN, Voss LD, Wilkin TJ. Contribution of early weight gain to childhood overweight and metabolic health: A longitudinal study (EarlyBird 36). *Pediatrics*. 2009;123(1):e67–73.

70. Sébert SP, Hyatt MA, Chan LL, et al. Influence of prenatal nutrition and obesity on tissue specific fat mass and obesity-associated (FTO) gene expression. *Reproduction*. 2010;139(1):265–74.

71. Bispham J, Gopalakrishnan GS, Dandrea J, et al. Maternal endocrine adaptation throughout pregnancy to nutritional manipulation: Consequences for maternal plasma leptin and cortisol and the programming of fetal adipose tissue development. *Endocrinology*. 2003;144(8):3575–85.

72. Fernandez-Twinn DS, Constância M, Ozanne SE. Intergenerational epigenetic inheritance in models of developmental programming of adult disease. *Semin Cell Dev Biol*. 2015;43:85–95.
73. de Boo HA, Harding JE. The developmental origins of adult disease (Barker) hypothesis. *Aust NZ J Obstet Gynaecol*. 2006;46(1):4–14.
74. Demicheva E, Crispi F. Long-term follow-up of intra uterine growth restriction: Cardiovascular disorders. *Fetal Diagn Ther*. 2014;36:143–53.

16

Long-Term Effects of Premature Birth

Grace Eunjin Lee and Kent Willis

Introduction

The World Health Organization defines birth under 37 weeks of gestational age as premature birth [1]. Every year more than 1 in 10 infants are born preterm, an estimated 15 million preterm births. The number of preterm births has increased over the last 20 years in nearly every country with reliable data. Preterm birth is also a global problem, with the 10 countries with the most preterm births widely distributed around the world, as can be seen in Figure 16.1 [1–4].

Three main conditions explain the majority of preterm births. Medically indicated (iatrogenic) preterm birth and preterm premature rupture of membranes each account for approximately a quarter of preterm births, respectively, with spontaneous (idiopathic) preterm births accounting for the remaining half of births [5]. Underlying these conditions, however, are heterogeneous multifactorial origins. Numerous etiologies and risk factors underlying each of these three categories have been described, but none can completely account for all preterm births, and some may underlay multiple categories [6]. Common etiologies are infections and chronic maternal conditions such as diabetes or hypertension. Multiple pregnancies are also a significant contributor to preterm births, and often have obstetrical, maternal, or fetal complications as well [7].

The financial impact of preterm birth is significant. In 2005, the average cost of a preterm birth in the United States was $32,325 as opposed to $3,325 for a term birth. This difference compounds to a estimated $26 billion economic cost to society due to premature birth in the United States. About 65% of this cost was related to medical care and 22% related to lost household income [8]. The cost of preterm birth is also inversely related to gestational age [9].

In this chapter we will review the data describing mortality and the long-term sequelae of preterm birth in higher-income countries. We will address a wide range of outcomes, particularly those related to the organ systems most specifically effected by prematurity—namely, the lungs and brain—but including development, growth, education, behavior, psychology, and health as well. We will describe how many of these outcomes exist along a continuum of increasing risk and decreasing gestational age at birth. We will also show how many of these outcomes are dependent on birth weight as well, with the worst outcomes in the smallest neonates. Because the vast majority of the extant literature examines the most preterm infants, we will focus primarily on their outcomes throughout the lifespan. Where the limited data describing the outcomes of more mildly premature infants exist, we will incorporate it as it pertains to the discussion.

Mortality

More than one million infants a year will die as a direct result of being born preterm. Globally, prematurity is the leading cause of death during the first month of life and the second leading cause after pneumonia for the remainder of the first 5 years of life. Combined, prematurity is the single leading cause of death for children under 5 years of age, as seen in Figure 16.2 [1–4]. In nearly all high- and

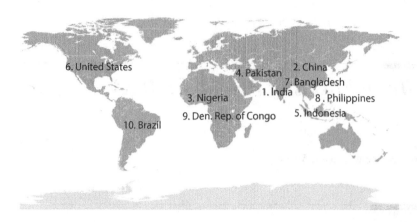

FIGURE 16.1   Ten countries account for 60% of preterm births.

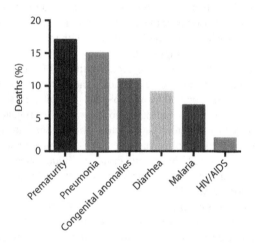

FIGURE 16.2   Causes of child death under 5 years of age.

middle-income countries preterm birth is the leading cause of child death [3]. There is also a tragic disparity in survival depending on where an infant is born. Less than 10% of extremely premature infants (<28 weeks of gestation) die in high-income countries, while greater than 90% of those born in low-income countries die within several days of birth. As many as three-quarters of deaths related to prematurity in low-income countries could be prevented with essential newborn care, even without access to neonatal intensive care [1,2].

Preterm birth is the leading cause of infant mortality in industrialized countries. Changing attitudes toward neonatal intensive care, the development and maturation of mechanical ventilation techniques, and the widespread use of surfactant and antenatal steroids have made a significant difference to neonatal mortality. Before the 1970s, very few neonates survived before 28 weeks of gestation, and mature neonates more frequently died from respiratory distress [10]. Striking improvements had resulted by the 1990s [11], with significantly more gradual improvement over the last 20 years [12].

Survival and mortality rates exhibit significant variability between countries, regionally within the same country, and by sex, race, and ethnicity [8,13–16]. In the United States, black preterm infants appear to have a survival advantage over white infants, but because the rate of premature black infant births is nearly double that of white or Hispanic neonates, the overall neonatal mortality rate for black preterms is significantly higher than for white preterms [17]. The racial disparity in the United States is also increasing. Racial disparity is most likely related to changes in mortality specific to birth weight and gestational age resulting from improvements in the survival of white preterm and low–birth weight infants. Survival of these infants probably reflects advances in and changing access to medical technology [18].

Most studies of preterm mortality have focused on infants born under 32 weeks of gestation. The mortality rates of late- (34–36 weeks of gestation) and moderate-preterm (32–33 weeks of gestation) infants are much lower than these more significantly preterm infants. The prevalence of late- and moderate-preterm birth is also significantly higher than early-preterm birth. Infants born after 32 weeks of gestation therefore contribute a significant portion of neonatal deaths [16].

Survival rates for infants of borderline viability vary significantly depending on the region being studied. Regional cohorts regularly show lower survival rates because they include deaths that do not reach the tertiary referral centers that primarily compose the populations of single and multihospital studies. It has been suggested that regional differences between higher-income countries can be primarily explained by differing attitudes toward offering intensive care to infants of borderline viability, both before and after birth [10]. Several studies have shown the benefit of a proactive attitude toward management [19] and the benefits of regionalization (transporting sick neonates from community to tertiary care and the transport of higher-risk mothers before delivery) to improve survival [20–22]. Proactive strategies in the United States resulted in an improved survival when compared with more selective practices in the Netherlands (24.1 infants per 100 live births), but resulted in an increase in cerebral palsy (CP) (7.2 cases per 100 live births) and an increase in the number of ventilator days (1372 ventilator days per 100 live births) [23].

Respiratory Outcomes

Neonatal mechanical ventilation techniques are one of the major advances in medicine in the last few decades. Improvements in respiratory outcomes are the most important contribution to reducing neonatal mortality. The respiratory-related contribution to mortality reduction is primarily due to the widespread use of exogenous surfactant antenatal steroids, and improvements in more physiologic ventilation technology and techniques. Fanaroff et al. [24] compared the survival rates of 501–1500 g infants born during three eras: presurfactant, postsurfactant, and after the widespread usage of antenatal steroids, demonstrating a reduction in mortality rates from 23% to 17% to 14% over these time periods. Survival free of significant morbidity, however, has not significantly changed over the same period, primarily due to a relative increase in the prevalence of chronic lung disease in very low birth weight (VLBW; <1500 g) infants [25,26].

Long-term respiratory outcomes are a moving target with a constantly shifting baseline. Due to the rapid evolution of respiratory therapies, by the time a cohort of infants has matured sufficiently to evaluate a particular intervention, the data produced may evaluate interventions that have already been abandoned for newer techniques. To clarify long-term respiratory outcomes of prematurity, we will need to examine chronic lung disease, the severity of neonatal lung disease, and the contribution of the degree of prematurity to pulmonary outcomes. Common adverse respiratory outcomes can be seen in Table 16.1.

TABLE 16.1

Summary of Adverse Respiratory Outcomes of Premature Birth

Respiratory Outcome
Bronchopulmonary dysplasia
Increased frequency and severity of viral respiratory illnesses
Decreased forced expiratory volume (FEV_1)
Reduced exercise capacity
Reduced peak oxygen uptake
Airway hyperresponsiveness
In severe BPD: Pulmonary hypertension

Lung Development

Preterm infants are born during the late-second and third trimesters when lung development should be at its maximum rate [27–29]. Preterm birth disrupts the normal progression of lung maturation, leading to lungs with reduced function and increased susceptibility to injury [30]. Preterms are primarily born during the saccular stage of lung development, during which the number of bronchi increases, saccule invaginate to form alveoli, capillaries cover the air sacs, and the surfactant and antioxidant systems develop [27,29]. These changes result in a rapid increase in lung volume and surface area [28].

Ventilatory support in neonates is complicated because it is imposed on an actively developing respiratory system. In order to provide support, the developing lungs must be exposed to forces that lead to both acute and chronic tissue injury. Tissue injury alters the way the lungs develop and respond to future stressors. The healing process further alters lung function and development. Early-preterm delivery alters subsequent alveolar development [31]. In addition, the lung may be injured due to a lack of surfactant, impaired gas exchange, and delayed intrapulmonary fluid absorption [32,33].

Lung function normally increases in healthy individuals until late adolescence to early adulthood then slowly declines throughout the rest of life. In preterms, early lung injury and maldevelopment may lead to a lower maximum lung function and potential earlier or more precipitous decline in lung function [34]. There is concern that this may mean that preterm children are at greater risk of significant pulmonary morbidity at earlier ages in adulthood, but there is a paucity of longitudinal data to evaluate this hypothesis.

Bronchopulmonary Dysplasia

Bronchopulmonary dysplasia (BPD) is the preferred term for chronic lung disease of infancy [31,35]. Despite the advances in more physiologic respiratory care, a small proportion of neonates will develop respiratory failure, and the interventions used to care for them will lead many to develop BPD. Prolonged exposure to oxygen and to mechanical ventilation at a time when the developing lungs should still be bathed in hypooxygenated fluid in utero leads to inflammatory and histological changes [36]. The original BPD as described by Northway et al. [37] and Stocker [38] was characterized by lung injury that resulted in bronchiolar squamous metaplasia, necrotizing bronchiolitis, and alveolar cell hyperplasia. The "healing" of this original injury resulted classically in a highly variable residual focal alveolar septal fibrosis that produced apparently normal lung lobes adjacent to hyperinflated or severely fibrous lobes. The literature suggests that BPD does not limit parenchymal lung growth [31,39–42], but evidence of small airway obstruction indicates that while there is normal lung volume, airway size is reduced [43]. Clinically, this results in infants with increased small airway resistance, maldistributed ventilation, airway hyperactivity, and increased functional residual capacity [31,38].

Today, advances in mechanical ventilation, and the modification of the definition to include all infants requiring mechanical ventilation or oxygen therapy for greater than 28 days or beyond 36 weeks post-conceptual age, has led to a "new" BPD characterized by relatively minimal alveolar septal fibrosis and more uniform inflation [31,44]. The primary insult is now thought to be mediated by reactive oxygen species resulting from prolonged respiratory therapy [45]. The development of BPD is now seen primarily as a consequence of lung inflammation that in addition to prolonged exposure to supplemental oxygen and mechanical ventilation may arise from intrauterine exposure in infection or inflammation [46–48]. The prematurely respired lung undergoes a disruption of saccular and alveolar development, an *acinar arrest*, precisely during the period when a term infant would be undergoing rapid alveolar development. The resulting lung contains simplified gas exchange structures with fewer and larger alveoli [31,36,45,46,48,49]. Severe cases of BPD may still result in pulmonary hypertension, abnormal pulmonary vascular development, and significant morbidity [50].

Respiratory Health

Preterm birth leaves underdeveloped lungs at increased risk of infection with viral illness. Infants born between 33 and 36 weeks were nearly twice as likely to be hospitalized for respiratory syncytial virus than term-born infants (57 per 1000 compared with 30 per 1000) [28]. A study by Gunville et al. [51] appears to indicate that preterm survivors have more severe respiratory illnesses, form a larger proportion of pediatric intensivecare unit admissions, and utilize a larger proportion of resources.

Survivors with BPD often experience asthma-like exacerbations due to viral illnesses characterized by airway hyperresponsiveness and impaired exercise capacity [52]. Because infants with BPD tend to have more severe viral respiratory illness, they unsurprisingly require more frequent hospital readmissions. Even asymptomatic BPD survivors may have persistent fibrotic changes detectable in adulthood [53]. Alterations in the pulmonary oxidative stress response have also been found persisting in adolescents as well [54].

Respiratory Function

Young children with a mental age lower than 5 years have difficulty producing reliable spirometry data. There is a paucity of data related to the pulmonary function of preschool-age children as a result. The limited data suggest that very preterm infants with BPD have persistent reductions in flow and higher airway resistance compared with controls without BPD. Friedrich et al. [55] examined infants born between 30 and 34 weeks of gestation and found decreased forced expiratory flow between 25% and 75% of forced vital capacity at 4 ($p = .022$) and 16 months ($p = .027$) of age. No difference in forced vital capacity was noted. Hoo et al. [56] suggested that early respiratory function tracks with time in premature infants after noting similar lung function at 3 weeks of age and 1 year.

Pulmonary function in older children and adolescents is better studied. Most studies demonstrate a significant reduction in airflow in preterms, as measured by the forced expiratory volume in 1 second (FEV_1). Meta-analysis by Gibson and Doyle [34] showed a reduction in the mean difference for FEV_1 by 0.8 standard deviations (SD). There was no obvious trend with time despite the introduction of surfactant. One regional cohort of children born <26 weeks had a 1.26 SD reduction in FEV_1 in the preterm group compared with controls [57]. They also appreciated that 23% of <26 week survivors and 66% of survivors who developed BPD had clinically significant impairments. Late-preterm outcomes are less well studied, but they may be impaired similarly to more preterm infants. The Avon Longitudinal Study of Parents and Children (ALSPAC) showed that 8–9 year olds born between 33 and 34 weeks of gestation had similarly reduced mean FEV_1 measurements as infants born between 25 and 32 weeks of gestation. Late-preterm infants born between 35 and 36 weeks of gestation had normal lung function at both ages [58].

Preterm survivors who developed BPD had greater reductions in FEV_1 compared with other preterms in most studies in a recent meta-analysis [34]. Overall differences approached 1 SD. The outcomes of infants who had BPD improved during the surfactant era, but the age at which survivors lung function was assessed did not appreciably change outcomes.

Lung function does not clearly improve with age in very preterm survivors. An Australian [59] and two Norwegian cohorts [60] that examined lung function in adolescence and young adulthood demonstrated insignificant change with time compared with controls. However, in contrast to other studies of very preterm infants, late-preterm infants in the ALSPAC trial had airway function similar to term children when reexamined between 14 and 17 years of age [58].

Preterms appear to have more reactive airways than controls, especially infants who developed BPD [57,61–63]. Preterms also have other abnormalities such as diffusion impairment and air trapping. In late preterms, however, Todisco et al. [64] found no significant difference in bronchial responsiveness compared with term-born children when examined at a mean age of 11.6 years.

Exercise Capacity

Preterms have a reduced exercise capacity. Eleven-year-olds born <800 g were found to have a reduced mean maximal oxygen consumption compared with controls [65]. A study of 10-year-olds born <1000 g and <32 weeks of gestation quantified a reduction of 3.9 (95% CI 2.6–5.2) mL/kg/min in the mean maximal oxygen consumption [66]. Another study of 11-year-olds born <26 weeks found very preterms had a reduced peak oxygen consumption as well [67]. Clemm et al. [68] was able to demonstrate that these effects persist at least into late adolescence by examining two cohorts of 18-year-olds, one born <28 weeks and another born <1000 g. Exercise capacity and peak oxygen uptake were moderately reduced compared with term-born controls, but did show improvement with physical activity. At 25 years of age, extreme preterms born in the 1980s had 10% less exercise capacity than term-born controls, but they were still within the normal range and similar to when they had been examined at 18 years of age. Preterms may eventually outgrow their exercise limitations with conditioning, as evidenced by a correlation with self-reported physical activity and exercise capacity and a lack of a strong correlation with neonatal factors [69]. Encouraging exercise in preterm survivors is likely important to promoting recovery in lung function.

Neuromotor Outcomes

CP is the most important motor impairment in premature survivors. CP is frequently used as a marker of the quality of neonatal care in studies of temporal trends, because the risk of CP is likely a constellation of multiple factors including, but not limited to, the aggressiveness of intervention, population characteristics, new therapies, and mortality. In addition to CP, premature infants are at risk of gross and fine motor impairments as well [70]. Common neuromotor outcomes in preterms can be seen in Table 16.2.

Neural Mechanisms

In premature infants, brain injuries have been found in the form of multiple lesions, principally germinal matrix-intraventricular hemorrhage, posthemorrhagic hydrocephalus, and periventricular leukomalacia (PVL) [71]. Of these injuries, PVL is the most important determinant of neurological morbidity. While the focal necrotic lesions of PVL located deep in cerebral white matter correlate with cerebral palsy, cognitive/behavioral deficits may be associated with the more diffuse white matter injury also often found with PVL. In studies using immunocytochemical markers in autopsies of premature infant brains, PVL was evidenced by focal necrosis deep in periventricular matter that usually evolved to cyst formation in addition to more diffuse noncystic injury in central cerebral white matter [72]. In such diffuse white matter injury, the preferential death of preoligodendrocytes and evidence for lipid peroxidation and protein nitration in the preoligodendrocytes was observed. This would suggest that the mode by which these cells are destroyed is reactive oxygen species and reactive nitrogen species. Additionally, the marked prevalence of activated microglia in the diffuse component of PVL suggests that these cells may be involved in generating reactive species found in the brain lesion [71]. Microglia have been shown to be activated by ischemia and to remain active for weeks after the injury [73]. Additionally, activated microglia release reactive oxygen and nitrogen species, which then results in cell death [74]. Preoligodendrocytes of the cerebral white matter in premature infants are particularly vulnerable to attack by reactive species [75,76], while mature oligodendrocytes that can produce myelin and are found primarily in post-term infants are resistant to such attack [75,76]. Brain microglia can also be activated by maternal intrauterine infection/ inflammation; thus, infection has been associated with the vulnerability of preoligodendrocytes [77,78].

In neuroimaging studies of cerebral palsy, abnormal neuroanatomical findings were found in 80%–90% of children with cerebral palsy. White matter damage is the most common finding, particularly in

TABLE 16.2

Summary of Adverse Neuromotor
Outcomes of Premature Birth

Neuromotor Outcome
Cerebral palsy
Developmental coordination disorder
Impaired balance
Impaired ball skills
Impaired manual dexterity
Deficits in fine and gross motor development

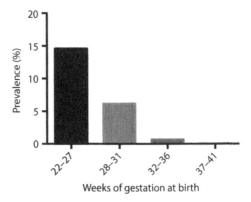

FIGURE 16.3   Prevalence of CP related to gestational age.

children with bilateral spasticity and athetosis. Isolated gray matter damage is rare. Hemiplegic children have more combined gray and white matter abnormalities. Neuroimaging suggests that about a third of cerebral palsy results from prenatal insults and about 40% from perinatal insults, with the remainder occurring postnatally [79].

Cerebral Palsy

CP is the umbrella term for a group of persistent but nonprogressing neurodevelopmental disorders of movement and posture due to a defect or lesion in the fetal or infant brain [80]. The prevalence of CP is inversely related to gestational age [81]. One meta-analysis conducted over 25 studies reported a prevalence of 14.6% at 22–27 weeks of gestation, compared with a prevalence of 6.2% at 28–31 weeks, 0.7% at 32–36 weeks of gestation, and 0.1% at term [81]. Regardless of whether the risk of developing CP has been declining in survivors or not, the absolute number of cases of CP is increasing because more early-preterm infants are surviving to discharge [82].

Motor Impairments without Cerebral Palsy

Children born without CP may still present with motor deficits in coordination, balance, gross and fine motor control, and visual integration. These deficits are often classified as developmental coordination disorder (DCD). A higher incidence of DCD has been reported in school-age children who are born preterm in contrast to that of the general population [83]. One meta-analysis found a prevalence of 19% for moderate and 40.5% for mild-to-moderate impairment in preterm children [84]. This is roughly three to four times the 5%–8% prevalence found in the general population [85], as can be seen in Figure 16.3 [84,85]. As shown in one study in Denmark, gestational age at birth is inversely related to the risk of growing up with DCD [86]. Non-CP motor problems found in preterm children include balance skills, ball skills, manual dexterity, and fine and gross motor development, with balance skills being reported as the most impaired [87]. Such children with mild-to-moderate motor impairment may have difficulties crawling, walking, and running during their early childhood years. For school-age children, motor impairments may make a variety of activities difficult that might hinder their social and academic life [88,89]. These motor deficits persist into adolescence and adulthood [87,89].

Neurocognitive Outcomes

Early-preterm infants have high rates of cognitive dysfunction in nonmotor cognitive domains, such as attention, visual processing, academic performance, and executive function [90]. Common adverse neurocognitive outcomes can be seen in Table 16.3. General cognitive ability as assessed by intelligence

TABLE 16.3

Summary of Adverse Neurocognitive Outcomes of
Premature Birth

Neurocognitive Outcome
Reduced IQ
Slower processing speed
Impairments in selecting, shifting, sustaining, and dividing attention
Visual sensory impairment
Impaired stereopsis
Impaired visual convergence
Impaired visual acuity and contrast sensitivity
Deficits in visual motor integration

quotient (IQ) is well studied in preterm survivors. One recent meta-analysis of 27 studies published between 1980 and 2009 found a mean difference of 11.9 points in IQ, with preterm children performing 0.8 SD below term controls [91]. Deficits in IQ have been associated with decreased gestational age [92]. One study estimated that for every week before 33 weeks an infant is born, IQ decreases by approximately 1.5 points [93]. These results did not seem to vary with the year of birth, suggesting that IQ measurements for preterm children have not significantly improved in the last 25 years [92].

Processing Speed

Processing speed is the cognitive ability that measures the speed at which elementary cognitive tasks are performed. Processing speed is a direct measurement of the time required to interpret and respond to visual stimuli, and is quantified by reaction time and decision time [94]. Processing speed plays an important role in the development of working memory capacity and, consequently, the development of intelligence [95].

Slower processing speed has been reported in very preterm children. A study compared processing speed in preterm infants (<1750 g birth weight) with their term counterparts [96] and reported that preterm infants needed about 30% more inspection time than term infants during the first year of life. Reduced processing efficiency may persist into toddlerhood [97] and middle childhood [98].

Attention

Attention is a multifaceted core cognitive ability consisting of the capacity to selectively focus, sustain, encode, shift, and divide attention [99]. One systematic review found that all these attention domains were delayed in young preterm children compared with term controls, and deficits became more apparent as the infants aged [100]. Another meta-analysis found that preterm children performed below their term peers at selective attention, sustained attention, and certain tasks requiring shifting attention [101]. Similarly, a cohort study of extremely preterm adolescents found persisting high rates of impairment in selective, shifting, and divided attention [102].

Visual Perception

Visual perceptual difficulties are commonly found in very preterm survivors [103]. One large cohort study found that among adolescents born extremely preterm, 43% had at least one visual sensory impairment (vs. 29% in controls), 26% had impaired stereopsis (vs. 10%), and 16% had impaired visual convergence (vs. 6%) [104]. Other visual problems often reported in preterm children include strabismus and impaired visual acuity and contrast sensitivity [105]. Additionally, very preterm children have been shown to frequently report visual motor integration deficits, as expressed by difficulty copying increasingly complex geometric designs [106].

Speech and Language Outcomes

Speech and language impairments are common in preterm survivors. Delays in articulation, receptive language processing, expressive language acquisition, and deficits in phonological short-term memory [107–111] may impair the development of crucial skills required for the development of joint attention, social interaction, and other aspects of appropriate communication [112]. Such limitations in preterms may arise from neonatal brain injury, other neurodevelopmental impairments such as neurosensory deficits and abnormal neural development due to too early exposure to the extrauterine environment. Poor linguistic outcomes may also be influenced by lower gestational age, longer hospitalization, gender, age at assessment, the developmental environment, and socioeconomic factors [113–116].

Immature Brains

The origins of speech development arise in utero at around 26 weeks of gestation. As the fetus perceives, reacts, and stores the sounds of the maternal voice and body, a progressive maturation of the auditory cortex occurs [117]. Preterm birth distorts this process as the infant is thrust into an abnormally noisy nursery with limited access to their mother's voice [117–119]. Deprivation from maternal speech has a profound impact on the development of the auditory system and eventual language and speech patterns [120,121].

Language Outcomes

The separation of the Bayley III into separate language and cognitive composite scores has generated considerable research into the language outcomes of preterms. Preterm infants have been constantly shown to exhibit an increased risk of speech and language delays compared with term infants. A meta-analysis by van Noort-van der Spek et al. [108] showed that preterms scored significantly lower on tests of both simple and complex language function, and that they had progressive difficulty with complex language as they aged, even after controlling for the presence of disabilities and socioeconomic confounders. Brain injury in preterms is a significant factor in producing lower language outcomes. Neonatal severe brain injury as measured by cranial ultrasound has been shown to be the strongest predictor of outcomes on language test scores [111].

The Indomethacin Trial tracked longitudinal data on language outcomes as an outcome measure, which has provided valuable data on the language function of preterms in contrast to term controls. In general, the trial showed that the simple language function of preterms improves between 3 and 12 years of age. Lower-level language functions such as phonological processing and phonemic decoding showed greater improvements in lower–birth weight infants than did higher-level language functions such as syntax, semantics, and verbal language memory. Despite these demonstrated improvements, deficits in language function as measured by the Peabody Picture Vocabulary Test and Clinical Evaluation of Language Fundamentals persisted in preterms compared with term controls, even after the exclusion of children with severe brain injury [111,122]. Catch-up continued into adolescence, but some deficits still persisted at age 16 for higher-level language functions [110].

General Health Outcomes

In recent years, the research into the long-term outcomes of premature survivors has progressed from crude measures of mortality and major morbidities, particularly respiratory and cognitive outcomes, to a more nuanced assessment of general health and qualitative outcomes such as the character of adult functioning and quality of life. Common adverse outcomes of premature birth can be seen in Table 16.4.

TABLE 16.4

Summary of General Health Outcomes of Premature Birth

Vision and Hearing	Infections	Bones	Quality of Life	Adult Functioning
Retinopathy of prematurity	Increased risk of sepsis	Reduced bone mass	Without disability: similar quality of life	Lower rate of school completion
Cerebral visual impairment	Early-onset sepsis: gram-negative organisms	Osteoporosis	With disability: quality of life slightly lower	Lower job income, partly due to disability
Myopia, hypermetropia	Late-onset sepsis: gram-positive organisms	Increased risk of bone fractures in adulthood	Impaired mental health	Lower rates of employment
Strabismus			Reduced socioeconomic function	Lower reproduction rates
Increased risk of retinal detachment			Reduced physical function and health	Female survivors: increased risk of recurrent preterm birth in offspring
Central auditory processing deficits				

Vision and Hearing

Sensorineural impairments are important morbidities of premature birth, with limitations of vision and hearing having profound effects during life. Visual sequelae of extremely premature birth most often involve retinopathy of prematurity and cerebral visual impairment [123]. The rate of blindness and severe visual impairment has been reported to increase with decreasing gestational age [124]. Infants born <25 weeks of gestation had rates of 4%–8%, compared with the 1%–2% occurrence in those born between 26 and 27 weeks [125]. However, the use of cryotherapy, beginning in the late 1990s as a treatment for severe retinopathy of prematurity, has reduced rates of blindness from 8%–10% to <2% [126].

Extremely preterm children are often at higher risk of refractive error and visual accommodation problems compared with term controls [123]. For such preterm children, the rates of myopia and hypermetropia have been reported in early childhood at around 20%–30% [105,127] and strabismus at rates of around 10%–30% [128,129]. As an additional adverse outcome, a high rate of retinal detachment (4%–5%) was reported in extremely low–birth weight (ELBW; <1000 g) individuals during late adolescence [124].

The rates of hearing impairment in preterm children and young adults have been reported to be relatively low, in the range of 1%–4% [126,127,130]. In a cohort of Canadian young adults, no differences in the use of hearing aids were found between ELBW subjects and their term controls [124]. However, significant central auditory processing deficits have been reported in ELBW adolescents compared with term controls [131]. These deficits were in turn associated with poorer behavioral, academic, and intellectual progress. Both impaired speech pattern recognition and sound discrimination have been reported in preterm children [132,133].

Infections

Moderate- and late-preterm infants are more likely to develop an infection than term neonates. A large cohort of late-preterm infants showed early-onset sepsis was diagnosed in 0.44% of late preterms and late-onset sepsis in 0.63% of late preterms. Gram-positive organisms accounted for the majority of cases of early sepsis (66%), followed by gram-negative organisms (27%). Late-onset sepsis was also primarily caused by gram-positive organisms (59%), followed by gram-negatives (30%), but there were more cases due to systemic yeast (7%) [134]. A large retrospective population-based study by McIntire and Leveno [135] found late preterms had an increased risk of sepsis (OR 2.18) and infectious workup (OR 1.73).

It is well known that VLBW and early premature infants are at increased risk of sepsis. In a study of 108,000 VLBW neonates, 0.96% of infants were diagnosed with early-onset sepsis and 11.3% experienced late-onset sepsis. Gram-negative organisms were most commonly isolated in early-onset sepsis, and gram-positive organisms in late-onset sepsis. Early- and late-onset sepsis were both associated with an increased risk of mortality after controlling for other confounders (OR 1.45, 95% CI 1.21–1.73, and OR 1.30, 95% CI 1.21–1.40, respectively) [136].

Bones

Early preterms have an increased risk of reduced bone mass and osteoporosis, which in turn translates into an increased risk of bone fractures in adulthood [137,138]. Up to 80% of the calcium in a term infant's body at birth is deposited in the third trimester. Preterms miss this crucial calcium deposition due to their shorter gestations, which would explain why early-preterm infants are often born with suboptimal bone development [139]. Longitudinal cohort studies following VLBW individuals have shown reduced femoral neck bone density and reduced lumbar spine density in adulthood compared with controls born at term [137].

Quality of Life

Young-adult survivors of prematurity without significant disability rate their quality of life similar or only slightly reduced compared with term-born individuals. Danish researchers found nonimpaired 18–20-year-old VLBW survivors had no significant difference in quality of life, but impaired individuals did rate their quality of life slightly lower [140,141]. A Swiss study using a mail-in questionnaire also found no significant difference [142]. However, two other studies using the same questionnaire reported reduced self-perception of mental health, socioeconomic function [143], physical function, and health [144].

Adult Functioning

Adult survivors of prematurity are as a whole functioning surprisingly well as adults. Where their functioning is limited as a whole, it is most often related to the presence of disabilities. Educational achievement is often used as a marker of successful transition to adult life. A Norwegian study observed a gestational-age gradient with regard to school completion in preterm individuals. A 68% high school completion and 25% bachelor's degree completion were observed for individuals born between 23 and 27 weeks of gestation, compared with 70% and 28%, respectively, for individuals born at 28–30 weeks of gestation, and 75% and 35%, respectively, for those born at normal birth weight (NBW) [145]. This same study showed that while rates for unemployment were comparable, young adults born between 23 and 27 weeks of gestation had lower job incomes (20%) compared with those born at term (23%). These differences were in part due to disability [145]. A higher proportion of Ontario ELBW adults than NBW adults were neither employed nor at school (26% vs. 15%), largely because of chronic illnesses or permanent disabilities [146]. In a Swedish national cohort study, overall, a significant proportion of those born between 24 and 28 weeks of gestation were employed, and more were paying taxes than receiving benefits [147].

A study drawn from the Norwegian Medical Birth Registry strongly suggests that for both men and women born very preterm, reproduction rates are lower than for those born at term [148]. Reproduction seems to increase with gestational age at birth until about 35 weeks of gestation. While 68% of women and 50% of men born at term had reproduced later in life, only 25% of women and 13.9% of men born between 22 and 27 weeks had subsequently reproduced [148]. Additionally, female but not male preterm participants had an increased risk of recurrent preterm birth in offspring. Women born at 22 and 27 weeks had a risk of preterm offspring of 14%, compared with women born at term with a risk of 6.4% [148].

CONCLUSIONS

There is substantial evidence that long-term outcomes have improved with neonatal intensive care. Significant improvements have been appreciated in the most preterm and small neonates in higher-income countries. Higher absolute rates of CP, developmental delay, cognitive impairment, and chronic respiratory conditions, however, have resulted from the improved survival of preterm neonates. At the same time, the majority of preterm infants now survive without major disabilities.

Despite some dire warnings to the contrary [149], as a whole, adult survivors of prematurity are doing better than we predicted. While unemployment was admittedly more prevalent among preterms with a disability, even among disadvantaged populations in the United States [130] and Europe [144,150], a significant majority had completed high school and were living independent productive lives. Among ELBW infants, about one-quarter have disabilities but generally enjoy a similar quality of life to their NBW peers [151]. Moving beyond the stringent usage of IQ and other tests of ability to more broader levels of functioning has allowed us to appreciate that while some functional differences and disabilities exist, for the most part preterms have no significant differences in behavioral functioning, self-esteem, or satisfaction with their lives [152]. In short, the neurodevelopmental and cognitive function of preterms during infancy and early childhood are valid assessments of current status and useful to providing intervention, but they may lack long-term validity to accurately predict adverse quality of life in adulthood [153].

From the data describing global preterm birth, two clear goals emerge: first, to narrow the survival gap for preterm infants in lower- and middle-income countries by implementing widely available improved obstetric and neonatal care; and second, to develop solutions to prevent premature birth globally. Narrowing the survival gap through such interventions will significantly alter the effects of prematurity on the global burden of disease. At the same time, further advances in neonatal intensive care are also required to improve the neurodevelopmental and respiratory outcomes of the youngest and smallest infants born on the cusp of viability. The long-term follow-up of preterm infants will be crucial to evaluating the efficacy of these interventions and their eventual impact on quality of life.

REFERENCES

1. March of Dimes, PMNCH, Save the Children, WHO. *Born Too Soon: The Global Action Report on Preterm Birth*. Eds. CP Howson, MV Kinney, JE Lawn. Geneva, Switzerland: World Health Organization; 2012. Available from: http://www.marchofdimes.org/mission/global-preterm.aspx.
2. Blencowe H, Cousens S, Oestergaard MZ, et al. National, regional, and worldwide estimates of preterm birth rates in the year 2010 with time trends since 1990 for selected countries: A systematic analysis and implications. *Lancet*. 2012;379(9832):2162–72. Available from: http://linkinghub.elsevier.com/retrieve/pii/S0140673612608204.
3. Liu L, Oza S, Hogan D, et al. Global, regional, and national causes of child mortality in 2000–13, with projections to inform post-2015 priorities: An updated systematic analysis. *Lancet*. 2015;385(9966):430–40. Available from: http://linkinghub.elsevier.com/retrieve/pii/S0140673614616986.
4. Liu L, Johnson HL, Cousens S, et al. Global, regional, and national causes of child mortality: An updated systematic analysis for 2010 with time trends since 2000. *Lancet*. 2012;379(9832):2151–61. Available from: http://linkinghub.elsevier.com/retrieve/pii/S0140673612605601.
5. Moutquin JM, Milot-Roy V. Preterm birth prevention: Effectiveness of current strategies. *Journal SOGC*. 1996;18(6):571–88. Available from: http://scholar.google.com/scholar?q=related:eMRZLSMR ohkJ:scholar.google.com/&hl=en&num=20&as_sdt=0,5.
6. Moutquin JM. Classification and heterogeneity of preterm birth. *BJOG: An Int J Obstet Gynaecol*. 2003;110:30–33. Available from: http://onlinelibrary.wiley.com/doi/10.1046/j.1471-0528.2003.00021.x/full.
7. Mattison DR, Damus K, Fiore E, Petrini J, Alter C. Preterm delivery: A public health perspective. *Paediatr Perinat Epidemiol*. 2001;15:7–16. Available from: http://onlinelibrary.wiley.com/doi/10.1046/j.1365-3016.2001.00004.x/full.
8. Institute of Medicine. *Preterm Birth: Causes, Consequences, and Prevention*. Washington, DC: National Academies Press; 2007. Available from: http://www.ncbi.nlm.nih.gov/books/NBK11362.
9. Gilbert W. The cost of prematurity: Quantification by gestational age and birth weight. *Obstet Gynecol*. 2003;102(3):488–92. Available from: http://linkinghub.elsevier.com/retrieve/pii/S0029784403006173.

10. Saigal S, Doyle LW. An overview of mortality and sequelae of preterm birth from infancy to adulthood. *Lancet*. 2008;371:261–9. Available from: http://eutils.ncbi.nlm.nih.gov/entrez/eutils/elink.fcgi?dbfrom= pubmed&id=18207020&retmode=ref&cmd=prlinks.
11. Doyle LW, Rogerson S, Chuang SL, James M, Bowman ED, Davis PG. Why do preterm infants die in the 1990s? *Med J Aust*. 1999;170:528–32. Available from: http://eutils.ncbi.nlm.nih.gov/entrez/eutils/ elink.fcgi?dbfrom=pubmed&id=10397043&retmode=ref&cmd=prlinks.
12. Fanaroff AA, Stoll BJ, Wright LL, et al. Trends in neonatal morbidity and mortality for very low birth-weight infants. *Am J Obstet Gynecol*. 2007;196(2):147.e1. Available from: http://linkinghub.elsevier. com/retrieve/pii/S0002937806012105.
13. Draper ES, Manktelow B, Field DJ, James D. Prediction of survival for preterm births by weight and gestational age: Retrospective population based study. *BMJ*. 1999;319:1093–7. Available from: http:// www.bmj.com/cgi/doi/10.1136/bmj.319.7217.1093.
14. Allen MC, Alexander GR, Tompkins ME, Hulsey TC. Racial differences in temporal changes in new-born viability and survival by gestational age. *Paediatr Perinat Epidemiol*. 2000;14:152–8. Available from: http://onlinelibrary.wiley.com/doi/10.1046/j.1365-3016.2000.00255.x/full.
15. Alexander GR, Kogan MD, Himes JH. 1994–1996 U.S. singleton birth weight percentiles for gesta-tional age by race, Hispanic origin, and gender. *Matern Child Health J*. 1999;3:225–31. Available from: http://link.springer.com/10.1023/A:1022381506823.
16. Kramer MS, Demissie K, Yang H, et al. The contribution of mild and moderate preterm birth to infant mortality. *JAMA*. 2000;284(7):843–9. Available from: http://jama.jamanetwork.com/article. aspx?doi=10.1001/jama.284.7.843.
17. Alexander GR, Kogan M, Bader D, Carlo W, Allen M, Mor J. US birth weight/gestational age-specific neonatal mortality: 1995–1997 rates for whites, Hispanics, and blacks. *Pediatrics*. 2003;111:e61. Available from: http://pediatrics.aappublications.org/cgi/doi/10.1542/peds.111.1.e61.
18. Alexander GR, Wingate MS, Bader D, Kogan MD. The increasing racial disparity in infant mortal-ity rates: Composition and contributors to recent US trends. *Am J Obstet Gynecol*. 2008;198:51.e1. Available from: http://linkinghub.elsevier.com/retrieve/pii/S0002937807007351.
19. Håkansson S, Farooqi A, Holmgren PA, Serenius F, Högberg U. Proactive management promotes out-come in extremely preterm infants: A population-based comparison of two perinatal management strate-gies. *Pediatrics*. 2004;114:58–64. Available from: http://pediatrics.aappublications.org/cgi/doi/10.1542/ peds.114.1.58.
20. McCormick MC, Escobar GJ, Zheng Z, Richardson DK. Place of birth and variations in management of late preterm ("near-term") infants. *Semin Perinatol*. 2006;30:44–7. Available from: http://linkinghub. elsevier.com/retrieve/pii/S0146000506000139.
21. Stolz JW, McCormick MC. Restricting access to neonatal intensive care: Effect on mortality and eco-nomic savings. *Pediatrics*. 1998;101:344–8. Available from: http://www.jstor.org/stable/1602506?origin =crossref.
22. McCormick MC, Richardson DK. Access to neonatal intensive care. *Future Child*. 1995;5:162. Available from: http://www.jstor.org/stable/1602513?origin=crossref.
23. Lorenz JM, Paneth N, Jetton JR, Ouden L den, Tyson JE. Comparison of management strategies for extreme prematurity in New Jersey and the Netherlands: Outcomes and resource expenditure. *Pediatrics*. 2001;108:1269–74. Available from: http://eutils.ncbi.nlm.nih.gov/entrez/eutils/elink.fcgi?dbfrom=pubm ed&id=11731647&retmode=ref&cmd=prlinks.
24. Fanaroff AA, Hack M, Walsh MC. The NICHD Neonatal Research Network: Changes in practice and outcomes during the first 15 years. *Semin Perinatol*. 2003;27(4):281–7. Available from: http://eutils. ncbi.nlm.nih.gov/entrez/eutils/elink.fcgi?dbfrom=pubmed&id=14510318&retmode=ref&cmd=prlinks.
25. Lemons JA, Bauer CR, Oh W, et al. Very low birth weight outcomes of the National Institute of Child Health and Human Development Neonatal Research Network, January 1995 through December 1996. *Pediatrics*. 2001;107(1):e1. Available from: http://pediatrics.aappublications.org/cgi/doi/10.1542/peds.107.1.e1.
26. Stoelhorst GMSJ, Rijken M, Martens SE, et al. Changes in neonatology: Comparison of two cohorts of very preterm infants (gestational age <32 weeks): The project on preterm and small for gesta-tional age infants 1983 and the Leiden follow-up project on prematurity 1996–1997. *Pediatrics*. 2005;115(2):396–405. Available from: http://pediatrics.aappublications.org/content/115/2/396.abstract.
27. Joshi S, Kotecha S. Lung growth and development. *Early Hum Dev*. 2007;83(12):789–94. Available from: http://www.earlyhumandevelopment.com/article/S037837820700165X/fulltext.

28. Resch B, Paes B. Are late preterm infants as susceptible to RSV infection as full term infants? *Early Hum Dev.* 2011;87(Suppl 1). Available from: http://linkinghub.elsevier.com/retrieve/pii/S037837821100020X.
29. Kotecha S. Lung growth: Implications for the newborn infant. *Arch Dis Child Fetal Neonatal Ed.* 2000;82(1). Available from: http://fn.bmj.com/content/82/1/F69.full.
30. Maritz GS, Morley CJ, Harding R. Early developmental origins of impaired lung structure and function. *Early Hum Dev.* 2005;81(9):763–71. Available from: http://www.earlyhumandevelopment.com/article/S0378378205001349/fulltext.
31. Niedermaier S, Hilgendorff A. Bronchopulmonary dysplasia: An overview about pathophysiologic concepts. *Mol Cell Pediatr.* 2015;2(1):2. Available from: http://www.molcellped.com/content/2/1/2.
32. Escobar GJ, Clark RH, Greene JD. Short-term outcomes of infants born at 35 and 36 weeks gestation: We need to ask more questions. *Semin Perinatol.* 2006;30(1):28–33. Available from: http://linkinghub.elsevier.com/retrieve/pii/S0146000506000061.
33. Jain L, Eaton DC. Physiology of fetal lung fluid clearance and the effect of labor. *Semin Perinatol.* 2006;30(1):34–43. Available from: http://linkinghub.elsevier.com/retrieve/pii/S0146000506000073.
34. Gibson AM, Doyle LW. Respiratory outcomes for the tiniest or most immature infants. *Semin Fetal Neonatal Med.* 2014;19(2):105–11. Available from: http://linkinghub.elsevier.com/retrieve/pii/S1744165X1300098X.
35. Ehrenkranz RA, Walsh MC, Vohr BR, et al. Validation of the National Institutes of Health consensus definition of bronchopulmonary dysplasia. *Pediatrics.* 2005;116(6):1353–60. Available from: http://pediatrics.aappublications.org/cgi/doi/10.1542/peds.2005-0249.
36. Hayes D, Meadows JT, Murphy BS, Feola DJ, Shook LA, Ballard HO. Pulmonary function outcomes in bronchopulmonary dysplasia through childhood and into adulthood: Implications for primary care. *Prim Care Respir J.* 2011;20(2):128–33. Available from: http://www.nature.com/articles/pcrj20112.
37. Northway WH Jr, Rosan RC, Porter DY. Pulmonary disease following respirator therapy of hyaline-membrane disease. *New Engl J Med.* 1967;276(7):357–68. Available from: http://www.nejm.org/doi/abs/10.1056/NEJM196702162760701.
38. Stocker JT. Pathologic features of long-standing "healed" bronchopulmonary dysplasia: A study of 28 3- to 40-month-old infants. *Hum Pathol.* 1986;17(9):943–61. Available from: http://eutils.ncbi.nlm.nih.gov/entrez/eutils/elink.fcgi?dbfrom=pubmed&id=3639056&retmode=ref&cmd=prlinks.
39. Northway WH, Moss RB, Carlisle KB, et al. Late pulmonary sequelae of bronchopulmonary dysplasia. *New Engl J Med.* 1990;323(26):1793–9. Available from: http://www.nejm.org/doi/abs/10.1056/NEJM199012273232603.
40. Hakulinen AL, Järvenpää AL, Turpeinen M, Sovijärvi A. Diffusing capacity of the lung in school-aged children born very preterm, with and without bronchopulmonary dysplasia. *Pediatr Pulmonol.* 1996;21(6):353–60. Available from: http://doi.wiley.com/10.1002/%28SICI%291099-0496%28199606%2921%3A6%3C353%3A A%3AAID-PPUL2%3E3.0.CO%3B2-M.
41. Kim YC, Wheeler W, Longmate J, Wohl M. Longitudinal study of lung function in children following bronchopulmonary dysplasia. 1988. Available from: http://scholar.google.com/scholar?q=related:elub-biHoTYJ:scholar.google.com/&hl=en&num=20&as_sdt=0,5.
42. Andreasen LA, Nilas L, Kjær MM. Operative complications during pregnancy after gastric bypass: A register-based cohort study. *Obes Surg.* 2014;24(10):1634–8. Available from: http://link.springer.com/10.1007/s11695-014-1232-z.
43. Chernick V. Long-term pulmonary function studies in children with bronchopulmonary dysplasia: An ever-changing saga. *J Pediatr.* 1998;133(2):171–2. Available from: http://eutils.ncbi.nlm.nih.gov/entrez/eutils/elink.fcgi?dbfrom=pubmed&id=9709697&retmode=ref&cmd=prlinks.
44. Husain AN, Siddiqui NH, Stocker JT. Pathology of arrested acinar development in postsurfactant bronchopulmonary dysplasia. *Hum Pathol.* 1998;29(7):710–17. Available from: http://eutils.ncbi.nlm.nih.gov/entrez/eutils/elink.fcgi?dbfrom=pubmed&id=9670828&retmode=ref&cmd=prlinks.
45. McCarthy K, Bhogal M, Nardi M, Hart D. Pathogenic factors in bronchopulmonary dysplasia. *Pediatr Res.* 1984;18(5):483–8. Available from: http://eutils.ncbi.nlm.nih.gov/entrez/eutils/elink.fcgi?dbfrom=pubmed&id=6610166&retmode=ref&cmd=prlinks.
46. Coalson JJ. Pathology of new bronchopulmonary dysplasia. *Semin Neonatol.* 2003;8(1):73–81. Available from: http://www.sfnmjournal.com/article/S1084275602001938/fulltext.
47. Baker CD, Accurso FJ. Preterm birth and airway inflammation in childhood. *J Pediatr.* 2012;161(6):979–80. Available from: http://linkinghub.elsevier.com/retrieve/pii/S0022347612009183.

48. Westover AJ, Moss TJ. Effects of intrauterine infection or inflammation on fetal lung development. *Clin Exp Pharmacol Physiol*. 2012;39(9):824–30. Available from: http://onlinelibrary.wiley.com/doi/10.1111/j.1440-1681.2012.05742.x/full.

49. Wong PM, Lees AN, Louw J, et al. Emphysema in young adult survivors of moderate-to-severe bronchopulmonary dysplasia. *Eur Respir J*. 2008;32(2):321–8. Available from: http://erj.ersjournals.com/cgi/doi/10.1183/09031936.00127107.

50. Baker CD, Abman SH. Impaired pulmonary vascular development in bronchopulmonary dysplasia. *Neonatology*. 2015;107(4):344–51. Available from: http://www.karger.com/?doi=10.1159/000381129.

51. Gunville CF, Sontag MK, Stratton KA, Ranade DJ, Abman SH, Mourani PM. Scope and impact of early and late preterm infants admitted to the PICU with respiratory illness. *J Pediatr*. 2010;157(2):209–14. Available from: http://linkinghub.elsevier.com/retrieve/pii/S0022347610001162.

52. Jobe AH. The new bronchopulmonary dysplasia. *Curr Opin Pediatr*. 2011;23(2):167–72. Available from: http://content.wkhealth.com/linkback/openurl?sid=WKPTLP:landingpage&an=00008480-201104000-00007.

53. Bhandari A, Panitch HB. Pulmonary outcomes in bronchopulmonary dysplasia. *Semin Perinatol*. 2006;30(4):219–26. Available from: http://linkinghub.elsevier.com/retrieve/pii/S0146000506000747.

54. Carraro S, Filippone M, Da Dalt L, et al. Bronchopulmonary dysplasia: The earliest and perhaps the longest lasting obstructive lung disease in humans. *Early Hum Dev*. 2013;89(Suppl 3). Available from: http://linkinghub.elsevier.com/retrieve/pii/S037837821300162X.

55. Friedrich L, Pitrez PMC, Stein RT, Goldani M, Tepper R, Jones MH. Growth rate of lung function in healthy preterm infants. *Am J Respir Crit Care Med*. 2007;176(12):1269–73. Available from: http://www.atsjournals.org/doi/abs/10.1164/rccm.200703-476OC.

56. Hoo AF, Dezateux C, Henschen M, Costeloe K, Stocks J. Development of airway function in infancy after preterm delivery. *J Pediatr*. 2002;141(5):652–8. Available from: http://www.jpeds.com/article/S0022347602001804/fulltext.

57. Fawke J, Lum S, Kirkby J, et al. Lung function and respiratory symptoms at 11 years in children born extremely preterm: The EPICure study. *Am J Respir Crit Care Med*. 2010;182(2):237–45. Available from: http://www.atsjournals.org/doi/abs/10.1164/rccm.200912-1806OC.

58. Kotecha SJ, Watkins WJ, Paranjothy S, Dunstan FD, Henderson AJ, Kotecha S. Effect of late preterm birth on longitudinal lung spirometry in school age children and adolescents. *Thorax*. 2012;67(1):54–61. Available from: http://thorax.bmj.com/cgi/doi/10.1136/thoraxjnl-2011-200329.

59. Doyle LW, Faber B, Callanan C, Freezer N, Ford GW, Davis NM. Bronchopulmonary dysplasia in very low birth weight subjects and lung function in late adolescence. *Pediatrics*. 2006;118(1):108–13. Available from: http://pediatrics.aappublications.org/cgi/doi/10.1542/peds.2005-2522.

60. Vollsæter M, Røksund OD, Eide GE, Markestad T, Halvorsen T. Lung function after preterm birth: Development from mid-childhood to adulthood. *Thorax*. 2013;68(8):767–76. Available from: http://thorax.bmj.com/cgi/doi/10.1136/thoraxjnl-2012-202980.

61. Halvorsen T, Skadberg BT, Eide GE, Røksund OD, Carlsen KH, Bakke P. Pulmonary outcome in adolescents of extreme preterm birth: A regional cohort study. *Acta Paediatrica*. 2004;93(10):1294–300. Available from: http://doi.wiley.com/10.1111/j.1651-2227.2004.tb02926.x.

62. Narang I, Rosenthal M, Cremonesini D, Silverman M, Bush A. Longitudinal evaluation of airway function 21 years after preterm birth. *Am J Respir Crit Care Med*. 2008;178(1):74–80. Available from: http://www.atsjournals.org/doi/abs/10.1164/rccm.200705-701OC.

63. Pelkonen AS, Hakulinen AL, Turpeinen M. Bronchial lability and responsiveness in school children born very preterm. *Am J Respir Crit Care Med*. 1997;156(4):1178–84. Available from: http://www.atsjournals.org/doi/abs/10.1164/ajrccm.156.4.9610028.

64. Todisco T, De Benedictis FM, Iannacci L, et al. Mild prematurity and respiratory functions. *Eur J Pediatr*. 1993;152(1):55–8. Available from: http://link.springer.com/10.1007/BF02072517.

65. Kilbride HW, Gelatt MC, Sabath RJ. Pulmonary function and exercise capacity for ELBW survivors in preadolescence: Effect of neonatal chronic lung disease. *J Pediatr*. 2003;143(4):488–93. Available from: http://linkinghub.elsevier.com/retrieve/pii/S002234760300413X.

66. Smith LJ, van Asperen PP, McKay KO, Selvadurai H, Fitzgerald DA. Reduced exercise capacity in children born very preterm. *Pediatrics*. 2008;122(2). Available from: http://pediatrics.aappublications.org/cgi/doi/10.1542/peds.2007-3657.

67. Clemm H, Røksund O, Thorsen E, Eide GE, Markestad T, Halvorsen T. Aerobic capacity and exercise performance in young people born extremely preterm. *Pediatrics*. 2012;129(1):e97. Available from: http://pediatrics.aappublications.org/cgi/doi/10.1542/peds.2011-0326.
68. Clemm H, Vollsæter M, Thorsen E, Røksund O, Halvorsen T. Exercise capacity at 18 years of age in two extremely preterm born cohorts from the 1980s and 1990s. *Eur Respir J*. 2014;44:P4875. Available from: http://erj.ersjournals.com/content/44/Suppl_58/P4875.abstract.
69. Clemm HH, Vollsæter M, Røksund OD, Eide GE, Markestad T, Halvorsen T. Exercise capacity after extremely preterm birth: Development from adolescence to adulthood. *Ann Am Thorac Soc*. 2014;11(4):537–45. Available from: http://www.atsjournals.org/doi/abs/10.1513/AnnalsATS.201309-311OC.
70. Spittle AJ, Orton J. Cerebral palsy and developmental coordination disorder in children born preterm. *Semin Fetal Neonatal Med*. 2014;19(2):84–9. Available from: http://linkinghub.elsevier.com/retrieve/pii/S1744165X13001145.
71. Volpe JJ. Neurobiology of periventricular leukomalacia in the premature infant. *Pediatr Res*. 2001;50(5):553–62. Available from: http://www.nature.com/doifinder/10.1203/00006450-200111000-00003.
72. Haynes RL, Folkerth RD, Keefe RJ, et al. Nitrosative and oxidative injury to premyelinating oligodendrocytes in periventricular leukomalacia. *J Neuropathol Exp Neurol*. 2003;62(5):441. Available from: http://journals.lww.com/jneuropath/Fulltext/2003/05000/Nitrosative_and_Oxidative_Injury_to_Premyelinating.2.aspx.
73. Ivacko JA, Sun R, Silverstein FS. Hypoxic-ischemic brain injury induces an acute microglial reaction in perinatal rats. *Pediatr Res*. 1996;39(1):39–47. Available from: http://www.nature.com/doifinder/10.1203/00006450-199604001-00241.
74. Chao CC, Hu S, Molitor TW, Shaskan EG, Peterson PK. Activated microglia mediate neuronal cell injury via a nitric oxide mechanism. *J Immunol*. 1992;149(8):2736–41. Available from: http://www.jimmunol.org/content/149/8/2736.abstract.
75. Back SA, Gan X, Li Y, Rosenberg PA, Volpe JJ. Maturation-dependent vulnerability of oligodendrocytes to oxidative stress-induced death caused by glutathione depletion. *J Neurosci*. 1998;18(16):6241–53. Available from: http://eutils.ncbi.nlm.nih.gov/entrez/eutils/elink.fcgi?dbfrom=pubmed&id=9698317&retmode=ref&cmd=prlinks.
76. Baud OF, Haynes R, Volpe JJ. Developmental upregulation of manganese superoxide dismutase (MnSOD) expression in oligodendrocytes (OLs) confers resistance to nitric oxide. 2003. Available from: http://scholar.google.com/scholar?q=related:zUT3S7aY06YJ:scholar.google.com/&hl=en&num=20&as_sdt=0,5.
77. Eklind S, Mallard C, Leverin AL, et al. Bacterial endotoxin sensitizes the immature brain to hypoxic: Ischaemic injury. *Eur J Neurosci*. 2001;13(6):1101–6. Available from: http://eutils.ncbi.nlm.nih.gov/entrez/eutils/elink.fcgi?dbfrom=pubmed&id=11285007&retmode=ref&cmd=prlinks.
78. Lehnardt S, Lachance C, Patrizi S, et al. The toll-like receptor TLR4 is necessary for lipopolysaccharide-induced oligodendrocyte injury in the CNS. *J Neurosci*. 2002;22(7):2478–86. Available from: http://eutils.ncbi.nlm.nih.gov/entrez/eutils/elink.fcgi?dbfrom=pubmed&id=11923412&retmode=ref&cmd=prlinks.
79. Korzeniewski SJ, Birbeck G, DeLano MC, Potchen MJ, Paneth N. A systematic review of neuroimaging for cerebral palsy. *J Child Neurol*. 2008;23(2):216–27. Available from: http://jcn.sagepub.com/cgi/doi/10.1177/0883073807307983.
80. Bax M, Goldstein M, Rosenbaum P, et al. Proposed definition and classification of cerebral palsy, April 2005. *Dev Med Child Neurol*. 2005;47(8):571–6. Available from: http://eutils.ncbi.nlm.nih.gov/entrez/eutils/elink.fcgi?dbfrom=pubmed&id=16108461&retmode=ref&cmd=prlinks.
81. Himpens E, Van den Broeck C, Oostra A, Calders P, Vanhaesebrouck P. Prevalence, type, distribution, and severity of cerebral palsy in relation to gestational age: A meta-analytic review. *Dev Med Child Neurol*. 2008;50(5):334–40. Available from: http://doi.wiley.com/10.1111/j.1469-8749.2008.02047.x.
82. Bhushan V, Paneth N, Kiely JL. Impact of improved survival of very low birth weight infants on recent secular trends in the prevalence of cerebral palsy. *Pediatrics*. 1993;91(6):1094–100. Available from: http://pediatrics.aappublications.org/content/91/6/1094.short.
83. Lingam R, Hunt L, Golding J, Jongmans M, Emond A. Prevalence of developmental coordination disorder using the DSM-IV at 7 years of age: A UK population-based study. *Pediatrics*. 2009;123(4). Available from: http://pediatrics.aappublications.org/cgi/doi/10.1542/peds.2008-1770.

84. Williams J, Lee KJ, Anderson PJ. Prevalence of motor-skill impairment in preterm children who do not develop cerebral palsy: A systematic review. *Dev Med Child Neurol*. 2010;52(3):232–7. Available from: http://doi.wiley.com/10.1111/j.1469-8749.2009.03544.x.

85. Barnhart RC, Davenport MJ, Epps SB, Nordquist VM. Developmental coordination disorder. *Phys Ther*. 2003;83(8):722–31. Available from: http://eutils.ncbi.nlm.nih.gov/entrez/eutils/elink.fcgi?dbfrom=pubmed&id=12882613&retmode=ref&cmd=prlinks.

86. Zhu JL, Olsen J, Olesen AW. Risk for developmental coordination disorder correlates with gestational age at birth. *Paediat Perinat Epidemiol*. 2012;26(6):572–7. Available from: http://doi.wiley.com/10.1111/j.1365-3016.2012.01316.x.

87. De Kieviet JF, Piek JP, Aarnoudse-Moens CS, Oosterlaan J. Motor development in very preterm and very low-birth-weight children from birth to adolescence: A meta-analysis. *JAMA*. 2009;302(20):2235–42. Available from: http://jama.jamanetwork.com/article.aspx?doi=10.1001/jama.2009.1708.

88. Zwicker JG, Harris SR, Klassen AF. Quality of life domains affected in children with developmental coordination disorder: A systematic review. *Child Care Health Dev*. 2013;39(4):562–80. Available from: http://doi.wiley.com/10.1111/j.1365-2214.2012.01379.x.

89. Msall ME. Optimizing neuromotor outcomes among very preterm, very low-birth-weight infants. *JAMA*. 2009;302(20):2257–8. Available from: http://jama.jamanetwork.com/article.aspx?doi=10.1001/jama.2009.1730.

90. Anderson PJ. Neuropsychological outcomes of children born very preterm. *Semin Fetal Neonatal Med*. 2014;19(2):90–96. Available from: http://linkinghub.elsevier.com/retrieve/pii/S1744165X13001212.

91. Kerr-Wilson CO, Mackay DF, Smith GCS, Pell JP. Meta-analysis of the association between preterm delivery and intelligence. *J Public Health (Oxf)*. 2012;34(2):209–16. Available from: http://jpubhealth.oxfordjournals.org/cgi/doi/10.1093/pubmed/fdr024.

92. Bhutta AT, Cleves MA, Casey PH, Cradock MM, Anand KJS. Cognitive and behavioral outcomes of school-aged children who were born preterm: A meta-analysis. *JAMA*. 2002;288(6):728–37. Available from: http://eutils.ncbi.nlm.nih.gov/entrez/eutils/elink.fcgi?dbfrom=pubmed&id=12169077&retmode=ref&cmd=prlinks.

93. Johnson S. Cognitive and behavioural outcomes following very preterm birth. *Semin Fetal Neonatal Med*. 2007;12(5):363–73. Available from: http://linkinghub.elsevier.com/retrieve/pii/S1744165X07000649.

94. Takeuchi H, Kawashima R. Effects of processing speed training on cognitive functions and neural systems. *Rev Neurosci*. 2012;23(3):289–301. Available from: http://www.degruyter.com/view/j/revneuro.2012.23.issue-3/revneuro-2012-0035/revneuro-2012-0035.xml.

95. Fry AF, Hale S. Relationships among processing speed, working memory, and fluid intelligence in children. *Biol Psychol*. 2000;54(1):1–34. Available from: http://eutils.ncbi.nlm.nih.gov/entrez/eutils/elink.fcgi?dbfrom=pubmed&id=11035218&retmode=ref&cmd=prlinks.

96. Rose SA, Feldman JF, Jankowski JJ. Processing speed in the 1st year of life: A longitudinal study of preterm and full-term infants. *Dev Psychol*. 2002;38(6):895–902. Available from: http://eutils.ncbi.nlm.nih.gov/entrez/eutils/elink.fcgi?dbfrom=pubmed&id=12428702&retmode=ref&cmd=prlinks.

97. Rose SA, Feldman JF, Jankowski JJ, Rossem RV. A cognitive cascade in infancy: Pathways from prematurity to later mental development. *Intelligence*. 2008;36(4):367–78. Available from: http://linkinghub.elsevier.com/retrieve/pii/S0160289607000980.

98. Rose SA, Feldman JF. Memory and processing speed in preterm children at eleven years: A comparison with full-terms. *Child Dev*. 1996;67(5):2005–21. Available from: http://eutils.ncbi.nlm.nih.gov/entrez/eutils/elink.fcgi?dbfrom=pubmed&id=9022226&retmode=ref&cmd=prlinks.

99. Mirsky AF, Anthony BJ, Duncan CC, Ahearn MB, Kellam SG. Analysis of the elements of attention: A neuropsychological approach. *Neuropsychol Rev*. 1991;2(2):109–45. Available from: http://eutils.ncbi.nlm.nih.gov/entrez/eutils/elink.fcgi?dbfrom=pubmed&id=1844706&retmode=ref&cmd=prlinks.

100. Van de Weijer-Bergsma E, Wijnroks L, Jongmans MJ. Attention development in infants and preschool children born preterm: A review. *Infant Behav Dev*. 2008;31(3):333–51. Available from: http://linkinghub.elsevier.com/retrieve/pii/S0163638308000040.

101. Mulder H, Pitchford NJ, Hagger MS, Marlow N. Development of executive function and attention in preterm children: A systematic review. *Dev Neuropsychol*. 2009;34(4):393–421. Available from: http://www.tandfonline.com/doi/abs/10.1080/87565640902964524.

102. Wilson-Ching M, Molloy CS, Anderson VA, et al. Attention difficulties in a contemporary geographic cohort of adolescents born extremely preterm/extremely low birth weight. *J Int Neuropsychol Soc*. 2013;19(10):1097–108. Available from: http://www.journals.cambridge.org/ abstract_S1355617713001057.

103. Hård AL, Niklasson A, Svensson E, Hellström A. Visual function in school-aged children born before 29 weeks of gestation: A population-based study. *Dev Med Child Neurol*. 2000;42(2):100–105. Available from: http://eutils.ncbi.nlm.nih.gov/entrez/eutils/elink.fcgi?dbfrom=pubmed&id=10698327&retmode=r ef&cmd=prlinks.

104. Molloy CS, Wilson-Ching M, Anderson VA, Roberts G, Anderson PJ, Doyle LW. Visual processing in adolescents born extremely low birth weight and/or extremely preterm. *Pediatrics*. 2013;132(3):e704. Available from: http://pediatrics.aappublications.org/cgi/doi/10.1542/peds.2013-0040.

105. O'Connor AR, Stephenson T, Johnson A, et al. Long-term ophthalmic outcome of low birth weight children with and without retinopathy of prematurity. *Pediatrics*. 2002;109(1):12–18. Available from: http://pediatrics.aappublications.org/cgi/doi/10.1542/peds.109.1.12.

106. Ornstein M, Ohlsson A, Edmonds J, Asztalos E. Neonatal follow-up of very low birthweight/extremely low birthweight infants to school age: A critical overview. *Acta Paediatr Scand*. 1991;80(8):741–8. Available from: http://eutils.ncbi.nlm.nih.gov/entrez/eutils/elink.fcgi?dbfrom=pubmed&id=172026 9&retmode=ref&cmd=prlinks.

107. Barre N, Morgan A, Doyle LW, Anderson PJ. Language abilities in children who were very preterm and/or very low birth weight: A meta-analysis. *J Pediatr*. 2011;158(5):766–74. Available from: http:// linkinghub.elsevier.com/retrieve/pii/S0022347610009236.

108. Van Noort-van der Spek IL, Franken M-CJP, Weisglas-Kuperus N. Language functions in preterm-born children: A systematic review and meta-analysis. *Pediatrics*. 2012;129(4):745–54. Available from: http://pediatrics.aappublications.org/cgi/doi/10.1542/peds.2011-1728.

109. Ortiz Mantilla S, Choudhury N, Leevers H, Benasich AA. Understanding language and cognitive deficits in very low birth weight children. *Dev Psychobiol*. 2008;50(2):107–26. Available from: http://doi. wiley.com/10.1002/dev.20278.

110. Luu TM, Vohr BR, Allan W, Schneider KC, Ment LR. Evidence for catch-up in cognition and receptive vocabulary among adolescents born very preterm. *Pediatrics*. 2011;128(2):313–22. Available from: http://pediatrics.aappublications.org/cgi/doi/10.1542/peds.2010-2655.

111. Luu TM, Vohr BR, Schneider KC, et al. Trajectories of receptive language development from 3 to 12 years of age for very preterm children. *Pediatrics*. 2009;124(1):333–41. Available from: http://pedi-atrics.aappublications.org/cgi/doi/10.1542/peds.2008-2587.

112. Durkin K, Conti-Ramsden G. Language, social behavior, and the quality of friendships in adolescents with and without a history of specific language impairment. *Child Dev*. 2007;78(5):1441–57. Available from: http://doi.wiley.com/10.1111/j.1467-8624.2007.01076.x.

113. Grunau RVE, Kearney SM, Whitfield MF. Language development at 3 years in pre-term children of birth weight below 1000 g. *Br J Disord Commun*. 2009;25(2):173–82. Available from: http://doi.wiley. com/10.3109/13682829009011972.

114. Williams TR, Alam S, Gaffney M, Centers for Disease Control and Prevention (CDC). Progress in identifying infants with hearing loss: United States, 2006–2012. *MMWR*. 2015;64(13):351–6. Available from: http://eutils.ncbi.nlm.nih.gov/entrez/eutils/elink.fcgi?dbfrom=pubmed&id=25856256&retmode= ref&cmd=prlinks.

115. Marston L, Peacock JL, Calvert SA, Greenough A, Marlow N. Factors affecting vocabulary acquisition at age 2 in children born between 23 and 28 weeks' gestation. *Dev Med Child Neurol*. 2007;49(8):591–6. Available from: http://doi.wiley.com/10.1111/j.1469-8749.2007.00591.x.

116. Clark CAC, Woodward LJ. Neonatal cerebral abnormalities and later verbal and visuospatial working memory abilities of children born very preterm. *Dev Neuropsychol*. 2010;35(6):622–42. Available from: http://www.tandfonline.com/doi/abs/10.1080/87565641.2010.508669.

117. McMahon E, Wintermark P, Lahav A. Auditory brain development in premature infants: The importance of early experience. *Ann NY Acad Sci*. 2012;1252(1):17–24. Available from: http://doi.wiley. com/10.1111/j.1749-6632.2012.06445.x.

118. Caskey M, Stephens B, Tucker R, Vohr B. Importance of parent talk on the development of preterm infant vocalizations. *Pediatrics*. 2011;128(5):910–16. Available from: http://pediatrics.aappublications. org/cgi/doi/10.1542/peds.2011-0609.

119. Doheny L, Hurwitz S, Insoft R, Ringer S, Lahav A. Exposure to biological maternal sounds improves cardiorespiratory regulation in extremely preterm infants. *J Matern Fetal Neonatal Med*. 2012;25(9):1591–4. Available from: http://www.tandfonline.com/doi/full/10.3109/14767058.2011.648237.

120. deRegnier R-A, Wewerka S, Georgieff MK, Mattia F, Nelson CA. Influences of postconceptional age and postnatal experience on the development of auditory recognition memory in the newborn infant. *Dev Psychobiol*. 2002;41(3):216–25. Available from: http://doi.wiley.com/10.1002/dev.10070.

121. Fifer WP, Moon CM. The role of mother's voice in the organization of brain function in the newborn. *Acta Paediatr Suppl*. 1994;397:86–93. Available from: http://eutils.ncbi.nlm.nih.gov/entrez/eutils/elink. fcgi?dbfrom=pubmed&id=7981479&retmode=ref&cmd=prlinks.

122. Luu TM, Ment LR, Schneider KC, Katz KH, Allan WC, Vohr BR. Lasting effects of preterm birth and neonatal brain hemorrhage at 12 years of age. *Pediatrics*. 2009;123(3):1037–44. Available from: http:// pediatrics.aappublications.org/cgi/doi/10.1542/peds.2008-1162.

123. Dutton GN. The spectrum of cerebral visual impairment as a sequel to premature birth: An overview. *Doc Ophthalmol*. 2013;127(1):69–78. Available from: http://link.springer.com/10.1007/s10633-013-9382-1.

124. Saigal S, Stoskopf B, Boyle M, et al. Comparison of current health, functional limitations, and health care use of young adults who were born with extremely low birth weight and normal birth weight. *Pediatrics*. 2007;119(3). Available from: http://pediatrics.aappublications.org/cgi/doi/10.1542/peds.2006-2328.

125. Farooqi A, Hägglöf B, Sedin G, Gothefors L, Serenius F. Chronic conditions, functional limitations, and special health care needs in 10- to 12-year-old children born at 23 to 25 weeks' gestation in the 1990s: A Swedish national prospective follow-up study. *Pediatrics*. 2006;118(5). Available from: http:// pediatrics.aappublications.org/cgi/doi/10.1542/peds.2006-1070.

126. Doyle LW, Roberts G, Anderson PJ, Victorian Infant Collaborative Study Group. Changing long-term outcomes for infants 500–999 g birth weight in Victoria, 1979–2005. *Arch Dis Child Fetal Neonatal Ed*. 2011;96(6). Available from: http://fn.bmj.com/cgi/doi/10.1136/adc.2010.200576.

127. Marlow N, Wolke D, Bracewell MA, Samara M, EPICure Study Group. Neurologic and developmental disability at six years of age after extremely preterm birth. *N Engl J Med*. 2005;352(1):9–19. Available from: http://www.nejm.org/doi/abs/10.1056/NEJMoa041367.

128. Haugen OH, Nepstad L, Standal OA, Elgen I, Markestad T. Visual function in 6 to 7 year-old children born extremely preterm: A population-based study. *Acta Ophthalmol*. 2012;90(5):422–7. Available from: http://doi.wiley.com/10.1111/j.1755-3768.2010.02020.x.

129. Darlow BA, Clemett RS, Horwood LJ, Mogridge N. Prospective study of New Zealand infants with birth weight less than 1500 g and screened for retinopathy of prematurity: Visual outcome at age 7–8 years. *Br J Ophthalmol*. 1997;81(11):935–40. Available from:/pmc/articles/PMC1722066/?report=abstract.

130. Hack M, Flannery DJ, Schluchter M, Cartar L, Borawski E, Klein N. Outcomes in young adulthood for very-low-birth-weight infants. *N Engl J Med*. 2002;346(3):149–57. Available from: http://www.nejm. org/doi/abs/10.1056/NEJMoa010856.

131. Davis NM, Doyle LW, Ford GW, et al. Auditory function at 14 years of age of very-low-birthweight. *Dev Med Child Neurol*. 2001;43(3):191–6. Available from: http://eutils.ncbi.nlm.nih.gov/entrez/eutils/elink. fcgi?dbfrom=pubmed&id=11263690&retmode=ref&cmd=prlinks.

132. Jansson-Verkasalo E, Ceponiene R, Valkama M, et al. Deficient speech-sound processing, as shown by the electrophysiologic brain mismatch negativity response, and naming ability in prematurely born children. *Neurosci Lett*. 2003;348(1):5–8. Available from: http://eutils.ncbi.nlm.nih.gov/entrez/eutils/elink. fcgi?dbfrom=pubmed&id=12893412&retmode=ref&cmd=prlinks.

133. Herold B, Höhle B, Walch E, Weber T, Obladen M. Impaired word stress pattern discrimination in very-low-birthweight infants during the first 6 months of life. *Dev Med Child Neurol*. 2008;50(9):678–83. Available from: http://onlinelibrary.wiley.com/doi/10.1111/j.1469-8749.2008.03055.x/full.

134. Cohen-Wolkowiez M, Moran C, Benjamin DK, Cotten CM, Clark RH, Smith PB. Early and late onset sepsis in late preterm infants. *Pediatr Infect Dis J*. 2009;28:1052–6. Available from:/pmc/articles/ PMC2798577/?report=abstract.

135. McIntire DD, Leveno KJ. Neonatal mortality and morbidity rates in late preterm births compared with births at term. *Obstet Gynecol*. 2008;111:35–41. Available from: http://content.wkhealth.com/linkback/ openurl?sid=WKPTLP:landingpage&an=00006250-200801000-00007.

136. Hornik CP, Fort P, Clark RH, et al. Early and late onset sepsis in very-low-birth-weight infants from a large group of neonatal intensive care units. *Early Hum Dev*. 2012;88:S69. Available from: http://www. earlyhumandevelopment.com/article/S0378378212700191/fulltext.

137. Hovi P, Andersson S, Järvenpää AL, et al. Decreased bone mineral density in adults born with very low birth weight: A cohort study. *PLoS Med.* 2009;6(8):e1000135. Available from: http://dx.plos.org/10.1371/journal.pmed.1000135.

138. Fewtrell MS, Williams JE, Singhal A, Murgatroyd PR, Fuller N, Lucas A. Early diet and peak bone mass: 20 year follow-up of a randomized trial of early diet in infants born preterm. *Bone.* 2009;45(1):142–9. Available from: http://linkinghub.elsevier.com/retrieve/pii/S8756328209012058.

139. Kovacs CS. Calcium and bone metabolism disorders during pregnancy and lactation. *Endocrinol Metab Clin North Am.* 2011;40(4):795–826. Available from: http://linkinghub.elsevier.com/retrieve/pii/S0889852911000673.

140. Bjerager M, Steensberg J, Greisen G. Quality of life among young adults born with very low birth-weights. *Acta Paediatr.* 1995;84(12):1339–43. Available from: http://eutils.ncbi.nlm.nih.gov/entrez/eutils/elink.fcgi?dbfrom=pubmed&id=8645947&retmode=ref&cmd=prlinks.

141. Dinesen SJ, Greisen G. Quality of life in young adults with very low birth weight. *Arch Dis Child Fetal Neonatal Ed.* 2001;85(3). Available from: http://fn.bmj.com/content/85/3/F165.full.

142. Baumgardt M, Bucher HU, Mieth RA, Fauchère JC. Health-related quality of life of former very preterm infants in adulthood. *Acta Paediatr.* 2012;101(2). Available from: http://doi.wiley.com/10.1111/j.1651-2227.2011.02422.x.

143. Natalucci G, Becker J, Becher K, Bickle GM, Landolt MA, Bucher HU. Self-perceived health status and mental health outcomes in young adults born with less than 1000 g. *Acta Paediatr.* 2013;102(3):294–9. Available from: http://onlinelibrary.wiley.com/doi/10.1111/apa.12102/full.

144. Cooke RWI. Health, lifestyle, and quality of life for young adults born very preterm. *Arch Dis Child.* 2004;89(3):201–6. Available from: http://adc.bmj.com/content/89/3/201.1.full.

145. Moster D, Lie RT, Markestad T. Long-term medical and social consequences of preterm birth. *N Engl J Med.* 2008;359(3):262–73. Available from: http://www.nejm.org/doi/abs/10.1056/NEJMoa0706475.

146. Saigal S, Stoskopf B, Streiner D, et al. Transition of extremely low-birth-weight infants from adolescence to young adulthood: Comparison with normal birth-weight controls. *JAMA.* 2006;295(6):667–75. Available from: http://jama.jamanetwork.com/article.aspx?doi=10.1001/jama.295.6.667.

147. Lindström K, Winbladh B, Haglund B, Hjern A. Preterm infants as young adults: A Swedish national cohort study. *Pediatrics.* 2007;120(1):70–77. Available from: http://pediatrics.aappublications.org/cgi/doi/10.1542/peds.2006-3260.

148. Swamy GK, Østbye T, Skjærven R. Association of preterm birth with long-term survival, reproduction, and next-generation preterm birth. *JAMA.* 2008;299(12):1429–36. Available from: http://jama.jamanetwork.com/article.aspx?doi=10.1001/jama.299.12.1429.

149. Walther FJ, Ouden AL den, Verloove-Vanhorick SP. Looking back in time: Outcome of a national cohort of very preterm infants born in the Netherlands in 1983. *Early Hum Dev.* 2000;59(3):175–91. Available from: http://linkinghub.elsevier.com/retrieve/pii/S0378378200000943.

150. Hille ETM, Weisglas-Kuperus N, van Goudoever JB, et al. Functional outcomes and participation in young adulthood for very preterm and very low birth weight infants: The Dutch Project on Preterm and Small for Gestational Age Infants at 19 years of age. *Pediatrics.* 2007;120(3). Available from: http://pediatrics.aappublications.org/cgi/doi/10.1542/peds.2006-2407.

151. Saigal S, Stoskopf B, Pinelli J, et al. Self-perceived health-related quality of life of former extremely low birth weight infants at young adulthood. *Pediatrics.* 2006;118(3):1140–48. Available from: http://pediatrics.aappublications.org/cgi/doi/10.1542/peds.2006-0119.

152. Saigal S, Stoskopf B, Pinelli J, Boyle M, Streiner D. Social functioning, peer, partner and family relationships and satisfaction with life. 2005. Available from: http://scholar.google.com/scholar?q=related:y-dGCUmFGisJ:scholar.google.com/&hl=en&oe=ASCII&as_sdt=0,5.

153. Saigal S, Rosenbaum P. What matters in the long term: Reflections on the context of adult outcomes versus detailed measures in childhood. *Semin Fetal Neonatal Med.* 2007;12(5):415–22. Available from: http://linkinghub.elsevier.com/retrieve/pii/S1744165X07000832.

17

Long-Term Health Outcomes for Children Born as a Result of In Vitro Fertilization Treatment

Jennifer M. Beale, Jennifer C. Pontré, and Roger Hart

Introduction

Following the first successful in vitro fertilization (IVF) pregnancy in 1976 and successful birth following IVF in 1978 [1], it is now estimated that in excess of 5 million children have been born as a result of IVF since the technique was developed in the early 1970s [2]. Europe currently leads the world in rates of IVF, taking responsibility for up to 55% of all IVF cycles, and in 2011 France, Germany, and Italy were the world's most active countries in this area. Approximately 1.5 million IVF cycles are performed each year worldwide. This number is predicted to rapidly increase in years to come. Currently, good data exists regarding pregnancy and short-term outcomes for children conceived via IVF [3,4]; however, there is a need for more to clearly establish long-term health and safety.

Overall, singletons born after IVF are known to be at risk of poorer perinatal outcomes compared with children born after natural conception [5]. In addition, there is an increased risk of congenital malformation [6,7] and potential increased risk of imprinting disorders [8,9]. These children are at risk of other health consequences that may not be evident early in life, highlighting the need for more study in this area. Given that the majority of children conceived through IVF are yet to reach adulthood or even middle age, we may not become aware for years to come of the true long-term health effects of this method of conception. The Barker hypothesis [10] established the relationship between adverse conditions during prenatal life and long-term adverse cardiometabolic outcomes [2]. Given the manipulation of the early prenatal environment that occurs within an IVF cycle, it is also possible that alterations made during this early phase of embryonic and fetal development may also influence later susceptibility to cardiometabolic disease [11,12,13].

There exist major inherent methodological challenges in studying and evaluating the effects of IVF [5]. It is difficult to control for the large number of potential confounding factors that may affect long-term health and development, and while some studies have successfully addressed this issue [14], others have failed in this area. Women undergoing assisted reproduction are often of an older age, and often have an older partner, with an accompanying increase in the risk of abnormal gametes from both parties, which may affect the outcomes of children conceived via IVF [15]. In addition, the full pathogenesis of infertility itself is yet to be understood in its entirety, and with unexplained infertility comes factors that may never be determined but which may influence results. Given the inherent difficulty in defining a "normal" fertile population, the identification of adequate and representative "controls" is also a challenging task. With emerging evidence that subtle details of the technology used can influence child health and development, and given the rapidly evolving technologies available, identifying all potential influencing factors is difficult. The health of the woman embarking on treatment, the use of ovarian stimulation, the use of testicular sperm, the type of embryo transfer (fresh or cryopreserved), intracytoplasmic sperm injection (ICSI), the number of embryos transferred, and the culture medium used may all influence outcomes [16–18]. IVF is associated with intrauterine growth restriction [19], and in turn intrauterine growth restriction is associated with several longer-term medical conditions of relevance

[20]. In evaluating the long-term effect of IVF on offspring, it is essential that this and other factors are controlled for.

As mentioned, there is concern that children conceived by IVF are at increased risk of imprinting disorders [21]. These are rare conditions affecting growth and neurodevelopment through aberrations in gene methylation arising during meiosis or fertilization. IVF itself may induce epigenetic alterations in IVF-conceived offspring [8] and as such this area is under increasing scrutiny [22,23].

This chapter aims to review the most up-to-date evidence available on the long-term health outcomes of children conceived through IVF.

Cardiovascular and Metabolic Effects

Body Mass Index

One of the earliest cohort studies following 173 IVF offspring into early adulthood found no significant differences in the prevalence of being overweight or obese when compared with a representative population conceived spontaneously [24]. However, increasingly, the literature suggests that the offspring of IVF treatment may be at increased risk of being overweight in later life [25]. When controlled for antenatal, maternal, and parental factors, IVF offspring in late childhood and adolescence have a significantly higher sum of peripheral deposition of adipose tissue and total body fat when compared with controls, despite minimal difference in body mass index (BMI) [26]. These findings are further supported by recent research that demonstrates the vulnerability of preimplantation embryos to environmental disturbance, confirming that conception by IVF can reprogram metabolic homeostasis through metabolic, transcriptional, and epigenetic mechanisms, with lasting effects on adult growth [27]. Given the potential adverse health implications of elevated BMI in adulthood, the follow-up of IVF children to monitor body fat pattern and potentially related health problems from adolescence into adulthood is of great importance [26].

Blood Pressure

It has been asserted for some time that children conceived through IVF are predisposed to developing high blood pressure recordings in late childhood [2]. Systolic and diastolic blood pressure levels have been found to be higher in IVF children than in controls, with these differences unable to be explained by factors such as birth weight, BMI, early life, and parental factors, including the cause of subfertility [2]. These conclusions are confirmed in a large Dutch paper investigating the cardiovascular and metabolic profiles of children conceived through IVF aged 5–6 years. Blood pressure was higher in the children of subfertile couples compared with that of the children of fertile couples (adjusted difference systolic blood pressure: 0.8 mmHg, 95% CI −0.2–1.8; diastolic blood pressure: 1.4 mmHg, 95% CI 0.6–2.3) [28]. While the evidence clearly points toward an adverse effect on the cardiovascular profiles of IVF offspring, the underlying mechanisms remain unclear [29]. It has been hypothesized that changes in the early environment of the oocyte and/or embryo possibly result in epigenetic modifications of key metabolic systems that are involved in blood pressure regulation [30], although it is possible that these differences may occur due to postnatal factors. Given the importance of cardiovascular disease and hypertension for lifelong health, further research is required in this area.

Vascular Dysfunction

Adverse events during early life are associated with an increased prevalence of cardiovascular disease and dysfunction later in life, as documented by Barker [10]. There is increasing evidence that, similarly, offspring conceived by IVF may be at risk due to alterations in the early environment of the oocyte or embryo. It has recently been observed that healthy children conceived by IVF display generalized vascular dysfunction, with a reduction in the flow-mediated dilation of the brachial artery, increased carotid-femoral pulse wave velocity, greater systolic pulmonary artery pressure, and greater carotid intima-media thickness [31]. This small study was controlled for multiple variables including parental and perinatal factors. Children born to women who develop ovarian hyperstimulation syndrome as a consequence of IVF may also be at increased risk of cardiovascular dysfunction [32]. Children conceived using IVF may also demonstrate premature subclinical atherosclerosis in the systemic circulation and pulmonary vascular dysfunction, predisposing them to exaggerated hypoxia-induced pulmonary hypertension [11]. A recent small study reported that antioxidant administration to IVF offspring improved systemic endothelial function, nitric oxide bioavailability, and vascular responsiveness in the systemic and pulmonary circulation, suggesting reversibility [33]. There is a need to further understand the responsible mechanisms potentially underpinning these processes.

Metabolic Profile and Glucose Metabolism

Given the concern that a suboptimal environment for the preimplantation embryo may lead to metabolic dysfunction later in life, insulin and lipid metabolism are an important focus of study with respect to IVF treatment. Higher fasting glucose levels have been observed in pubertal IVF offspring, with this difference persisting after controlling for multiple variables [2]. An obesogenic environment may be a trigger for this effect, as observed by a recent group comparing glucose metabolism in adult offspring conceived by natural conception, ovarian stimulation alone, or by IVF. Both ovarian stimulation and IVF resulted in impaired glucose metabolism, but the consumption of a high fat diet was required to unmask this effect [34]. The evidence for altered levels of serum insulin-like growth factor (IGF) 1 and 2 is somewhat less clear. One study found that despite a significant reduction in levels of serum IGF-1 in the first year of life, only subtle differences that were not clinically significant persisted at 5 years of age [35]. This is in contrast to the findings of another study in which IVF offspring were found to have elevated IGF-1 and IGF-2 levels and have a slightly more favorable lipid profile [36]. ICSI may be an independent risk factor for metabolic disorders in later life, with another paper noting lipid dysregulation in children conceived by IVF compared with the offspring of fertile controls [37]. Significantly higher levels of triglycerides and apolipoprotein B were observed in ICSI-conceived fetuses [37]. While these findings may suggest the use of testicular sperm or the process of ICSI itself may lead to these findings, it may well be the age and health of the man at the time of conception that is of most relevance. Further large prospective trials are clearly required.

Malignancy

There have been conflicting reports of a possible increase in the risk of malignancy in offspring conceived and born through IVF [38]. This concern is further supported by the hypothesis that epigenetic phenomena may have a role to play in the later development of some childhood cancers, as human embryos created using IVF may demonstrate an altered epigenetic profile [8,39]. However, increasingly, the evidence points away from an elevated overall cancer risk when compared with children born as a result of spontaneous conception [40–43]. A small but increased risk of specific cancers including leukemias, neuroblastomas, and retinoblastomas was suggested by a systematic review and meta-analysis [38], although the absolute excess risks were small [43]. A large population-based Scandinavian cohort study, controlled for country, maternal age, parity, sex, gestational age, and birth defects, demonstrated no overall increase in cancer rates, but a specific increase in central nervous system tumors (adjusted HR 1.44, 95% CI 1.01–2.05) and malignant epithelial neoplasms (adjusted HR 2.03, 95% CI 1.06–3.89); the absolute risks were 0.46/1000 and 0.15/1000 children, respectively, corresponding to an absolute increased risk of 0.14/1000 and 0.08/1000 children, respectively [42]. This study did not control for other factors such as socioeconomic status and perinatal factors (e.g., Apgar score) [42]. Other rarer cancers have been reported, but an association cannot be confirmed due to the paucity of cases [44]. Large, population-based studies are required to elucidate the effect of these reproductive techniques on the occurrence of specific congenital tumors. Controlling for confounding factors remains a complex task, with one recent analysis noting no correlation between IVF and childhood leukemia, but a positive association with maternal factors such as the use of third-generation oral contraceptives, a history of stillbirth, and miscarriage [45]. Overwhelmingly, the literature to date confirms that overall cancer risk in IVF offspring is not increased, although an increase in some specific cancers is greater, with the absolute risk of each cancer remaining low.

Respiratory and Allergy Disorder: Asthma, Allergy, and Atopy

The evidence for an association between subfertility, IVF, and allergic disorders is growing. One earlier case-controlled study of IVF offspring found that the prevalence of asthma, allergic rhinitis, and atopic dermatitis were similar when compared with non-IVF-conceived controls [46]. However, the UK Millennium Cohort Study found that children born to subfertile parents were significantly more likely to experience asthma and wheezing and to be taking antiasthmatics at 5 years of age. This was mainly due to an increase among children born after IVF, with the association persisting to 7 years of age [47]. However, this study included a relatively small number of singletons and as such data must be extrapolated with caution. Another paper found that the link between IVF and the future development of asthma remained after adjustment for an extensive list of potential confounding factors [48]. A systematic review published in 2015 concluded that children conceived by assisted reproductive technology (ART) are at increased risk of asthma [49]. This risk potentially persists, with an association found between controlled ovarian hyperstimulation IVF/ICSI and the use of asthma medication in the 4-year-old offspring of subfertile couples [50].

Endocrine Disorders

Limited data are available investigating the effect of IVF conception on future susceptibility to endocrine disease. One study investigated a total of 106 IVF-conceived children and compared these with 68 children conceived spontaneously. The findings suggested a significantly increased susceptibility to subclinical hypothyroidism, with seven IVF children but none of the controls demonstrating persistently elevated serum thyroid stimulating hormone (TSH) levels and no differences in serum T3 or T4 [51]. These differences were not due to the presence of antithyroid autoantibodies. A recent Chinese paper found that elevated maternal serum oestrogen levels in the first trimester due to controlled ovarian hyperstimulation (COH) correlated with an altered thyroid hormone profile in the offspring. Significant increases in T4, fT4, and TSH levels were recorded in newborns and in children aged 3–10 years of age [52].

A third and final paper also found an increase in "combined endocrine, nutritional, and metabolic disease" (OR 2.16, 95% CI 1.01–4.64). This was a heterogeneous list of conditions, individually only making up very small numbers, including type 1 diabetes [13].

The limited data available do suggest that IVF conception is associated with future thyroid dysfunction in offspring; however, further research is required.

Ophthalmological and Auditory Disorders

There are few published data investigating the long-term effect of IVF on ophthalmological and auditory health in IVF offspring. Despite the finding that ocular anomalies are more frequently observed in children conceived with IVF [53], one of the largest follow-up studies followed 1515 children to the age of 5 years and found no significant difference in hearing or vision assessments [54]. Another previously published prospective, controlled, and blinded study followed children to the age of 4–6 years and also found no significant difference in vision or hearing test results between controls and ICSI children [55]. Interestingly, significantly more children in the control group were wearing glasses, compared with the ICSI children. Other small studies have reported similar findings [54,56]. While the small amount of available evidence is reassuring, more is required in the future. Table 17.1 summarizes the long-term health outcomes of IVF-conceived children.

TABLE 17.1

Summary of Long-Term Health Outcomes of IVF-Conceived Children

Health Outcome	Effect of IVF Treatment
BMI	No effect
	Note: Emerging evidence showing trend to increased body fat
Blood pressure	Increased
Vascular dysfunction	Increased
Fasting glucose levels	Possible increase
Lipid dysregulation	Possible increase
Malignancy	No effect
(Leukemia Retinoblastoma Neuroblastoma)	*(Very small possible increase in these three cancers)*
Asthma	Possible increase
Thyroid dysfunction	Possible increase
Ophthalmological disorder	No effect
Auditory disorder	No effect
Hospital admissions	Increased
Chronic illness	No effect

Growth and Pubertal Development

Growth

Although previous studies have identified IVF as a risk factor for low birth weight [4], several cohort studies have addressed the subject of growth and development with reassuring results, suggesting appropriate catch-up growth [3,35,57]. One trial interestingly found that singleton females conceived using ICSI had a slightly lower birth weight than IVF conceptions [35]. A recent prospective follow-up study investigating long-term growth in IVF offspring reviewed 1773 singletons at the age of 5 and compared them with spontaneously conceived children born to fertile parents [58]. No significant differences were observed for body weight, height, BMI, or head circumference. Another case-controlled longitudinal study of 438 IVF children between 5 and 10 years of age examined growth curves and influencing factors and found no difference between the growth curves of IVF, ICSI, and spontaneously conceived children at 10 years of age [59]. This study suggested that while fetal malformation, maternal BMI, and neonate hospitalization influence weight gain during the first year, from age 1 to 10 years weight gain is affected by familial affluence, socioeconomic status, and education level. The embryo culture media used is another potential influence on fetal growth [60]. Another small study found that IVF children were significantly taller and, in addition, demonstrated higher IGF-1 and IGF-2 levels [36]. While the data are generally reassuring, longer-term follow-up studies are required to ensure this increased height and catch-up growth do not translate into longer-term health risks [15,61].

Puberty and Timing of Puberty

A longitudinal study published in 2012 reported no difference in pubertal development as assessed by Tanner staging and the onset of menarche in children at age 14 years conceived via ICSI versus spontaneously conceived controls [62]. In this paper, the age of menarche, genital development, and pubic hair development were similar, although breast development was found to be less advanced in the ICSI group of girls. These reassuring findings are further supported by the Dutch OMEGA study, which found no significant difference in pubertal stage and the age of menarche when comparing IVF-conceived children with spontaneously conceived controls [63]. However, this retrospective cohort study found that IVF-conceived girls demonstrated advanced bone age and significantly higher DHEAS and LH levels

TABLE 17.2

Pubertal Development of IVF-Conceived Children

Pubertal Development	ART Mean (SD)	Non-ART Mean (SD)	Unadjusted Mean Diff. (95% CI); *p* Value	Adjusted Mean Diff (95% CI); *p* Value
Female	*n* = 303	*n* = 306		
Mean age at menarche (years, SD)	12.98 (1.39)	12.89 (1.57)		
Composite score	−0.005 (0.05)	0.005 (0.05)	−0.01 (−0.16–0.14); *p* = .89	0.01 (−0.15–0.17); *p* = .91
Male	*n* = 244	*n* = 243		
Mean age at voice break (years, SD)	13.60 (1.30)	13.71 (1.27)		
Composite score	−0.003 (0.7)	0.003 (0.7)	−0.006 (−0.12–0.11); *p* = .92	−0.06 (−0.21–0.08); *p* = .37

Source: Halliday J, et al., *Fertil Steril*, 101(4), 1055–63, 2014.
Abbreviation: ART: assisted reproductive technology.

compared with the control group. A recent cohort study evaluating children conceived via IVF also addressed pubertal development [13]. Even after adjustment for confounders, no difference in measures of sexual maturation between groups was found (Table 17.2). Follow-up studies are required to ensure that subsequent progression through the stages of pubertal development are normal.

Testicular Function

There are limited but reassuring data available on the gonadal development of men and boys conceived via IVF. One longitudinal cohort study assessed morphological and functional gonadal parameters in boys conceived via ART and correlated these results with paternal sperm characteristics [64]. Penile length, testicular size, and Sertoli cell function, as assessed by serum inhibin B and anti-Mullerian hormone levels, were found to be normal. When followed to age 14 years, a group of boys in this cohort were also found to have age-appropriate levels of inhibin B [65]. More research into the testicular function of male offspring born as a result of IVF is required, due to the very limited amount of data that exist.

Mental Health and Socioemotional Development

General Health and Well-Being

Various cohort studies of children conceived via IVF have shown increased rates of hospital admissions compared with non-IVF-conceived children. An Australian study showed increased hospital admissions in the first 5 years of life in singletons born following IVF [66]. Following on from this, another Australian study showed the same findings through to adulthood, with a significantly greater number of hospital admissions up until the age of 18 in the IVF-conceived population compared with the non-IVF-conceived population [13]. Reasons for this increase may be due to factors such as complications from the neonatal period extending into childhood, and attitude and access to health care. A small cross-sectional study of IVF-conceived children up to the age of 21 from the United States reported no increased rates of chronic disease [24].

Quality-of-life scores have shown equal results between children born from IVF, ICSI, and natural conception [67]. Similar results were found in another study of young adults using the self-reporting of quality of life, showing an increased quality of life reported in IVF-conceived young adults, but no statistical difference after adjusting for confounding factors [13].

Neuromotor Development

A comprehensive systematic review has shown no increase in neuromotor development problems in children conceived after IVF, although most studies did not review children beyond infancy [68]. This systematic review has been helpful in interpreting the data on the neurodevelopment of IVF-conceived children as the available studies have been of variable methodological quality, thus making comparison between them challenging. More recent studies have shown variable results in the motor development of IVF-conceived children. No motor development differences were seen in a comparison of over 800 children in a Japanese study comparing three groups at 18 months of age: those conceived with IVF, non-IVF ART, and spontaneous conception [69]. A small study comparing singleton children born as a result of ICSI treatment with spontaneous conception showed impaired motor development in the ICSI group at age 5–6 years old [70]. These results must be interpreted with some caution, however, as the study was underpowered.

Cerebral Palsy

Cerebral palsy rates in IVF-conceived children appear to be greater than that of the general population. A systematic review and meta-analysis showed cerebral palsy rates were significantly increased in children born as a result of IVF treatment (adjusted OR 1.81, 95% CI 1.52–2.13) after controlling for singleton pregnancies [71]. There is a suggestion that the increased rate of cerebral palsy in IVF-conceived children is in fact related to multiple pregnancies, preterm birth, and low birth weight, hence obstetric complications and neonatal morbidity are the causative factors related to cerebral palsy, rather than the IVF treatment itself. A large Swedish study reviewing over two million children born between 1982 and 2007 would also appear to support this assertion [72]. Initial results in this Swedish study showed increased risk of cerebral palsy on analysis overall, but when analyzing singleton births alone the risk was no longer significant. The study also found that rates of multiple births decreased over time, with a corresponding decrease in cerebral palsy rates. Over the final 3 years of the study (2004–2007), the rate of multiple births was lowest (less than 10%), and no increased risk of cerebral palsy was demonstrated (OR 0.97, 95% CI 0.57–1.66). A case-control study from Australia looking at only singleton pregnancies did not show an association between cerebral palsy and IVF-conceived children [73], further supporting the theory that multiple births and the associated obstetric and neonatal morbidity are the main risk factors in developing cerebral palsy in the IVF-conceived population.

Cognitive Function and Intelligence Quotient

No difference has been seen in the cognitive function of children conceived after IVF and those spontaneously conceived [15]. The highest predictor of a child's intelligence quotient (IQ) has been shown to be maternal education level [74]. A Danish prospective follow-up study also supported these findings, with no significant difference in intelligence, attention, and executive functions at age 5 in spontaneous or ART-conceived children. This study found that maternal IQ and parental education level were important covariates in determining the child's IQ and consequently adjusted for this variable [75]. The results were separated into three groups: the children of fertile couples, subfertile couples taking more than 12 months to conceive (but not requiring IVF treatment), and the offspring of those couples that required IVF treatment, thereby accounting for the confounding factors of subfertility alone on cognitive function [75,76]. IVF-conceived children, and also children born of subfertile couples who spontaneously conceived, have shown significantly lower birth weights compared with fertile couples. While low birth weight is associated with future mental development, there was no significant difference in IQ scores in the Danish study [77].

The risk of mental retardation in children conceived after IVF was shown with a small but significant increased risk in a Swedish prospective cohort study [78]. However, the risk was no longer significant when including only singleton pregnancies.

School Performance

Children born as a result of IVF appear to do as well at school as spontaneously conceived children. A study reviewing the school functioning of IVF-conceived children showed no educational limitations, including comparable rates of performance in primary school and into secondary school in a Dutch population [79]. This is supported by a systematic review of the literature that has concluded that IVF does not appear to have a negative effect on school performance at the preschool age [74]. Completion rates of high school and tertiary education are comparable between IVF-conceived and non-IVF-conceived children [13].

Socioemotional Development and Psychological Disorders

The concept of psychosocial well-being is broad and can be difficult to quantify, making it a more complex area to evaluate than other medical conditions. The stress of IVF treatment and the desire for a family may have an impact on parental behavior and attitude, quite possibly impacting on the IVF-conceived child. The majority of studies investigating the socioemotional and psychological development of children born from IVF have shown normal psychosocial well-being.

A large Danish cohort study of over 30,000 ART-conceived children found no increase in mental health disorders in children born following IVF/ICSI treatment [77]. There was seen to be a small increase in the prevalence of tic disorders in the IVF-conceived group compared with the spontaneously conceived population. This finding was concluded after taking into account confounding factors. ICSI treatment did not seem to change psychosocial development compared with IVF or natural conception [67].

Limited research has been conducted into the development of depression. A study from the Netherlands reported higher rates of self-withdrawal-type behavior in IVF-conceived children as reported by parents and teachers [80]. A follow-up study of the same cohort revealed no difference in self-reporting for these behaviors compared with the general population. This may have been due to there being less respondents in the self-reporting cohort compared with the parent/teacher reporting cohort. Young adults in a small cross-sectional study from the United States demonstrated higher rates of depression compared with the general population [24].

Autism Spectrum Disorders

Studies exploring the association between children born as a result of IVF treatment and autism spectrum disorder (ASD) have revealed conflicting evidence. This may be related to some studies involving smaller sample sizes and variable diagnostic criteria for ASD between the studies. Two systematic reviews both concluded there was not enough evidence to prove a link between IVF and ASD [71,81].

A large population-based follow-up study from Denmark reviewed the offspring of women undergoing ART (including ovulation induction and IVF) and found no link between ASD and ART as a whole when confounding factors were adjusted for. These factors included maternal age, smoking, parity, education level, birth weight, and multiplicity [82].

The largest observational cohort study to date (from the United States) reviewed over five million live births, including over 48,000 children born as a result of IVF treatment, and found an increased risk between IVF and the diagnosis of ASD [83]. However, the same cohort study found the risk of ASD was not significantly increased among singleton births of children conceived through IVF. The highest rates of autism were found among triplets and higher-order multiples in the study. This suggests that multiple births and the related complications (such as preterm birth and low birth weight) are confounding factors and play an important role in the link between IVF and autism. This finding supports the judicious use of single-embryo transfer in IVF treatment.

Further, a retrospective cohort study found the incidence of autism significantly increased with the use of ICSI [84]. There has been debate surrounding this finding as being an association rather than causation, given the etiology of autism is still largely unknown [85,86]. A Swedish prospective cohort study found, overall, no significant increase in ASD with IVF, but in an ICSI population (generally with a male cause of subfertility) demonstrated an increased risk of ASD [78]. Other studies have demonstrated the same association and noted that parents undergoing ICSI had higher rates of stress, combined with medication use, which may explain these findings [67,87]. A study examining the genetic events associated with autism in children born from IVF showed no increased rate of autism-linked genetic abnormalities in this population [88]. Overall. there is not enough current evidence to support a definite link between IVF treatment and ASD, but emerging evidence suggests ICSI is related to an increased risk of ASD in the offspring (Table 17.3).

Attention Deficit Hyperactivity Disorder

Most studies looking at the association between attention deficit hyperactivity disorder (ADHD) and ART have shown no compelling link. A large cohort study from Sweden showed a weak association between drug-treated ADHD and IVF-conceived children (OR 1.18, 95% CI 1.03–1.36) [89]. The study looked at over 28,000 children born from IVF, comparing them with over two million spontaneously conceived children, and identifying those with ADHD from a prescription register of drugs used to treat the condition. When the duration of subfertility was taken into account as a cofounding factor, the result was no longer statistically significant. Girls conceived through IVF were also shown to be more likely to develop ADHD than boys (OR 1.4 vs. OR 1.11) although this may have been due to chance. The study also found the following factors increased the risk of drug-treated ADHD: young maternal age, high parity, smoking, a period of unwanted childlessness, high BMI, the presence of preeclampsia, cesarean section, non-cohabitation, and low maternal education, indicating a multifactorial etiology.

Smoking, Drinking, and Physical Activity

Given the population of IVF-conceived children worldwide are still relatively young, it is understandable that very few studies have reported on rates of smoking, drinking, and addiction in the IVF-conceived population. One small cross-sectional study of young adults born as a result of IVF reported increased rates of female binge drinking compared with the general population. Smoking behaviors were comparable to the general population, and physical activity was reported as greater than expected [24]. Due to the small, mostly Caucasian population and limited response rate of the participants of this study, the results should be interpreted with some caution. Larger prospective cohort studies may be able to address this topic with more conviction.

TABLE 17.3

Summary of Long-Term Complications Including Quality of Life, Neuromotor Mental Development, School Performance, and Autism of IVF-Conceived Children

Health Outcome	Effect of IVF Treatment
Quality of life (self-reported)	No effect
Neuromotor development	No effect
Cerebral palsy	Possible increase overall *Note*: No effect demonstrated in singleton pregnancies
IQ	No effect
Mental retardation	Possible increase overall *Note*: No effect demonstrated in singleton pregnancies
School performance	No effect
Mental health disorders	No effect overall *Note*: Possible small increase in tic disorders and depression
ASD	Possible increase in ICSI *Note*: No effect demonstrated in singleton pregnancies of IVF
ADHD	No effect or possible trend to increase

CONCLUSION

The studies to date have suggested an increase in cardiometabolic problems in later life in IVF-conceived children, but overall most studies do not reveal any major cause for concern. Deriving the true etiology to these possible increases in health disorders is more difficult. Further studies are needed to help differentiate whether the effects are due to an underlying predisposition in the subfertile couple, the IVF technology itself, or an obstetric or neonatal complication.

At the time of writing this chapter, the oldest IVF-conceived individual is less than 40 years of age [1]. While it is too premature to know the full extent of the long-term health implications of those born from IVF, more information will come to light as the population continues to age. The overall impact of IVF on the individual, and also on public health, is a vitally important area that needs continued research. It has been eloquently noted that the outcome of "success" in IVF does not just hinge on pregnancy or live birth rates, but the lifelong health of the offspring born as a result of this technology [90].

REFERENCES

1. Steptoe PC, Edwards RG. Birth after the reimplantation of a human embryo. *Lancet.* 1978;2(8085):366.
2. Ceelen M, van Weissenbruch MM, Vermeiden JP, et al. Cardiometabolic differences in children born after in vitro fertilization: Follow-up study. *J Clin Endocrinol Metab.* 2008;93(5):1682–8.
3. Epelboin S, Patrat C, Luton D. Health and development of children conceived through assisted reproductive technologies. [French]. *Revue du Praticien.* 2014;64(1):102–5.
4. Qin J, Wang H, Sheng X, et al. Pregnancy-related complications and adverse pregnancy outcomes in multiple pregnancies resulting from assisted reproductive technology: A meta-analysis of cohort studies. *Fertil Steril.* 2015;103(6):1492–508.
5. Romundstad LB. Increased morbidity and mortality after ART: Related to the infertility or the reproductive technology? *Hum Reprod.* 2015;30:i90.
6. Seggers J, de Walle HE, Bergman JE, et al. Congenital anomalies in offspring of subfertile couples: A registry-based study in the northern Netherlands. *Fertil Steril.* 2015;103(4):1001–10.
7. Sellers F, Ten J, Moliner B, Guerrero J, et al. Congenital anomalies after assisted reproduction techniques (ART) and their correlation with embryo quality. *Hum Reprod.* 2014;29:i278–9.
8. Hiura H, Okae H, Chiba H, et al. Imprinting methylation errors in ART. *Reprod Med Biol.* 2014;13(4):193–202.
9. Vincent RN, Dong KB, Chan Wong E, et al. Investigation into methylation of imprinted genes in children conceived via assisted reproductive technologies (ART) compared to naturally conceived (NC) controls. *Fertil Steril.* 2014;102(3 Suppl):e83.
10. Barker DJ. The fetal and infant origins of disease. *Eur J Clin Invest.* 1995;25(7):457–63.
11. Rimoldi SF, Sartori C, Rexhaj E, et al. Vascular dysfunction in children conceived by assisted reproductive technologies: Underlying mechanisms and future implications. *Swiss Med Wkly.* 2014;144:w13973.
12. Scherrer U, Rexhaj E, Allemann Y, et al. Cardiovascular dysfunction in children conceived by assisted reproductive technologies. *Eur Heart J.* 2015;36(25):1583–9.
13. Halliday J, Wilson C, Hammarberg K, et al. Comparing indicators of health and development of singleton young adults conceived with and without assisted reproductive technology. *Fertil Steril.* 2014;101(4):1055–63.
14. Wijers CH, van Rooij IA, Rassouli R, et al. Parental subfertility, fertility treatment, and the risk of congenital anorectal malformations. *Epidemiology.* 2015;26(2):169–76.
15. Fauser BC, Devroey P, Diedrich K, et al. Health outcomes of children born after IVF/ICSI: A review of current expert opinion and literature. *Reprod Biomed Online.* 2014;28(2):162–82.
16. Zhu J, Li M, Liu P, Qiao J. Culture media influence on birthweight of newborns following IVF. *Hum Reprod.* 2014;29:i285.
17. Dumoulin J. Critical periods of human development: ART effects? *Hum Reprod.* 2015;30:i59–60.
18. Perez Martinez N, Suarez-Gil P, Garcia S, et al. Perinatal results after IVF/ICSI: A prospective study. *Hum Reprod.* 2015;30:i183–4.
19. Society of Obstetricians and Gynaecologists of Canada, Okun N, Sierra S. Pregnancy outcomes after assisted human reproduction. *JOGC.* 2014;36(1):64–83.

20. Hart R, Norman RJ. The longer-term health outcomes for children born as a result of IVF treatment: Part I; General health outcomes. *Hum Reprod Update*. 2013;19(3):232–43.
21. Lazaraviciute G, Kauser M, Haggarty P, Bhattacharya S. A systematic review and meta-analysis of DNA methylation levels and imprinting disorders in children conceived by IVF/ICSI compared with children conceived spontaneously. *Hum Reprod Update*. 2014;20(6):840–52.
22. Chen Z, Hagen DE, Elsik CG, et al. Characterization of global loss of imprinting in fetal overgrowth syndrome induced by assisted reproduction. *Proc Natl Acad Sci USA*. 2015;112(15):4618–23.
23. Vincent R, Louie K, Chan Wong E, Ma S. Altered expression of imprinted genes in cord blood but not placenta from babies conceived via assisted reproductive technologies. *Hum Reprod*. 2015;30:i86.
24. Beydoun HA, Sicignano N, Beydoun MA, et al. A cross-sectional evaluation of the first cohort of young adults conceived by in vitro fertilization in the United States. *Fertil Steril*. 2010;94(6):2043–9.
25. Heilbronn L, Chen M, Wu L, Wittert G, et al. Long term consequences of in-vitro fertilisation (IVF) on adiposity and glucose metabolism in adult mice and humans. *Obes Rev*. 2014;15:124–5.
26. Ceelen M, van Weissenbruch MM, Roos JC, et al. Body composition in children and adolescents born after in vitro fertilization or spontaneous conception. *J Clin Endocrinol Metab*. 2007;92(9):3417–23.
27. Feuer SK, Liu X, Donjacour A, et al. Use of a mouse in vitro fertilization model to understand the developmental origins of health and disease hypothesis. *Endocrinology*. 2014;155(5):1956–69.
28. Pontesilli M, Painter RC, Grooten IJ, et al. Subfertility and assisted reproduction techniques are associated with poorer cardiometabolic profiles in childhood. *Reprod Biomed Online*. 2015;30(3):258–67.
29. Gao Q, Pan HT, Lin XH, et al. Altered protein expression profiles in umbilical veins: Insights into vascular dysfunctions of the children born after in vitro fertilization. *Biol Reprod*. 2014;91(3):71.
30. La Bastide-Van Gemert S, Seggers J, Haadsma ML, et al. Is ovarian hyperstimulation associated with higher blood pressure in 4-year-old IVF offspring? Part II: An explorative causal inference approach. *Hum Reprod*. 2014;29(3):510–17.
31. Scherrer U, Rimoldi SF, Rexhaj E, et al. Systemic and pulmonary vascular dysfunction in children conceived by assisted reproductive technologies. *Circulation*. 2012;125(15):1890–96.
32. Xu GF, Zhang JY, Pan HT, et al. Cardiovascular dysfunction in children born to women with ovarian hyperstimulation syndrome: A retrospective cohort study and proteomics analysis. *Fertil Steril*. 2014;102(3 Suppl):e23–4.
33. Rimoldi SF, Sartori C, Rexhaj E, et al. Antioxidants improve vascular function in children conceived by assisted reproductive technologies: A randomized double-blind placebo-controlled trial. *Eur J Prev Cardiol*. 2015;22(11):1399–407.
34. Chen M. Metabolic phenotyping of young adults and mice born through in vitro fertilization (IVF). PhD thesis, University of Adelaide, Australia; 2014.
35. Kai CM, Main KM, Andersen AN, et al. Serum insulin-like growth factor-I (IGF-I) and growth in children born after assisted reproduction. *J Clin Endocrinol Metab*. 2006;91(11):4352–60.
36. Miles HL, Hofman PL, Peek J, et al. In vitro fertilization improves childhood growth and metabolism. *J Clin Endocrinol Metab*. 2007;92(9):3441–5.
37. Lou H, Le F, Zheng Y, et al. Assisted reproductive technologies impair the expression and methylation of insulin-induced gene 1 and sterol regulatory element-binding factor 1 in the fetus and placenta. *Fertil Steril*. 2014;101(4):974–80.e2.
38. Hargreave M, Jensen A, Toender A, et al. Fertility treatment and childhood cancer risk: A systematic meta-analysis. *Fertil Steril*. 2013;100(1):150–61.
39. Santos F, Hyslop L, Stojkovic P, et al. Evaluation of epigenetic marks in human embryos derived from IVF and ICSI. *Hum Reprod*. 2010;25(9):2387–95.
40. Hyrapetian M, Loucaides EM, Sutcliffe AG. Health and disease in children born after assistive reproductive therapies (ART). *J Reprod Immunol*. 2014;106:21–6.
41. Bradbury K, Sutcliffe A. The health of children born following assisted reproductive technologies. *Paediatr Child Health (Oxford)*. 2014;24(4):172–6.
42. Sundh KJ, Henningsen AKA, Kallen K, et al. Cancer in children and young adults born after assisted reproductive technology: A Nordic cohort study from the Committee of Nordic ART and Safety (CoNARTaS). *Hum Reprod*. 2014;29(9):2050–57.
43. Williams CL, Bunch KJ, Stiller CA, et al. Cancer risk among children born after assisted conception. *New Engl J Med*. 2013;369(19):1819–27.

44. Tempe A, Singh N, Sharma I, Agarwal S. The case of sacrococcygeal teratoma in an IVF pregnancy: Is there any association between congenital tumors and assisted reproduction techniques? *J Reprod Infertil*. 2014;15(2):109–12.

45. Ajrouche R, Rudant J, Orsi L, et al. Maternal reproductive history, fertility treatments and folic acid supplementation in the risk of childhood acute leukemia: The ESTELLE Study. *Cancer Causes Control*. 2014;25(10):1283–93.

46. Cetinkaya F, Gelen SA, Kervancioglu E, Oral E. Prevalence of asthma and other allergic diseases in children born after in vitro fertilisation. *Allergol Immunopathol (Madr)*. 2009;37(1):11–13.

47. Carson C, Sacker A, Kelly Y, et al. Asthma in children born after infertility treatment: Findings from the UK Millennium Cohort Study. *Hum Reprod*. 2013;28(2):471–9.

48. Guibas GV, Moschonis G, Xepapadaki P, et al. PD44: In vitro fertilisation is positively associated with prevalence of asthma in childhood. *Clin Transl Allergy*. 2014;4:66.

49. Kettner LO, Henriksen TB, Bay B, et al. Assisted reproductive technology and somatic morbidity in childhood: A systematic review. *Fertil Steril*. 2015;103(3):707–19.

50. Kuiper DB, Seggers J, Schendelaar P, et al. Asthma and asthma medication use among 4-year-old offspring of subfertile couples: Association with IVF? *Reprod Biomed Online*. 2015;31(5):711–14.

51. Sakka SD, Malamitsi-Puchner A, Loutradis D, et al. Euthyroid hyperthyrotropinemia in children born after in vitro fertilization. *J Clin Endocrinol Metab*. 2009;94(4):1338–41.

52. Lv PP, Meng Y, Lv M, et al. Altered thyroid hormone profile in offspring after exposure to high estradiol environment during the first trimester of pregnancy: A cross-sectional study. *BMC Med*. 2014;12(1):240.

53. Anteby I, Cohen E, Anteby E, BenEzra D. Ocular manifestations in children born after in vitro fertilization. *Arch Ophthalmol*. 2001;119(10):1525–9.

54. Bonduelle M, Wennerholm UB, Loft A, et al. A multi-centre cohort study of the physical health of 5-year-old children conceived after intracytoplasmic sperm injection, in vitro fertilization and natural conception. *Hum Reprod*. 2005;20(2):413–19.

55. Ludwig AK, Katalinic A, Thyen U, et al. Physical health at 5.5 years of age of term-born singletons after intracytoplasmic sperm injection: Results of a prospective, controlled, single-blinded study. *Fertil Steril*. 2009;91(1):115–24.

56. Sutcliffe AG, Taylor B, Saunders K, et al. Outcome in the second year of life after in-vitro fertilisation by intracytoplasmic sperm injection: A UK case-control study. *Lancet*. 2001;357(9274):2080–84.

57. Ceelen M, van Weissenbruch MM, Vermeiden JP, et al. Growth and development of children born after in vitro fertilization. *Fertil Steril*. 2008;90(5):1662–73.

58. Bay B, Mortensen EL, Kesmodel US. Is subfertility or fertility treatment associated with long-term growth in the offspring? A cohort study. *Fertil Steril*. 2014;102(4):1117–23.

59. Boyer Gervoise M, Meddeb L, Pauly V, et al. IVF conceived children health: A retrospective growth study. *Hum Reprod*. 2014;29:i282–3.

60. Kleijkers SH, van Montfoort AP, Smits LJ, et al. IVF culture medium affects post-natal weight in humans during the first 2 years of life. *Hum Reprod*. 2014;29(4):661–9.

61. Brison DR, Smith H, Kimber SJ. The impact of IVF on embryonic and long term health. *Chromosome Res*. 2014;22(4):587–8.

62. Belva F, Roelants M, Painter R, et al. Pubertal development in ICSI children. *Hum Reprod*. 2012;27(4):1156–61.

63. Ceelen M, van Weissenbruch MM, Vermeiden JP, et al. Pubertal development in children and adolescents born after IVF and spontaneous conception. *Hum Reprod*. 2008;23(12):2791–8.

64. De Schepper J, Belva F, Schiettecatte J, et al. Testicular growth and tubular function in prepubertal boys conceived by intracytoplasmic sperm injection. *Horm Res*. 2009;71(6):359–63.

65. Belva F, Bonduelle M, Painter RC, et al. Serum inhibin B concentrations in pubertal boys conceived by ICSI: First results. *Hum Reprod*. 2010;25(11):2811–14.

66. Chambers GM, Lee E, Hoang VP, et al. Hospital utilization, costs and mortality rates during the first 5 years of life: A population study of ART and non-ART singletons. *Hum Reprod*. 2014;29(3):601–10.

67. Knoester M, Helmerhorst FM, van der Westerlaken LA, et al. Matched follow-up study of 5 8-year-old ICSI singletons: Child behaviour, parenting stress and child (health-related) quality of life. *Hum Reprod*. 2007;22(12):3098–107.

68. Middelburg KJ, Heineman MJ, Bos AF, Hadders-Algra M. Neuromotor, cognitive, language and behavioural outcome in children born following IVF or ICSI: A systematic review. *Hum Reprod Update*. 2008;14(3):219–31.
69. Kojima J, Suzuki K, Shimada H, et al. Long term prognosis of children born through assisted reproductive technologies in Japan. *Fertil Steril*. 2015;104(3):e244.
70. Winter C, Van Acker F, Bonduelle M, et al. Cognitive and psychomotor development of 5- to 6-year-old singletons born after PGD: A prospective case-controlled matched study. *Hum Reprod*. 2014;29(9):1968–77.
71. Hvidtjorn D, Schieve L, Schendel D, et al. Cerebral palsy, autism spectrum disorders, and developmental delay in children born after assisted conception: A systematic review and meta-analysis. *Arch Pediatr Adolesc Med*. 2009;163(1):72–83.
72. Kallen AJ, Finnstrom OO, Lindam AP, et al. Cerebral palsy in children born after in vitro fertilization. Is the risk decreasing? *Eur J Paediatr Neurol*. 2010;14(6):526–30.
73. Reid SM, Jaques AM, Susanto C, et al. Cerebral palsy and assisted reproductive technologies: A case-control study. *Dev Med Child Neurol*. 2010;52(7):e161–6.
74. Abdel-Mannan O, Sutcliffe A. I was born following ART: How will I get on at school? *Semin Fetal Neonatal Med*. 2014;19(4):245–9.
75. Bay B, Mortensen EL, Kesmodel US. Fertility treatment and child intelligence, attention, and executive functions in 5-year-old singletons: A cohort study. *BJOG*. 2014;121(13):1642–51.
76. Carter RC, Jacobson JL, Jacobson SW. Fertility treatments, maternal intelligence, and child cognition. *BJOG*. 2014;121(13):1652.
77. Bay B. Fertility treatment: Long-term growth and mental development of the children. *Dan Med J*. 2014;61(10):B4947.
78. Sandin S, Nygren KG, Iliadou A, et al. Autism and mental retardation among offspring born after in vitro fertilization. *JAMA*. 2013;310(1):75–84.
79. Wagenaar K, Ceelen M, van Weissenbruch MM, et al. School functioning in 8- to 18-year-old children born after in vitro fertilization. *Eur J Pediatr*. 2008;167(11):1289–95.
80. Wagenaar K, van Weissenbruch MM, van Leeuwen FE, et al. Self-reported behavioral and socioemotional functioning of 11- to 18-year-old adolescents conceived by in vitro fertilization. *Fertil Steril*. 2011;95(2):611–16.
81. Conti E, Mazzotti S, Calderoni S, et al. Are children born after assisted reproductive technology at increased risk of autism spectrum disorders? A systematic review. *Hum Reprod*. 2013;28(12):3316–27.
82. Hvidtjorn D, Grove J, Schendel D, et al. Risk of autism spectrum disorders in children born after assisted conception: A population-based follow-up study. *J Epidemiol Community Health*. 2011;65(6):497–502.
83. Fountain C, Zhang Y, Kissin DM, et al. Association between assisted reproductive technology conception and autism in California, 1997–2007. *Am J Public Health*. 2015;105(5):963–71.
84. Kissin DM, Zhang Y, Boulet SL, et al. Association of assisted reproductive technology (ART) treatment and parental infertility diagnosis with autism in ART-conceived children. *Hum Reprod*. 2015;30(2):454–65.
85. Barad DH, Kushnir VA, Albertini D, Gleicher N. CDC analysis of ICSI/autism: Association is not causation. *Hum Reprod*. 2015;30(7):1745–6.
86. Kissin DM, Zhang Y, Boulet SL, et al. Reply: CDC analysis of ICSI/autism; Association is not causation. *Hum Reprod*. 2015;30(7):1746.
87. Boukhris T, Sheehy O, Mottron L, Bérard A. Antidepressant use during pregnancy and the risk of autism spectrum disorder in children. *JAMA Pediatr*. 2016;170(2):117–24.
88. Ackerman S, Wenegrat J, Rettew D, et al. No increase in autism-associated genetic events in children conceived by assisted reproduction. *Fertil Steril*. 2014;102(2):388–93.
89. Kallen AJ, Finnstrom OO, Lindam AP, et al. Is there an increased risk for drug treated attention deficit/hyperactivity disorder in children born after in vitro fertilization? *Eur J Paediatr Neurol*. 2011;15(3):247–53.
90. Lewis SE, Kumar K. The paternal genome and the health of the assisted reproductive technology child. *Asian J Androl*. 2015;17:1–7.

18

Long-Term Impact of Antidepressant Exposure in Pregnancy: A Window into Developmental Outcomes in the Child

Salvatore Gentile

Introduction

Approximately 13% of pregnant women are actually prescribed antidepressant medications [1], selective serotonin reuptake inhibitors (SSRIs) being the class of medications most frequently used in pregnancy that influence serotonin (5-HT) regulation. Because 5-HT is critical to fetal brain development, concerns have arisen regarding prenatal exposure to SSRIs. Indeed, recent information suggests that antenatal exposure to psychotropics may impair child neurodevelopment. Thus, this chapter explores children's long-term developmental outcomes following antenatal antidepressant exposure.

Placenta, Serotonin, Selective Serotonin Reuptake Inhibitors, and the Developing Fetal Brain

The placenta is essential for ensuring the growth and survival of the fetus during its development. In fact, the placenta not only supports fetal homeostatic functions, but also serves as an essential source of 5-HT for the fetal forebrain during a transient, critical period of embryonic development.

5-HT is a phylogenetically ancient neurotransmitter widely distributed throughout the brain [2]. 5-HT plays two key roles: (1) during early developmental periods, 5-HT acts as a growth factor, regulating the development of its own and related neural systems [3]; (2) in its role as a trophic factor, 5-HT regulates diverse and developmentally critical processes such as cell division, differentiation, migration, myelination, synaptogenesis, and dendritic pruning [4]. Thus, all drugs used during pregnancy that modulate 5-HT levels act by impacting on placental functions. SSRIs are the class of medications most frequently used in pregnancy that influence 5-HT regulation.

Since the fetal brain acquires placenta-derived 5-HT during a critical period of widespread axonal outgrowth, the effects of SSRIs on brain development may be due to an indirect pathway that affects proper placental physiology, thus resulting in downstream effects on the fetus [5]. The impact of SSRIs on the developmental brain may therefore result from direct actions on the fetal central nervous system, indirect actions on placental or maternal physiology, or, more likely, a combination of both routes [6]. The transient disruption of essential signaling events during critical developmental periods may have lasting effects that are expressed throughout life [6]. Hence, the key placental function of maintaining fetal homeostasis may be compromised by such drugs, resulting in long-term effects on fetal forebrain development [5]. Drugs active on the serotonergic system may also impair the role of the placenta in attenuating the teratogenic effects (either structural and/or behavioral) of medications during the gestational period [7].

5-HT Receptors and 5-HTT in Human Fetal Brain

In the adult human brain, serotonin transporter (5-HTT) expression is limited to the 5-HT-producing neurons of the raphe nuclei [8].

However, a much broader expression has been observed and extensively described in developing rodents [4]. At mid-gestation, expression of the 5-HTT gene begins in the 5-HT neurons of the raphe nuclei, but expression soon extends to nonserotonergic neurons, including the principal projection neurons of the sensory systems and the corticolimbic pathways. However, 5-HTT expression in nonserotonergic neurons ends rapidly during the second postnatal week, coinciding with the maturation of neural circuits [9].

Although studies in humans are limited, they have provided further evidence for the broad developmental expression of 5-HTT. In embryos 8–11 gestational weeks old, 5-HTT is expressed in the fiber tracts of the internal capsule and the optic tract. These fibers do not correspond to raphe projections [10].

In animal studies, the elevation of 5-HT reduces depressive symptoms in adults, while exposure early in development may have the opposite consequence when examined long term. Behaviorally, acute fluoxetine (FLX) treatment attenuates depressive-like symptoms in immature rats [11]. In contrast, the long-term effects of early-life exposure are different. Postnatal exposure to FLX or the tricyclic antidepressant (TCA) clomipramine actually increases depressive- and anxiety-like behaviors in adulthood [12,13]. These effects are hence labeled *paradoxical* [7].

Moreover, new and emerging findings detected in human studies and highlighted by research in the field of perinatal psychiatry [14,15] suggest the risk of SSRI-induced neonatal behavioral disturbances, whose severity is associated with reduced levels of 5-HT and 5-hydroxyindoleacetic acid (5-HIAA) in cord blood, reflecting altered central 5-HT activity [16]. Moreover, antenatal SSRI exposure may also have specific, long-lasting developmental effects in children and adolescents [17].

Data Source

Data were collected from a computerized Medline/Pub Med/TOXNET/EMBASE search covering the period between January 1973 and September 2015. The following keywords were used: *pregnancy, child/infant development/neurodevelopment, mood disorders*, and *antidepressants*. Resultant articles were cross-referenced for other relevant articles not identified in the initial search. An extensive manual review of pertinent journals and textbooks was also performed. However, the evidence from research and practice in early childhood assessment indicates that the issue of technical adequacy is more difficult to address with young preschool children who have short attention spans and go through periods of variable and rapid development [18,19]. Hence, in this chapter, articles that assessed at least a proportion of children who had reached the age for compulsory education (60 months) were considered.

Studies That Demonstrated No Effects on Long-Term Developmental Outcomes following Antenatal Antidepressant Exposure

A preliminary report, published as abstracts, found no signs of neurodevelopmental teratogenicity in infants whose mothers had been treated with FLX [20].

A prospective controlled study [21] investigated school-age and younger children exposed in utero to a wide range of maternal daily doses of FLX because their mothers were diagnosed with major unipolar depression and were found to require pharmacotherapy. This group was matched with other two groups exposed to TCAs and unexposed to medications, respectively. The research failed to demonstrate any unwanted consequence of FLX exposure on cognitive, language, and behavioral development. Nevertheless, eventual relationships between maternal daily dosages of FLX and the quality of children's performances in neurodevelopmental tests were not investigated, whereas the following factors were entered as independent variables: the mother's IQ and socioeconomic status, ethanol and nicotine use, the duration and severity of depression, the number of depressive episodes after delivery, and the medications used for depression treatment.

The study by Oberlander et al. [22] concluded that the main clinical features characterizing impaired internalizing behaviors (such as emotional hyperreactivity, anxiety, depression, irritability, and withdrawal) were not affected by prenatal exposure to antidepressant medications. Symptoms associated with poor externalizing behaviors (including noncompliance, verbal/physical aggression, disruptive acts, and emotional outbursts) were also found to be unaffected by maternal treatment. Such findings were confirmed in an analogous study performed by the same group of researchers.

A cohort study of all singleton live births (from 1996 to 2005 with follow-up through 2009) used Danish population registries to link information on the maternal use of SSRIs before and during pregnancy, autism spectrum disorders (ASDs) diagnosed in the offspring, and a range of potential confounders [23]. In the fully adjusted analysis, the use of SSRIs during pregnancy (including use both before and during pregnancy and use only during pregnancy) was not associated with a significantly increased risk of ASDs in the offspring.

To investigate whether in utero exposure to antidepressants was associated with an increased risk of attention deficit hyperactivity disorder (ADHD), a cohort study used data extrapolated from several Danish medical registries [24]. The strengths of this study include a large study population with a long and virtually complete follow-up. Moreover, data from population-based databases in a setting of universal healthcare reduces the risk of recall and selection biases. The main study finding was that there was no evidence to support a causal association between in utero exposure to antidepressants and the risk of ADHD.

Santucci et al. [25] examined the impact of prenatal exposure to SSRIs/selective serotonin reuptake inhibitors (SNRIs) and major depressive disorder on infant functioning through a longitudinal study. Children were assessed up to early-school age. The study did not find any impact of antenatal antidepressant exposure on the main psychomotor, cognitive, and behavioral neurodevelopmental milestones. To examine the associations between prenatal exposure to SSRIs and intelligence, assessed with a standard clinical intelligence test at age 5, a longitudinal follow-up study [26] was performed in Denmark between 2003 and 2008. No consistent association between IQ and fetal exposure to antidepressants was observed.

Another population-based study identified children born to depressed women who took antidepressants during pregnancy or to depressed women who did not take any antidepressants during pregnancy [27]. A group of children to mothers with no psychiatric disorders was used as control group. No associations were observed between prenatal antidepressant exposure and abnormal behaviors.

A recent study [28] was focused to define the impact of antenatal SSRI/SNRI exposure on the child's neurodevelopment. To refine the study results, the analysis excluded potential genetic and environmental confounders by using a sibling design. The authors reported that in utero exposure to SSRIs/SNRIs is devoid of neurotoxic developmental effects (Table 18.1).

Studies that Opened a New Window into the Developmental Risks Associated with Antenatal Antidepressant Exposure

Children exposed in utero to antidepressants are at increased risk of developing prenatal antidepressant exposure syndrome (PAES), a complex constellation of neonatal problems characterized by neurological, gastrointestinal, metabolic, respiratory, and cardiac symptoms. Body temperature instability may also occur [29]. However, just two studies have investigated the potential long-term consequences of PAES [30,31]. The first found that children diagnosed at birth with PAES do not show evidence of impaired intelligence. Nevertheless, such children frequently exhibit abnormalities in behavior and social adaptability. The second study compared the effects of prenatal exposure to venlafaxine (VEN; an SNRI), SSRIs, and maternal depression on child neurodevelopment. Children of healthy women had higher IQs than those exposed to antidepressants. There were 14 children with PAES who did not differ in intelligence from the other exposed children, showing that these transient neonatal signs did not have a long-lasting impact on child cognitive development.

TABLE 18.1

Studies that Demonstrated No Long-Term Developmental Effects of In Utero Exposure to Antidepressants

Study; Study Design; Sample (n)	Age at Assessment (Months)	Drug(s)	Assessment	Findings
Mattson et al. 1999 [20]; prospective cohort; n = 66	48–72	FLX	1. Wechsler Preschool and Primary Scale of Intelligence	No difference in IQ between children antenatally exposed to FLX and unexposed children.
Nulman et al. 2002 [21]; prospective cohort control; n = 40	15–71	FLX TCAs	1. Bayley Scales of Infant and Toddler Development for children up to 30 months 2. McCarthy Scales of Children's Abilities for older children 3. Toddler Temperament Scale or Achenbach Child Behavior Checklist	Prenatal exposure to TCAs or FLX has no adverse effects on the cognition, language, development, or temperament of early-school children.
Oberlander et al. 2007 [22]; prospective cohort control; n = 36	48–60	PAR FLX SER SSRI plus clonazepam	1. Child Behavior Checklist	No difference from medication exposure. Maternal depression and anxiety at 4 years old was associated with externalizing behaviors.
Hviid et al. 2013 [23]; cohort; n = 626,875	Mean age of children at end of follow-up: 120	SSRI	1. ICD-10	SSRI use during pregnancy was not associated with a significantly increased risk of ASDs in the offspring.
Laugesen et al. 2013 [24]; cohort; n = 877,778	Mean age of children at end of follow-up: 96	SSRIs SNRIs TCAs Others	1. ICD-8	No association between in utero exposure to antidepressants and risk of ADHD.
Santucci et al. 2014 [25]; longitudinal; n = 27	Up to 79	SSRIs SNRIs	1. Bayley Scales of Infant and Toddler Development II	Children prenatally exposed to antidepressants did not differ from unexposed control in cognitive, behavioral, and psychomotor development.
Eriksen et al. 2015 [26]; longitudinal, follow-up: n = 13	60	SSRIs	1. Wechsler Preschool and Primary Scale of Intelligence, Revised	Prenatal exposure to SSRIs was not associated with a negative effect on intelligence.
Grzeskowiak et al. 2015 [27]; population-based cohort; n = 210	84	SSRIs SNRIs TCAs	1. Strengths and Difficulties Questionnaire	Prenatal antidepressant exposure was not associated with an increased risk of behavioral difficulties in children.
Nulman et al. 2015 [28]; prospective, sibling design; n = 45	36–132	SSRIs SNRIs	1. Wechsler Preschool and Primary Scale of Intelligence III 2. Child Behavior Checklist 3. Conners' Parent Rating Scale, Revised	Children prenatally exposed to antidepressants did not differ from their unexposed siblings in cognitive, behavioral, and physical development.

Abbreviations: FLX: fluoxetine; PAR: paroxetine; SER: sertraline; SSRIs: selective serotonin reuptake inhibitors; TCAs: tricyclic antidepressants; SNRIs: serotonin norepinephrine reuptake inhibitors; ASDs: autism spectrum disorders; ADHD: attention deficit hyperactivity disorder; ICD: *International Classification of Diseases*.

Nevertheless, one-fifth of these children had clinically significant behavior problems, suggesting that these signs may be a risk factor for future psychopathology.

A cohort study that linked data from several Finnish Health Registers compared the prevalence of psychiatric and neurodevelopmental outcomes in offspring exposed prenatally to SSRIs with offspring exposed to prenatal depression and unexposed to SSRIs. The cumulative incidence of registered psychiatric or neurodevelopmental disorders was particularly high among all offspring born during the study period and antenatally exposed to SSRIs [32].

Sorensen et al. [33] conducted a large population-based cohort study to investigate the association between the maternal use of antidepressant medication during pregnancy and the risk of ASDs in the offspring. This cohort study linked data from several Danish Health Registers. After adjusting for potential confounding factors, such as parental age at conception, parental psychiatric history at birth, gestational age, birth weight, the child's sex, and parity, an association between prenatal maternal antidepressant use and later ASD in the child was found, albeit weaker than that reported in other recent epidemiologic studies. This association was found for high- as well as low-dose levels, and risk estimates were comparable regardless of the timing of exposure.

To investigate the association between parental depression and maternal antidepressant use during pregnancy and ASDs in offspring, a population-based nested case-control study was conducted in Sweden from 2001 to 2007 [34]. A history of maternal depression was associated with an increased risk of ASDs. This association was confined to women reporting antidepressant use during pregnancy irrespective of whether these were SSRIs or non-SSRIs. All associations were higher in cases of autism without intellectual disability, there being no evidence of an increased risk of autism with intellectual disability.

The study by El-Marroun et al. [35] was embedded in an ongoing population-based cohort, the Generation R Study. In total, 8880 mothers were enrolled during pregnancy. Of the 69 women who used SSRIs during pregnancy, 35 women used SSRIs in the first trimester only and 34 women used them in the first and also in one or two other trimesters. Based on maternal depressive symptoms and SSRI use, children were classified into three groups: (1) no exposure to SSRIs and a low score of maternal depressive symptoms (92.5%, $n = 5531$), referred to as the "reference group"; (2) exposure to clinically relevant depressive symptoms and no maternal SSRI use (6.3%, $n = 376$), referred to as "exposed to depression"; and (3) exposure to SSRIs during pregnancy (1.2%, $n = 69$), referred to as "exposed to SSRIs." The study suggested an association between prenatal SSRI exposure and autistic traits in children. Prenatal depressive symptoms without SSRI use were also associated with autistic traits, albeit this was weaker and less specific. A case-control study [36] investigated whether there was an association between an increased risk of ASDs and SSRI use during pregnancy. This study used Denmark's health and population registers to obtain information regarding prescription drugs, ASD diagnosis, and health and socioeconomic status. The study found that 1.5% of cases and 0.7% of controls were exposed to SSRIs during the pregnancy period and observed higher effect estimates with longer use. The authors concluded that there was evidence that in utero exposure to SSRIs increases a child's risk of developing ASDs. The study included children ranging in age from 0 to 216 months (Dr. Gidaya, personal communication).

Hanley et al. [37] recruited women in their second trimester of pregnancy from primary maternity care providers in Vancouver, BC, in Canada. The authors compared the internalizing, externalizing, and the anxious and attention subscales of the internalizing behavior scores of children exposed to SSRIs and children not exposed to SSRIs at age 3 and age 6. The main study results suggested that developmental exposure to maternal depression or anxiety and to the medications used to treat maternal mood disturbances both were associated with increased levels of internalizing behaviors and anxiety at school entry age. Children who were exposed to SSRIs/SNRIs in utero were reported to have more anxious and internalizing behaviors at 3 years of age, and this pattern persisted at 6 years of age.

A single, unreplicated study [38] found that male children with prenatal SSRI exposure were more likely to be overweight than male children of mothers with a psychiatric illness but no SSRI use. Interestingly, no increased risk of childhood overweight was observed among female children with prenatal SSRI exposure (Table 18.2).

TABLE 18.2

Studies that Demonstrated Detrimental Long-Term Developmental Effects of In Utero Exposure to Antidepressants

Study; Study Design; Sample (*n*)	Age at Assessment (Months)	Drug(s)	Assessment	Findings
Klinger et al. 2011 [30]; prospective cohort; *n* = 82	12–60	SSRIs	1. DDST-II 2. Wechsler Preschool and Primary Scale of Intelligence II 3. Stanford–Binet Intelligence Scales 4. Bayley Scale of Infant and Toddler Development II (as age appropriate) 5. Connors' Parent Rating Scale	In children who suffered from PAES there was a threefold-increased risk of anomalies in the social component of the DDST-II (behavior and social adaptability, independence in self-help skills, social imitative play, and the ability to clearly communicate personal needs and desires).
Nulman et al. 2012 [31]; prospective cohort; *n* = 172	12–60	VEN SSRIs	1. Wechsler Preschool and Primary Scale of Intelligence III 2. Child Behavior Checklist 3. Conners' Parent Rating Scale 4. DSM-IV total symptom subscales	Children of healthy women had higher IQs than those exposed to antidepressants. One in five PAES children showed clinically significant behavior problems.
Malm et al. 2012 [32]; retrospective; *n* = 845,345	0–168	SSRIs SNRIs TCAs	1. ICD-10	The cumulative incidence of any registered psychiatric or neurodevelopmental disorder in the exposed population was 6.9% when considering the 0–14 age range and 12.9% among the oldest offspring cohort (age 14).
Sorensen et al. 2012 [33]; cohort; *n* = 655,615	Mean age of children at end of follow-up: 104	SSRIs SNRIs TCAs	1. ICD-10	Prenatal maternal antidepressant exposure was associated with an increased risk of later ASDs in children.
Rai et al. 2013 [34]; case-control; *n* = 4,429 (cases)	0–204	SSRIs TCAs	1. ICD-10	Antidepressant use during pregnancy explained 0.6% of the cases of ASDs.
El-Marroun et al. 2014 [35]; prospective; *n* = 69	73	SSRIs	1. Child Behavior Checklist for ages 1.5–5.0 (for reasons of continuity)	Prenatal SSRI exposure was associated with autistic traits.
Gidaya et al. 2014 [36]; case-control; *n* = 5,215	0–216	SSRIs	1. ICD-10	Increased risk of ASD associated with in utero exposure to SSRIs. The effect was present in all exposure windows considered.
Hanley et al. 2015 [37]; longitudinal; *n* = 44	72	SSRIs SNRIs	1. MacArthur Health and Behavior Questionnaire	In utero antidepressant exposure was associated with significantly higher scores on the internalizing behavior and anxious behavior subscales.
Grzeskowiak et al. 2013 [38]; ongoing, follow-up; *n* = 127	84	SSRIs	1. Overweight classified as body mass index >85th percentile	Male children with prenatal SSRI exposure were more likely to be overweight.

Abbreviations: SSRIs: selective serotonin reuptake inhibitors; SNRIs: serotonin norepinephrine reuptake inhibitors; VEN: venlafaxine; TCAs: tricyclic antidepressants; PAES: prenatal antidepressant exposure syndrome; ASDs: autism spectrum disorders; DDST-II: Denver Developmental Screening Test II; ICD: *International Classification of Diseases*; DSM: *Diagnostic and Statistical Manual of Mental Disorders*.

Discussion

Why some children are affected by prenatal SSRI exposure and others are not remains a pressing question [39]. SSRI exposure and maternal mood likely interact with genetic factors to affect serotonergic tone during development and/or disease susceptibility later in life. A moderating role for genetic variables is beginning to emerge, but not all alleles carry the same risk [39].

Among SSRI-exposed neonates, 5-minute Apgar scores are lower and the risk of neuromotor symptoms is higher in carriers of short (*s*) promoter alleles of the 5-HTT gene, *SLC6A4*, which is associated with reduced *SLC6A4* expression [40]. In contrast, the risk of respiratory distress is higher in SSRI-exposed neonates with two copies of the long (*l*) allele [39,40]. Infants with two high-activity *MAO-A* alleles have higher withdrawal symptom scores than infants with at least one low-activity allele [41]. Together, these findings may reflect "fetal serotonergic programming" arising from altered early levels of central 5-HT [1,39–41].

Even with prenatal SSRI exposure, changes in 5-HT signaling cannot be attributed to single causal factors. Development and behavior in this setting represent an ongoing interplay between psychological, molecular, genetic, and social factors inherent to both the mother and her child across the fetal and postnatal periods. Rather than being a case where 5-HT levels are "too high" or "too low," this is a setting where 5-HT levels are "finely tuned" over critical periods to meet developmental demands [1].

However, a more detailed expression map of 5-HTT gene expression during human development is needed for the determination of the critical developmental phases during which SSRI exposure could be harmful [8]. Impaired 5-HT regulation associated with in utero exposure to SSRIs was found not only in the central nervous system, but also in platelets. However, the decreased 5-HT uptake that was described in the platelets of fetuses exposed to SSRIs through the placenta [42] is of uncertain clinical significance [43]. Given this background, the finding that the majority of reviewed studies show opposite, discordant results is not unexpected.

Several teams of researchers actually failed to demonstrate the detrimental effects of antenatal antidepressant exposure on the child's intelligence [20,26,28], behaviors [23,25,27,28], or physical development [28]. Also, no association was found between antenatal antidepressant exposure and ADHD onset later in childhood [24].

On the other hand, children who have suffered from antidepressant-induced neonatal complications seem to be likely to show impaired social skills, low IQ, and behavioral problems overall [21,22].

In children who did not develop any neonatal iatrogenic complications, just two studies suggested that antenatal exposure to several classes of antidepressants may induce neurodevelopmental problems, such as internalizing behaviors, and even psychiatric disorders, including anxiety disorders [34,37].

A deeper discussion must be reserved for the potential association between prenatal SSRI exposure and an increase in the risk of ASDs. Further research into potential associations between maternal depression and childhood autism is actually needed. It may be that there are certain (genetic) traits predisposing individuals to both depression and autism [44]. A recent study of 60,000 individuals using whole-genome analysis found evidence for four common genetic variants that increase the risk of five different psychiatric disorders, including depression and autism [45]. It may be that maternal depression itself (prenatal as well as postnatal) triggers childhood autism, but let us not jump to any firm conclusions yet. However, it has been recently hypothesized that increased serotonergic activity during brain development may increase the risk of autism [46,47]. In fact, 5-HT has long been of interest in autism. Repeated findings of elevated platelet 5-HT levels in approximately one-third of children with autism has led some to believe that dysfunctional 5-HT signaling may be a causal mechanism for the disorder [48]. Low maternal plasma 5-HT may be a risk factor for autism through its effects on fetal brain development [49]. However, whether 5-HT is an etiologic factor in ASDs remains unclear [46]. Nevertheless, four studies (performed with different methodological designs, such as case-control, prospective, and cohort evaluation) demonstrated an association between antenatal antidepressant exposure and increased risks of developing autistic traits or full-blown ASDs [33–36]. This risk is not limited to SSRIs, but also involve SNRIs and TCAs, both classes of antidepressants having various degrees of impact on 5-HT receptors. Just one study did not confirm this association [23]. Thus, more than a few safety signals [50]

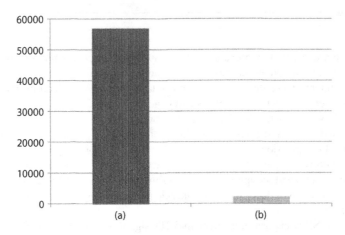

FIGURE 18.1   (a) Number of SSRI-exposed children in reviewed studies with no autistic symptoms. (b) Number of SSRI-exposed children with ASDs. (Adapted from Laugesen K, et al., *BMJ Open*, 3, 1–7, 2013; Sørensen MJ, et al. *Clin Epidemiol*, 5, 449–459, 2013; Rai D, et al., *BMJ*, 346, f2059, 2013; El Marroun H, et al., *BJP*, 205, 95–102, 2014; Gidaya NB, et al., *J Autism Dev Disord*, 44, 2558–2567, 2014.)

exist suggesting that antenatal exposure to SSRIs may increase the risk of ASDs [51]. It is noteworthy that recent research has suggested that the increased frequency of diagnoses of ASDs could be caused in part by nonetiologic factors such as changes in diagnosis reporting practices and diagnostic criteria [52] (Figure 18.1).

CONCLUSIONS

It seems that an association exists between SSRI exposure through the placenta and ASDs in children. Meanwhile, when choosing between starting or not starting, or continuing or withdrawing SSRI treatment in pregnant mothers, clinicians should balance the hypothesized risk of ASDs against the ascertained risks associated with untreated maternal depression. The clinician must take into account the consequences of worsening depressive symptoms, which may lead to tragic events for the mother–fetus dyad [53]. Since SSRIs have been considered the first-choice agents for treating antenatal depression, there is an urgent need for further larger, well-designed studies finalized to definitively assess the existence and the magnitude of this association.

REFERENCES

1. Friedman SH, Hall RCW. Antidepressant use during pregnancy: How to avoid clinical and legal pitfalls. *Curr Psychiatry*. 2013;12(2). Available from: http://www.currentpsychiatry.com/home/article/anti-depressant-use-during-pregnancy-how-to-avoid-clinical-and-legal-pitfalls/7b2ba0f17ac723309ffdae-f6770368e0.html (accessed September 25, 2015).
2. Oberlander TF. Fetal serotonin signaling: Setting pathways for early childhood development and behavior. *J Adol Health*. 2012; 51:S9–16.
3. Whitaker-Azmitia PM, Druse M, Walker P, Lauder JM. Serotonin as a developmental signal. *Behav Brain Res*. 1996;73:19–29.
4. Gaspar P, Cases O, Maroteaux L. The developmental role of serotonin: News from mouse molecular genetics. *Nat Rev Neurosci*. 2003;4:1002–12.
5. Velasquez JC, Golden N, Bonnin A. Placental serotonin: Implications for the developmental effects of SSRIs and maternal depression. *Fron Cell Neurosci*. 2013;7:1–7.
6. Bonnin A, Levitt P. Placental source for 5-HT hat tunes fetal brain development. *Neuropsychopharmacology*. 2012;37:299–300.

7. Bonnin, A, Goeden N, Chen K, et al. A transient placental source of serotonin for the fetal forebrain. *Nature*. 2011;472:347–50.

8. Homberg JR, Schubert D, Gaspar P. New perspectives on the neurodevelopmental effects of SSRIs. *Trends Pharmacol Sci*. 2010;31:60–65.

9. Narboux-Nême N, Pavone LM, Avallone L, et al. Serotonin transporter transgenic (SERTcre) mouse line reveals developmental targets of serotonin specific reuptake inhibitors (SSRIs). *Neuropharmacology*. 2008;55:994–1005.

10. Verney C, Lebrand C, Gaspar C. Changing distribution of monoaminergic markers in the developing human cerebral cortex with special emphasis on the serotonin transporter. *Anat Rec*. 2002;267:87–93.

11. Bylund DB, Reed AL. Childhood and adolescent depression: Why do children and adults respond differently to antidepressant drugs? Neurochem Int. 2007:51:246–53.

12. Mirmiran M, Van De Poll NE, Corner MA, et al. Suppression of active sleep by chronic treatment with chlorimipramine during early postnatal development: Effects upon adult sleep and behavior in the rat. *Brain Res*. 1981;204:129–46.

13. Vogel G, Neill D, Hagler M, Kors D. A new animal model of endogenous depression: A summary of present findings. *Neurosci Biobehav Rev*. 1990;14:85–91.

14. Gentile S. Neurodevelopmental effects of prenatal exposure to psychotropic medications. *Depress Anx*. 2010;27:675–86.

15. Gentile S. On categorizing gestational birth, and neonatal complications following late in utero exposure to antidepressants: The Prenatal Antidepressant Exposure Syndrome. *CNS Spectr*. 2010;15:167–85.

16. Laine K, Heikkinen T, Ekblad U, Kero P. Effects of exposure to selective serotonin reuptake inhibitors during pregnancy on serotonergic symptoms in newborns and cord blood monoamine and prolactin concentrations. *Arch Gen Psychiatry*. 2003;60:720–26.

17. Ruchkin V, Martin A. SSRIs and the developing brain. *Lancet* 2005;365:451–3.

18. AACAP. Practice parameters for the psychiatric assessment of infant and toddlers (0–36 months). *J Am Acad Child Adolesc Psychiatry*. 1997;36:S21–S36.

19. Meisels SJ, Provence S. *Screening and Assessment: Guidelines for Identifying Young Disabled and Developmentally Vulnerable Children and Their Families*. Washington, DC: Zero to Three/National Center for Clinical Infants Program; 1989.

20. Mattson SA, Eastvold V, Jones K, et al. Neurobehavioral follow-up of children prenatally exposed to fluoxetine. *Teratology*. 1999;59:376 [Abstract].

21. Nulman, I, Rovet J, Stewart DE, et al. Child development following exposure to tricyclic antidepressants or fluoxetine throughout fetal life: A prospective, controlled study. *Am J Psychiatry*. 2002;159:1889–95.

22. Oberlander TFP, Reebye P, Misri S, et al. Externalizing and attentional behaviors in children of depressed mothers treated with a selective serotonin reuptake inhibitor antidepressant during pregnancy. *Arch Pediatr Adolesc Med*. 2007;161:22–9.

23. Hviid A, Melbye M, Pasternak B. Use of selective serotonin reuptake inhibitors during pregnancy and risk of autism. *N Engl J Med*. 2013;69:2406–15.

24. Laugesen K, Olsen MS, Telén Andersen AB, et al. In utero exposure to antidepressant drugs and risk of attention deficit hyperactivity disorder: A nationwide Danish cohort study. *BMJ Open*. 2013;3:1–7.

25. Santucci AK, Singer LT, Wisniewski SR, et al. Impact on prenatal exposure to serotonin reuptake inhibitors or maternal depressive disorders on infant developmental outcomes. *J Clin Psychiatry*. 2014;55:1088–95.

26. Eriksen HLF, Kesmodel US, Pedersen LH, Mortensen EL. No association between prenatal exposure to psychotropics and intelligence at age five. *Acta Obstet Gynecol Scand*. 2015;94:501–7.

27. Grzeskowiak LE, Morrison JL, Henriksen TB, et al. Prenatal antidepressant exposure and child behavioural outcomes at 7 years of age: A study within the Danish National Birth Cohort. *BJOG*. 2016; (in press) doi:10.1111/1471-0528.13611.

28. Nulman I, Koren G, Rovet J, et al. Neurodevelopment of children prenatally exposed to selective reuptake inhibitor antidepressants: Toronto Sibling Study. *J Clin Psychiatry*. 2015;76:e842–7.

29. Gentile S. On categorizing gestational birth, and neonatal complications following late in utero exposure to antidepressants: The prenatal antidepressant exposure syndrome. *CNS Spectrums*. 2010;15:167–85.

30. Klinger G, Frankenthal D, Merlob P, et al. Long-term outcome following selective serotonin reuptake inhibitor induced neonatal abstinence syndrome. *J Perinatol*. 2011;31:615–20.

31. Nulman I, Koren G, Rovet J, et al. Neurodevelopment of children following prenatal exposure to ven-
    lafaxine, selective serotonin reuptake inhibitors, or untreated maternal depression. *Am J Psychiatry*.
    2012;169:1165–74.
32. Malm H, Artama M, Brown AS, et al. Infant and childhood neurodevelopmental outcomes following
    prenatal exposure to selective serotonin reuptake inhibitors: Overview and design of a Finnish Register-
    Based Study (FinESSI). *BMC Psychiatry*. 2012;12:217.
33. Sørensen MJ, Grønborg TK, Christensen J, et al. Antidepressant exposure in pregnancy and risk of
    autism spectrum disorders. *Clin Epidemiol*. 2013;5:449–59.
34. Rai D, Lee BK, Dalman C, et al. Parental depression, maternal antidepressant use during pregnancy,
    and risk of autism spectrum disorders: Population based case-control study. *BMJ*. 2013;346:f2059.
35. El Marroun H, White TJH, van der Knaap NJF, et al. Prenatal exposure to selective serotonin reuptake
    inhibitors and social responsiveness symptoms of autism: Population-based study of young children.
    BJP. 2014;205:95–102.
36. Gidaya NB, Lee BK, Burstyn I, et al. In utero exposure to selective serotonin reuptake inhibitors and
    risk for autism spectrum disorder. *J Autism Dev Disord*. 2014;44:2558–67.
37. Hanley GE, Brain U, Oberlander TF. Prenatal exposure to serotonin reuptake inhibitor antidepressants
    and childhood behaviors. *Pediatr Res*. 2015;78:174–80.
38. Grzeskowiak LE, Gilbert AL, Sørensen TIA, et al. Prenatal exposure to selective serotonin reuptake
    inhibitors and childhood overweight at 7 years of age. *Ann Epidemiol*. 2013;23:e681–7.
39. Oberlander TF, Gingrich JA, Ansorge MS. Sustained neurobehavioral effects of exposure to SSRI anti-
    depressants during development: Molecular to clinical evidence. *Clin Pharmacol Ther*. 2009;10:1–6.
40. Oberlander TF, Bonaguro RJ, Misri S, et al. Infant serotonin transporter (SLC6A4) promoter genotype
    is associated with adverse neonatal outcomes after prenatal exposure to serotonin reuptake inhibitor
    medications. *Mol Psychiatry*. 2008;13:65–73.
41. Hilli J, Heikkinen T, Rontu R, et al. MAO-A and COMT genotypes as possible regulators of perinatal
    serotonergic symptoms after in utero exposure to SSRIs. *Eur Neuropsychopharmacol*. 2009;19:363–70.
42. Anderson GM, Czarkowski K, Ravski N, Epperson CN. Platelet serotonin in newborns and infants:
    Ontogeny, heritability, and effect of in utero exposure to selective serotonin reuptake inhibitors. *Pediatr Res*.
    2004;56:418–22.
43. Gentile S. SSRIs in pregnancy and lactation with emphasis on neurodevelopmental outcome. *CNS
    Drugs*. 2005;19:623–33.
44. Petersen I, Evans S, Nazareth I. Prenatal exposure to selective serotonin reuptake inhibitors and autistic
    symptoms in young children: Another red herring? *Br J Psychiatry*. 2014;205:105–6.
45. Cross-Disorder Group of the Psychiatric Genomics Consortium, Genetic Risk Outcome of Psychosis
    (GROUP) Consortium. Identification of risk loci with shared effects on five major psychiatric disorders:
    A genome-wide analysis. *Lancet* 2013;381:1371–9.
46. Harrington RA, Lee LC, Crum RM, et al. Serotonin hypothesis of autism: Implications for selective
    serotonin reuptake inhibitor use during pregnancy. *Autism Res*. 2013;6:149–68.
47. Whitaker-Azmitia PM. Behavioral and cellular consequences of increasing serotonergic activity during
    brain development: A role in autism? *Int J Dev Neurosci*. 2005;23:75–83.
48. Stahl SM. The human platelet: A diagnostic and research tool for the study of biogenic amines in psy-
    chiatric and neurologic disorders. *Arch Gen Psychiatry*. 1977;34:509–16.
49. Anderson GM. Measurement of plasma serotonin in Autism. *Pediatr Neurol*. 2007;36:138.
50. Trontell A. Expecting the unexpected: Drug safety, pharmacovigilance, and the prepared mind. *N Engl
    J Med*. 2004;351:1385–7.
51. Gentile S. Prenatal antidepressant exposure and the risk of autism spectrum disorders in children: Are
    we looking at the falls of gods? *J Affect Disord*. 2015;182:132–7.
52. Hansen SN, Diana E, Schendel DE, et al. Explaining the increase in the prevalence of autism spectrum
    disorders: The proportion attributable to changes in reporting practices. *JAMA Pediatr*. 2015;169:56–62.
53. Gentile S. Untreated maternal depression during pregnancy: Short- and long-term effects in off-
    spring; A systematic review. *Neuroscience*. 2015;pii:S0306–4522(15)00811–8. doi: 10.1016/j.neurosci-
    ence.2015.09.001. [Epub ahead of print.]

Index

A

Abnormal placentation, 28, 177
ACOG, *see* American Congress of Obstetricians and Gynecologists
ADH, *see* Antidiuretic hormone
ADHD, *see* Attention deficit hyperactivity disorder
ADM, *see* Antidepressant medication
AHA, *see* American Heart Association
Alkaline phosphatase (ALP), 125
Alloimmune theories, 63
ALP, *see* Alkaline phosphatase
ALSPAC, *see* Avon Longitudinal Study of Parents and Children
American College of Obstetricians and Gynecologists, 62
American Congress of Obstetricians and Gynecologists (ACOG), 8–9
American Diabetes Association, 21
American Heart Association (AHA), 1, 8, 17
American Society for Reproductive Medicine (ASRM), 61
Amniotic fluid, 79, 80
Anatomic factors, 65
Angiogenic pathways, 154
Angiotensin II, 92
Animal models, 182–183
Antenatal and Postnatal Mental Health, 103
Antenatal depression, 103, 104, 105–106
    and fetal stress, 105
    pathophysiology of obstetrical complications, 105
    treatment of, 106
Antepartum, and postpartum VTE, 119
Antiangiogenic factors, 7–8
Antiangiogenic protein, 155
Antidepressant exposure, in pregnancy, 225–230
    data source, 226–230
        developmental risks associated with, 227–230
        no effects on developmental outcomes, 226–227
    5-HT receptors and 5-HTT in human fetal brain, 226
    placenta and serotonin, 225
Antidepressant medication (ADM), 106
Antidiuretic hormone (ADH), 93
Antiphospholipid syndrome (APLS), 63, 66, 117
Aortic pressure, 6
APLS, *see* Antiphospholipid syndrome
ART, *see* Assisted reproductive technology
Arterial stiffness, 6
ASD, *see* Autism spectrum disorder
ASRM, *see* American Society for Reproductive Medicine
Assisted reproductive technology (ART), 50, 131, 133, 214, 219
Atherosclerotic morbidity, 18, 96–99

Attention deficit hyperactivity disorder (ADHD), 219, 227, 219
Augmentation index, 6
Autism spectrum disorders (ASDs), 165, 218–219, 227, 229, 231
Autoimmune disorder, 63
Avon Longitudinal Study of Parents and Children (ALSPAC), 40, 195

B

Bariatric surgery, 141, 142
Barker, and thrifty phenotype hypotheses, 178–179
Bayley III, 199
Behavioral counseling, 146
Bennewitz, H. G., 15
Beta cells, 181
Biochemical profile, 93–94
    creatinine and urea, 93
    glucose and organic substance, 94
    osmolality and sodium, 93
    potassium, 93
    and pregnancy
        GDM and gestational hypertension, 94–95
        late atherosclerotic morbidity, 96–99
        uric acid, 95–96
    uric acid, 93
Birth weight, and insulin resistance, 40
Blood pressure, 212
Body mass index (BMI), 32, 140, 164, 212
Bone mass, and osteoporosis, 201
BPD, *see* Bronchopulmonary dysplasia
Brain injury, 199
Brain-sparing effect, 182
Breast cancer, 50, 51, 55, 133
British Women's Heart and Health Study, 32
Bronchopulmonary dysplasia (BPD), 194, 195
Bupropion, 148

C

Calcium deposition, 201
California Child Health and Development Study, 5
California Health and Development Study, 3
Cancer
    breast, 50, 51, 55
    cervical, 52, 55
    endometrial, 48–49, 51, 52
    female, 47
    ovarian, 49–50, 51, 55
    pregnancy and, 47–48
    uterine, 55
Cancer Prevention Study II, 48
Cardiovascular, and metabolic effects, 212–215

angiotensin II and norepinephrine, 92
    relaxin, 92
VEGF, *see* Vascular endothelial growth factor
VEINES, *see* Venous Insufficiency Epidemiological and
    Economic Study
Venous Insufficiency Epidemiological and Economic
    Study (VEINES), 119
Venous thromboembolism (VTE), 113, 115, 116, 117,
    119–120
    distribution across pregnancy and postpartum, 114
    pregnancy-related incidence of, 113–114
    recurrence, 119–120
    risk factor distribution in early- vs. late-
        postpartum, 118
Very low birth weight (VLBW), 201
Vision, and hearing, 200
Visual perception, 198–199

VLBW, *see* Very low birth weight
VTE, *see* Venous thromboembolism

W

Weight control, techniques for, 141–145
    cesarean delivery of obese woman, 142–144
    effects of smoking on pregnancy, 144–145
White, Priscilla, 15
White matter damage, 196
WHO, *see* World Health Organization
WHO Ad Hoc Diabetes Report Group, 16
World Health Organization (WHO), 15, 36, 115,
    140, 191

Y

Young Age Obesity, 48